Gynecological Endoscopy Simplified
Practical Tips by Experts

Gynecological Endoscopy Simplified
Practical Tips by Experts

Editor
Sunita R Tandulwadkar
MD, FICS, Dip. in Endo. (USA and Germany)
Head, Department of Obstetrics and Gynecology, Ruby Hall Clinic, Pune
Chief, Ruby Hall IVF and Endoscopy Center, Ruby Hall Clinic, Pune
Gynae Endoscopist, Poona Hospital and Research Center, Pune, India

Co-editors
(Ruby Hall IVF and Endoscopy Team)
Poonam Jagiasi
Amit Shah
Rakhi Sarda
Mugdha Joshi
Rahul A Gore
Pooja Lodha

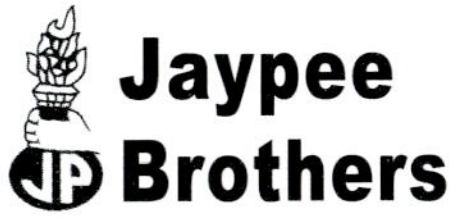

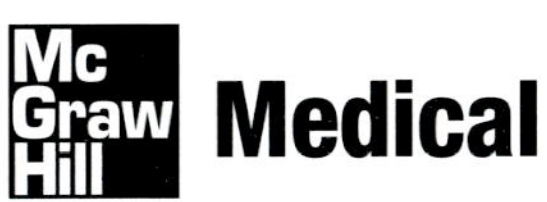

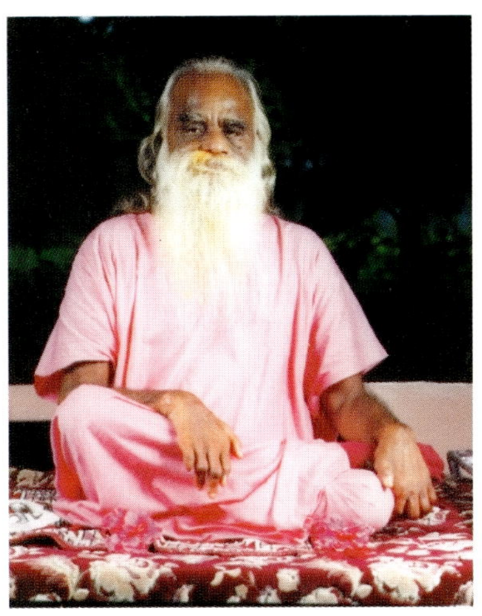

गुरू: ब्रह्म: गुरु: विष्णु: गुरु: देवमहेश्वर:।
गुरु: साक्षात् परं ब्रह्म: तस्मै श्रीगुरुवे नम:॥

CONTRIBUTORS

Dr Ajay Rane
Dr Kannan K, Dr Fiadjoe P
James Cook University
Townsville
Australia

Dr PG Paul, Dr Renuka Borisa
Dr P Biju
Paul's Hospital and Cochin
Gynecological Endoscopy
Training Centre
Cochin, Kerala, India

Dr Sanjay Patel
Dr Yogendra Jhala
Mayflower Hospital
Ahmedabad, India

Dr Pravin Patel
Advanced Fertility and
Endoscopic Centre
Melbourne IVF
Ahmedabad, India

Dr Bandana Sodhi
Dept of Obstetrics and Gynecology
Armed Forces Medical College
Pune, India

Dr Prakash Trivedi
Chief Gynaecological Endoscopist and
ART Consultant, NILES, Mumbai
Scientific Director, AKAR, IVF-ICSI
Center, Mumbai
Head of Department, Obstetrics and
Gynaecology, VC Gandhi Rajawadi
Municipal Hospital
Hon. Prof. Pd. DY Patil Medical College
Mumbai, India

Dr Sanjay Gupte
Gupte Hospital and Centre for
Research in Production
Hon. Professor, Sassoon General
Hospital
BJ Medical College
Pune, India

Dr JP Rath
Consultant, Critical Care Obstetrics
and Gynecology
Pune, India

Dr Girija Wagh
Dr S Puntambekar
Galaxy Laparoscopy Institute
Pune, India

FOREWORD

It gives me great pleasure to write the Foreword to this book Gynecological Endoscopy Simplified as it brings back memories of starting our IVF and Endoscopy Centre at the Ruby Hall Clinic with the help of Dr Sunita Tandulwadkar. The staff who helped Dr. Tandulwadkar have worked with determination to bring it to a top-level Endoscopic 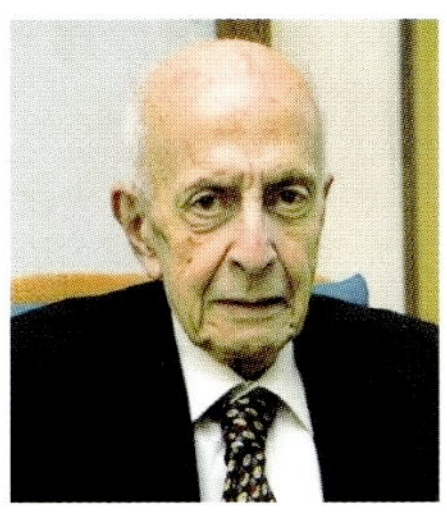
Centre in the city of Pune and made Dr. Tandulwadkar amongst the best in this field.

This book vividly recalls her journey from humble beginnings and challenges and provides state-of-the-art facilities to obtain the best result. It makes interesting reading and I am sure it will be a great source to all young doctors and entrepreneurs who wish to make their endoscopic centres as good as the present one.

Dr K.B. Grant
Chairman and Managing Trustee
Ruby Hall Clinic
Pune, India

FOREWORD

Endoscopy is a technology-driven dynamic discipline that has challenged conventional open surgery, introduced innovative advances and opened up numerous options for the treatment of infertility. In the past decade, gynecologic surgery, because of endoscopic surgery, has undergone a tremendous revolution. There 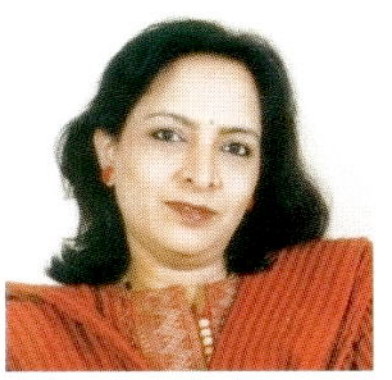 are few cases in the gynecologist's surgical armamentarium that cannot be carried out through an endoscopic approach. Gynecological endoscopic surgeries have changed and continued to evolve rapidly. Several procedures considered difficult are now being successfully done laparoscopically.

As a diagnostic tool, a combined laparoscopic and hysteroscopic examination is the gold standard for the evaluation of infertility.

I am glad that Dr. Sunita Tandulwadkar is bringing out *Gynecological Endoscopy Simplified—Practical Tips by Experts.* This book presents the entire gamut of all possible gynecological surgical procedures which can be carried out by endoscopy. Books such as these give us the opportunity of educating, advocating, training as well as developing quality output. The updated material has been presented in an articulate and precise manner making reading immensely satisfying accomplishment. I am sure that this helpful and practical handbook will be an essential resource for all clinicians dealing with this difficult subject.

Dr Kamini A Rao
Medical Director
Bangalore Assisted Conception Centre
Bengaluru, India

PREFACE

In this "Information Age", an interested reader can easily locate information on everything from movies to the medical care. When it comes to health and disease, the quality of information is vital.

Many standard books have been published on endoscopy during the last two to three decades to meet the needs of beginners in the field of endoscopy. *Gynecological Endoscopy Simplified—Practical Tips by Experts* covers important surgeries related to laparoscopy and hysteroscopy in gynecology and will be of great help to beginners as well as practising endoscopists. All the practical tips to enhance the surgical performance have been given in an absolutely simplified way.

I am extremely pleased and gratified to present this book, which, I presume will be read by tens of thousands of medical students and medical practitioners. One likes to think that the clinical practice of these practioners will be influenced by the book and that patient care will be a little more humane, a little more gentle and perhaps a little more effective because some of the practical tips in this book will take root.

A thorough reader of this book will have very little trouble in starting an endoscopy set-up with least complication rates. In order to make the book as useful as possible, other than the practical tips and footnotes at the end of the chapters, the salient feature of the book remains its self illustrative color figures.

Although this book will be useful for the medical students as well as the practising Endoscopists, Professors in training programmes will also find its content germane to their students. We have worked hard to make this book clinically relevant and almost all the chapters include the application of the principles being discussed. Every case draws on the clinical experience and expertise of the authors and illustrates how the principles of the book can be applied in a clinical setting. I am sure you will get an experience as if you are performing surgery while going through the steps of the surgery and the color figures. Also, apart from the practical tips that have been given, each endoscopist can individualize the steps of the surgery to enhance the performance.

I wish to thank Dr Girija Wagh who has given me this suggestion of pen suing down years of experience and come out with a book which will help to decrease the learning curve of beginners.

I wish to thank all my colleagues (Dr Poonam Jagiasi, Dr Amit Shah and Dr Rakhi Sarda) and students (Dr Mugdha Joshi, Dr Rahul Gore and Dr Pooja Lodha), in the Department of IVF and Endoscopy, Ruby Hall Clinic, Pune, for providing valuable suggestions, which have been indispensable to the accomplishment of my task.

Most of all thanks go to my family. My husband, Dr. Rajesh Tandulwadkar, Surgeon gastro-enterologist and GI Endoscopist and my son Rishi, all took notes for me that found their way into the pages of my book. And, as for my earlier writings, my husband continues to be my first reader and key critic apart from my great assistant in difficult situations.

Sunita R Tandulwadkar

CONTENTS

SECTION FOUR: VAGINAL SURGERY

SECTION FIVE: UNUSUAL CASES

GENERAL GUIDELINES FOR BEGINNERS

1. Good patient selection.
2. Good preoperative preparation.
3. Plan the surgery ahead.
4. Competent assistance: it is teamwork.
5. Check instrumentation and equipments ahead as it is; technologically driven surgical modality.
6. Handle all equipment with utmost care.
7. Maintenance of all equipment is the secret of their longevity.
8. All instruments should be cleaned with a brush and water to remove all clots. Ultrasonic cleaners and chemicals are also available to remove all the clots.
9. Instruments should be dried thoroughly before being replaced in their chambers.
10. Sterilization can be achieved as follows:
    - Metal instruments can be autoclaved.
    - Rapid sterilization can be done by placing in Cidex solution for 20 minutes.
    - Other instruments (like tubings and cables) can be placed in formalin chambers
11. Safe port access.
12. Safe use of energy.
13. Gentle dissection, tissue respect.
14. Always remember: limited view, only two-dimensional visions, no depth perception, therefore, always work under vision.
15. Review your own videos and you will understand your own mistakes which can be subsequently improved.
16. Endoscopic surgery should not be used as a technical gimmick to avoid laparotomy and attract patients. The goal of endoscopic surgery should not be to avoid laparotomy but to achieve highest surgical skills.
17. Quality of surgery inside is much more important than recovery one or two weeks later.
18. Every surgeon should pioneer his own technique in such a way that it gives the best of the results.
19. Every gynecologist should himself or herself decide which surgery he/she can do endoscopically.
20. With experience, the comfort level will definitely expand.
21. The flexible surgeon is familiar with all available techniques so that the best approach is selected for the individual patient.
22. Endoscopic surgeries are good both for the patient and the surgeon, it must always be remembered:

"First do no harm!"

DO'S AND DON'T

DO's

Surgeon

"I think It's OK" – Syndrome

Be aware of the words "I think it's OK".

The surgeon must determine whether the organ in question is or is not injured. If the conclusion is that it is injured, proper steps are taken to deal with it. The matter should not be put aside for period of observation.

- Be aware of any changes taking place in the operating room during the procedure or between the cases.
1. Personnel
2. Equipment not working
3. Running out of critical supplies
4. In fact, just about any thing that can have an effect on operating surgeon or his/her performance.

Assistant

Assisting is a very special part of any operative procedures.

The purpose of the assistance is not only to assist, but to enhance the performance of operating surgeon.

A good assistant can make a good case even Better
A bad assistant can turn a good case into a Disaster

Make suggestions that might help the procedure.

The surgeon and assistant should wok as a team, and each team member has his/her task to do.

DONT's

Assistant

Don't try to do the procedure.

In operative laparoscopy two surgeons can make great team if they work together. Remember the more you work together the more you will actually

"WORK TOGETHER"

A good operative Laparoscopy is four handed procedure

Don't let your mind wonder back to Mayo's stand or back table. If you are trying to assist someone and you let your attention drawn away from that person, you break line of communication.

"freeze, don't move !"

During the actual procedure your best move as an assistant is sometimes.

"No move at all !"

Basic
Endoscopy

How to Set-up an Ideal Endoscopic Operation Theater

1

- Well-equipped, well-organized and well-spaced operating room is essential for successful laparohysteroscopic procedures.
- The arrangement of instruments and equipments is important for safety and efficiency.
- Ceiling mounted instrument carts avoid gas tubing and electrical wires on the floor.
- Electrosurgical generator and suction irrigation device are kept on a separate trolley for avoiding spill of irrigation fluid on other equipments.
- Ideally operation theater should be square in shape with minimum measurement of 20 × 20 square foot and should be large enough to accommodate all the equipments (Fig. 1.1).
- The OT table should have capability for Trendelenberg and reverse Trendelenberg positions with right and left tilt. The table should have adjustment to go as below as 2 feet so that one can operate comfortably even with very obese patients. The height of the table should be below the waist of the surgeon for maximum efficacy. For short surgeons, use of stepping platforms is extremely valuable.
- To avoid fatigue and further consequences of the shoulder joint, surgeons should take precautions to see that his/her patient's position is in such a way that he/she does not have to abduct the upper extremity beyond 45° angle unless he/she is using contralateral port.
- A well-equipped Boyle's apparatus for general endotracheal anesthesia is essential to maintain proper oxygenation and relaxation during the procedure along with an ET CO_2 and pulse oximeter monitoring.
- The surgeon stands by the patients left side at an angle facing the patient's contralateral foot. Usually the first assistant stands opposite the surgeon, i.e. on the right side of the patient, while a second assistant sits between the legs of the patient and helps in uterine manipulation.

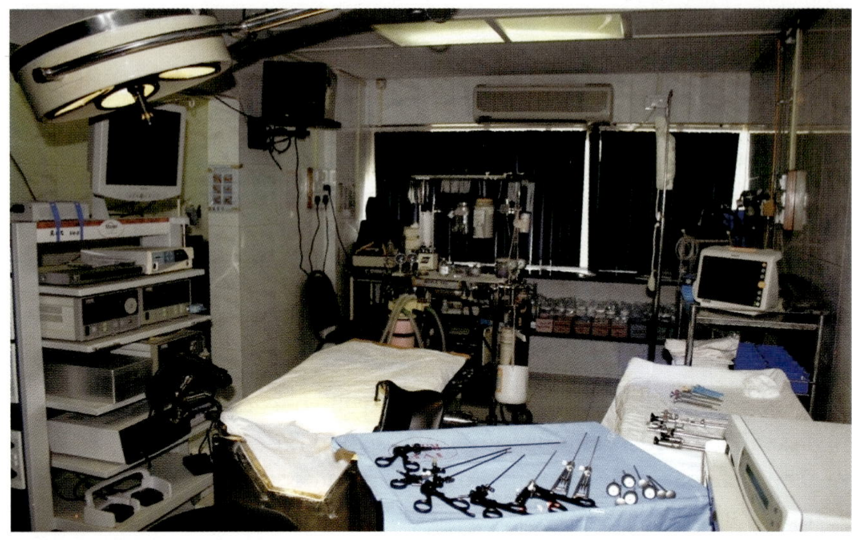

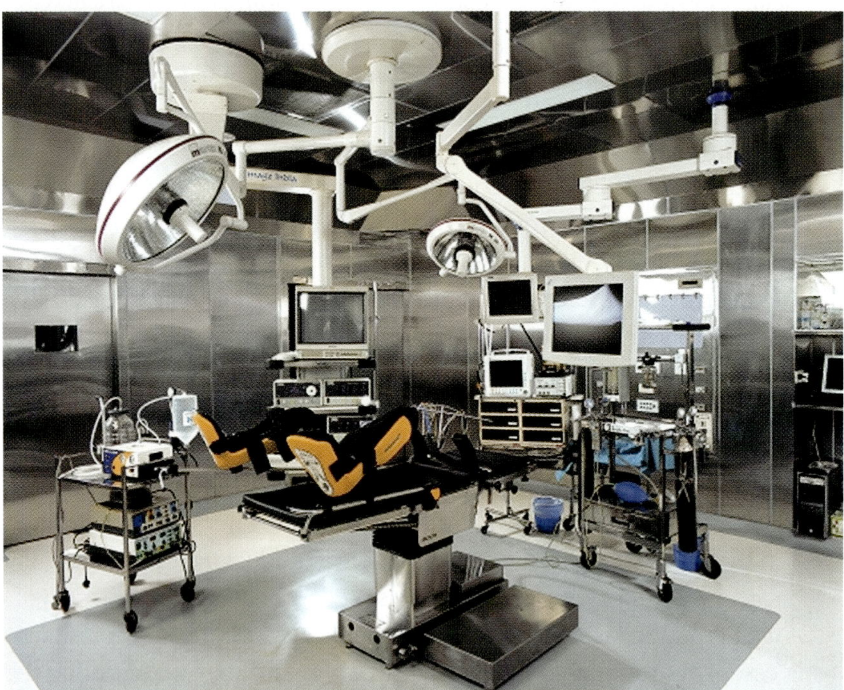

Fig. 1.1: OT layout

Rarely in cases of advanced surgery, where even first assistant is using two ipsilateral ports, one more assistant is needed to hold the camera, who can stand at the head end, next to the anesthetist.

- The nurse and the instrument table are positioned on the left side of the surgeon for easy accessibility.
- Second trolley is arranged on the foot end of the patient, easily accessible to the left hand of the sister and the right hand of the second assistant.
- Endoscopic equipment cart (Fig. 1.2) should carry.
  — Main video monitor
  — Endovision camera
  — Recording system
  — Light source
  — The CO_2 insufflator to allow continuous monitoring of inflation rate and intra-abdominal pressure
  — Electrosurgical generators/Harmonic/other energy sources
  — Endomat/Hysteromat
  — Morcellator

One can also have hanging unit which can carry monitor, camera, recording system, light source and CO_2 insufflator.

If its mobile cart ensure that wheels are good for easy mobility of the unit.

- For laparoscopic surgery this cart with monitor should be placed at the foot end of the table, usually at the patients right foot while for hysteroscopic surgery the monitor is placed towards the patient's right shoulder.
- Another monitor should be placed at the head end of the patient, which benefits the second assistant and the nurse/technician.
- It is not only the surgeon but assistants, nursing staff and even ward boys who should be familiar with the functioning of all the equipments for better outcome.
- The place of each and every equipment and instrument should be fixed and everyone should be aware of their placement.
- Sterilization system for the instrument could be either autoclaving, gassing of individual

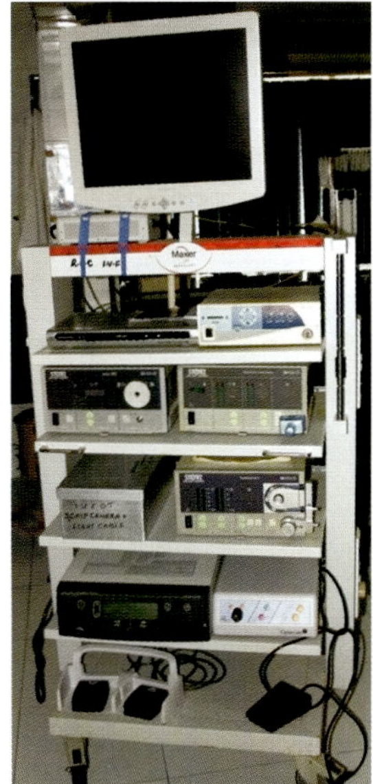

Fig. 1.2: Mobile cart

instrument or formalin sterilization by keeping in formalin chambers. It depends on individual's choice as long as it gives 100% assurance of sterility.

- One of the video monitors should have facility to record in Multisystem form. One of the most important aspects in endoscopy setup is the facility of proper documentation. The DVD recording is the most easiest and simplest installable modality. Many computer soft wares are available to record the live surgery as well as for the data base maintenance, which helps in quick analysis of the total patient information.

TIPS

- These are the minimum required gadgets for safe and hastle free environment in the operation theaters that one needs to have.
- One can keep on enhancing the operation theater with more gadgets (e.g. extra monitors, large monitors, other energy sources, back up equipments, etc.) with time.
- As the surgeon spends more time in the operation theater, other advancements in each gadget happen over the period.

(Photographs courtesy: Dr PG Paul/Ruby Hall IVF and Endoscopy Centre)

2 Equipments and Instruments in Endoscopic Surgery

Gynecologic endoscopic surgery has been evolving continuously and rapidly.

Goal of this chapter is to describe the basic equipment required for endoscopic surgery as well give an overview of the equipments required for advanced laparoscopic surgery.

So acquire the basic equipment and embark on your journey with full enthusiasm after acquiring training in the field of course.

The following equipments are a part of the video tower cart:

Anesthesia Work Station

Following are essential for all general anesthesia cases
- Good quality Boyle's apparatus with fresh soda lime.

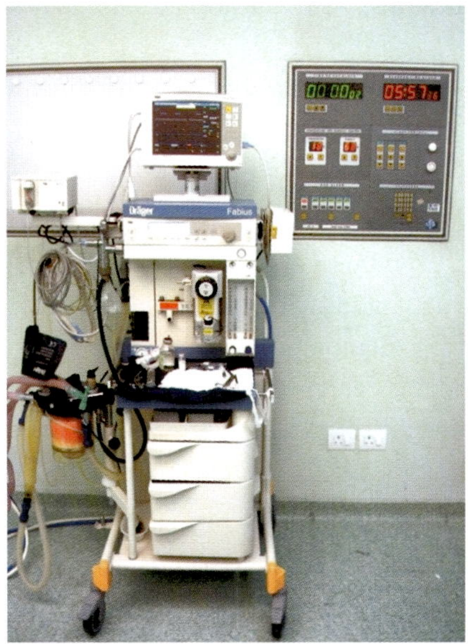

Fig. 2.1: Boyle's machine

- Electrocardiogram tracing
- Noninvasive arterial pressure monitor
- Airway pressure
- Pulse oxymeter
- End tidal carbon dioxide (ET CO_2) which detects drop in the oxygen level.
- Capnograph shows CO_2 retention.
- Defibrillators are essential for all general anesthesia cases.

CO_2 Insufflator

CO_2 insufflator allows regularized flow and maintenance of optimum intra-abdominal pressure with adjustable pressure and gas flow.

It consists of:

- CO_2 insufflators with jumbo CO_2 cylinders
- CO_2 filter is essential for generating pure CO_2 and thereby reducing postoperative pain
- Thermoflator—is used to decrease peritoneal irritation by providing warm CO_2 and prevents continuous fogging of the optics.

Endoscopic Camera with Camera Control Unit (CCU)

The picture should be at low lux/low intensity.

Glare should be reduced when the light intensity is high.

Available in two types, both are acceptable:

- Single chip
- Three chip – better picture quality useful in finer work like tuboplasty, severe endometriosis, etc.

Light Source

- Most commonly used bulbs are xenon bulbs and halogen bulbs. Xenon bulbs generate high intensity of pure white light, which lasts longer and gives best color production but is expensive.
- An ideal endoscopy center should have one good light source with another standby light source.

Light Cables

- Advanced endoscopic surgeries require fiber-optic cables of at least 4-5 mm diameter.
- Light carrying capacity of the cable depends on the number of fiber-optic bundles.

Endomat/Hysteromat

- It is useful in centers where operative hysteroscopies are done routinely.
- It has three settings – Inflow rate, pressure and suction pressure.
- For hysteroscopic surgeries, normally pressure of 100-150 mm of Hg, with flow rate of 300 ml/min and suction pressure of 50 mm of Hg is optimum. Pressure bags can be used as an alternative.
- They should have a Y tube connection for uninterrupted flow.

Suction Irrigation System

- It is a must for every endoscopic theater.
- It can also be used for aqua dissection.

Electrosurgical Generator (Fig. 2.2)

- A separate electro surgical unit with separate bipolar and monopolar foot switches is essential for endoscopic surgery.
- Placement of cautery foot switch is very important to avoid accidental injuries (Fig. 2.3).

Leg Stirrups (Fig. 2.4)

- Padded Allen stirrups provide good support and proper position.
- Disadvantage is the cost.
- Ordinary leg stirrups with 45° angle can be used, but care has to be taken when surgery is extended.

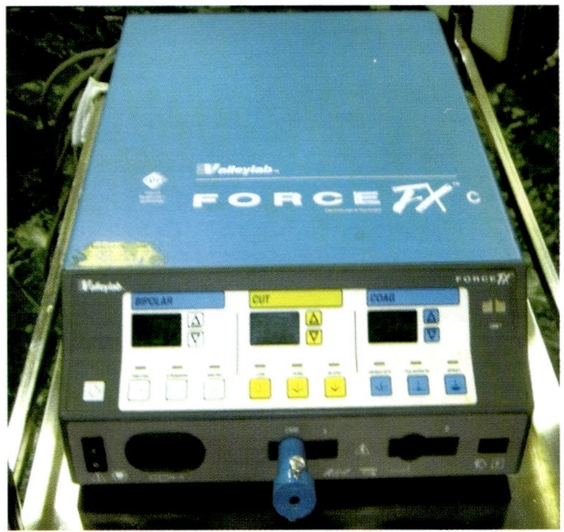

Fig. 2.2: Electrosurgical generator

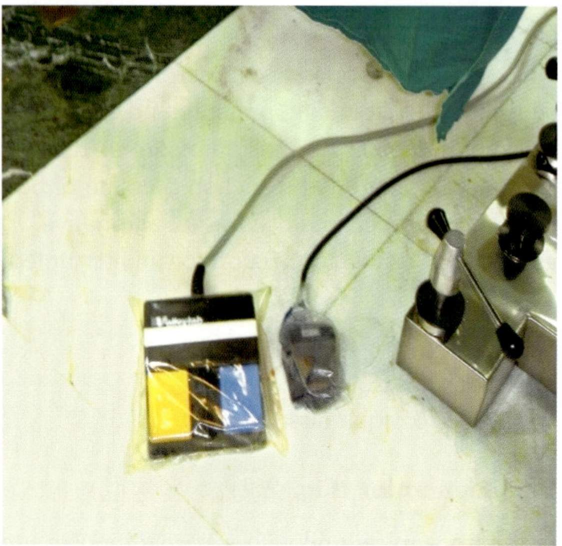

Fig. 2.3: Placement of foot switches in relation to operation table

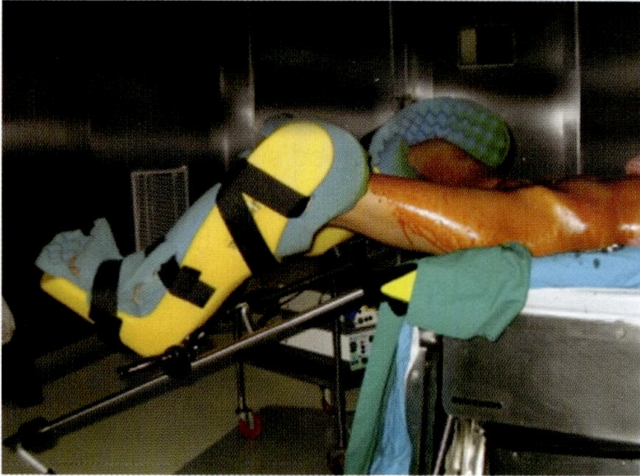

Fig. 2.4: Leg stirrups

Hand Instruments

Veress Needle (Fig. 2.5)

- It is used to create pneumoperitoneum.
- It has a spring mechanism, which protects the viscera from the sharp needle edge.

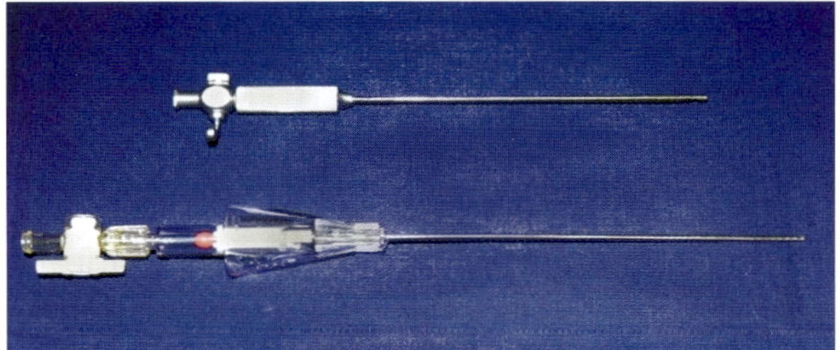

Fig. 2.5: Veress needle – disposable and reusable

Trocars (Figs 2.6 and 2.7)

- Various trocars are available in the market.
- Trocars usually have 2 types of valves to prevent the escape of gas. Trumpet valves are airtight but it grips the instruments and prevents smooth movement of telescope as well as operating instruments. So flap valve trocars are preferred.
- Pyramidal shape trocar is easy to insert.
- The conical trocar tip requires a stronger thrust to insert.
- Introduction of auxiliary trocars is always carried out under vision.
- Trocars come in different diameters 3 mm, 5 mm, 10 mm and 12 mm.

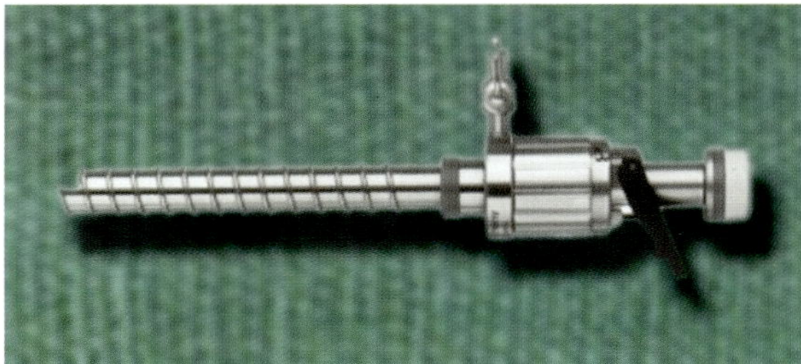

Fig. 2.6: Endotip

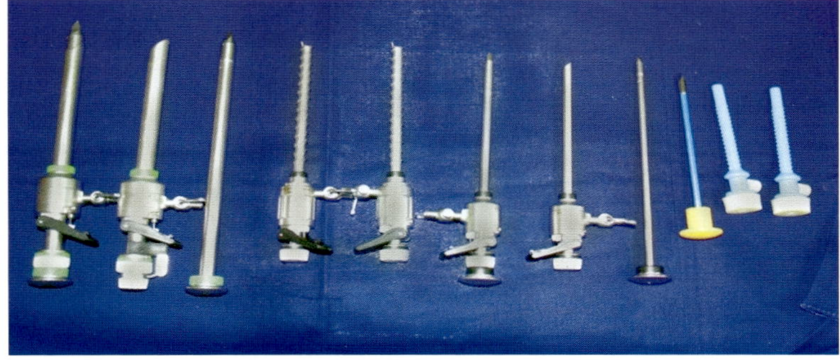

Fig. 2.7: Trocars and cannulae

Endoscopes (Figs 2.8 and 2.9)

- Most commonly used laparoscopes are 0° and 30°, 5 mm and 10 mm.
- In 0° scope, the direction of view corresponds to natural approach and facilitates orientation.
- 30° laparoscope is advantageous during dissection in the pouch of Douglas and in case of multiple fibroids where one has to see beyond the fibroids.

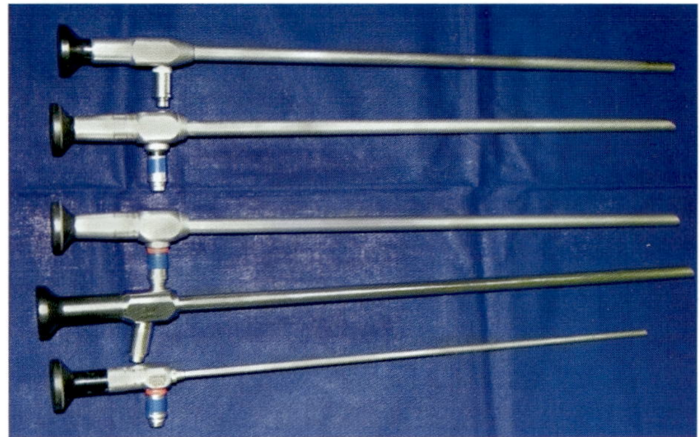

Fig. 2.8: Laparoscopes

Fig. 2.9: 10 mm laparoscopes 0° and 30°

Forceps/Graspers (Figs 2.10 and 2.11)

- They are available in different sizes and shapes.
- Ideal grasper should be medium sized with a rounded tip and serrated jaws so that it can grasp tissue and act as a blunt probe with jaws closed.
- **Maryland dissector** resembles the curved artery of open surgery.
- **Serrated traumatic tissue graspers** are designed for holding structures such as cyst wall, while **claw forceps** are useful for holding tough tissues like cervix at the time of hysterectomy or small myomas.

- **Tenaculum** are used along with morcellators for holding myoma and are available as 5 mm and 10 mm.
- **Bipolar forceps** are the key to success of endoscopic surgery. Everyone should have a good pair of these forceps. We recommend bipolar forceps with good grip and dissector type, so that it can be used as dissector and grasper which accelerates surgical speed.

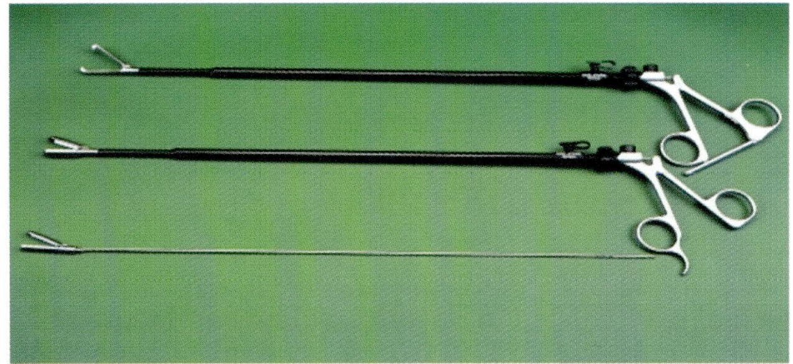

Fig. 2.10: 10 mm claw and spoon forceps

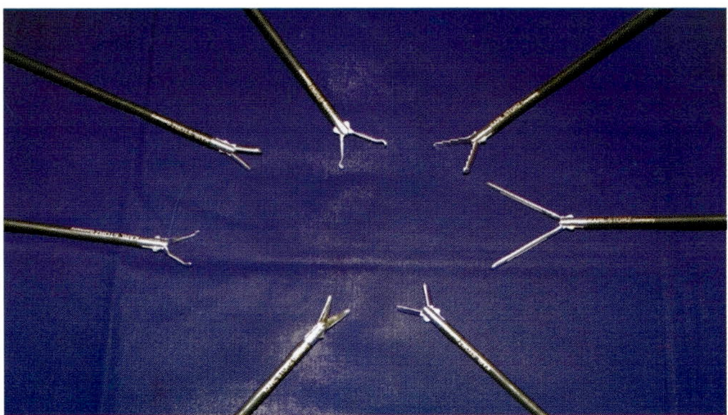

Fig. 2.11: Graspers – traumatic and atraumatic

Scissors (Fig. 2.12)

- Can be curved, straight or hooked.
- Some have electrical adapters.

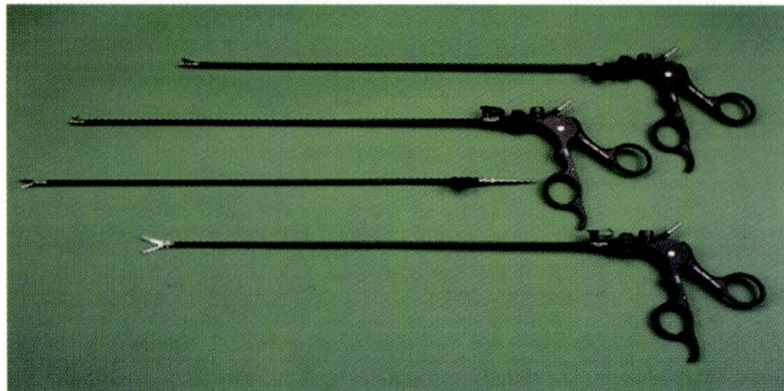

Fig. 2.12: Scissors

Suction Irrigation Cannula (Fig. 2.13)

- Available in 5 mm and 10 mm.
- The one end is connected to irrigation where as other end to the suction tube.
- It can also be used for aqua dissection.
- The suction tip can have single or multiple holes as per the individual's choice.

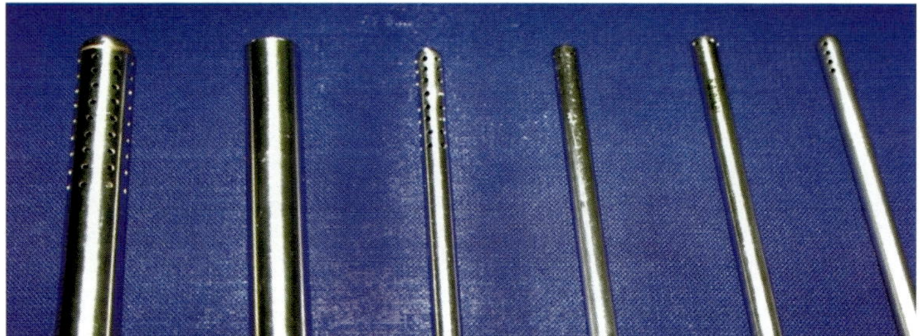

Fig. 2.13: Suction irrigation cannulae – 5 mm and 10 mm with different tips

Monopolar Needle (Fig. 2.14)

- It has a very fine needle with pin control used in cases of PCO drilling, puncturing of cysts and to take a fine incision for salpingostomy in cases of unruptured ectopic pregnancy, tubo-tubal anastamosis, etc.

Monopolar Spatula/Hook

- It can be used to make a precise incision.

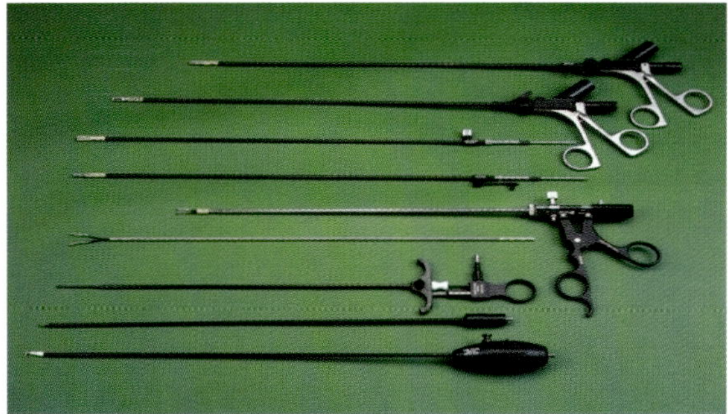

Fig. 2.14: Bipolar and unipolar forceps

Needle Holders (Fig. 2.15)

- One should definitely have a pair of excellent quality needle holders, we recommend left handed curve needle holders so that suture loops can be glided off easily.
- In case of myomectomy and hysterectomy during vault closure, left handed tooth forceps helps to have good grip of uterine flaps.

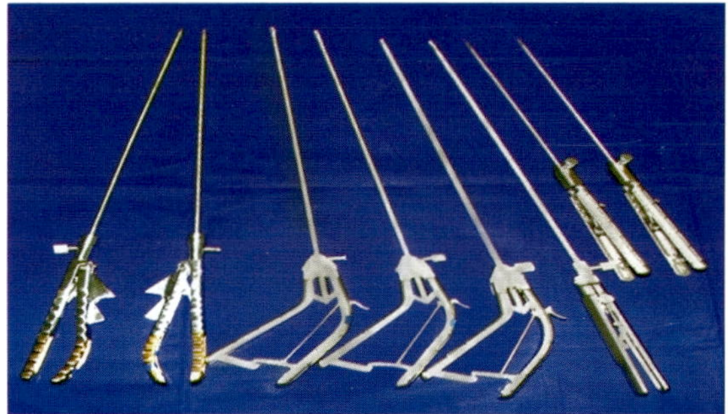

Fig. 2.15: Laparoscopic needle holders

Myoma Screw

- They are introduced into the myomas, which allow stabilizing the myoma, maneuvering it and applying traction to improve visibility, access and better performance of surgery.
- Some use it in total laparoscopic hysterectomy for uterine manipulation (instead of vaginal manipulator).

Clip Applicator

- They are used for hemostasis of medium sized vessels. One can have 3 mm and 5 mm clip applicators.

Uterine Manipulator

- It is used to mobilize or stabilize the uterus during surgery.

Self Designed (Fig. 2.16)

It has a handle with notch for the thumb to know internal curvature of the instrument—
- Notch anterior — curve anterior.
- Notch posterior — curve posterior.
- Handle makes the job of the vaginal assistant easy.

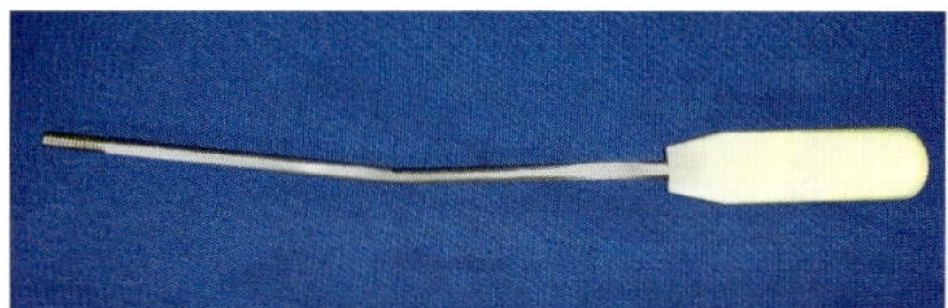

Fig. 2.16: Self designed manipulator

Long Sturdy Rod with Angle

Long sturdy rod with angle helps to manipulate bulky uterus even of 18 weeks easily.

TIPS

Tip is serrated to avoid perforation of uterus with manipulator.
- Same handle if put in the posterior fornix in reverse way can be used for taking posterior colpotomy incisions, as it does not conduct electricity.

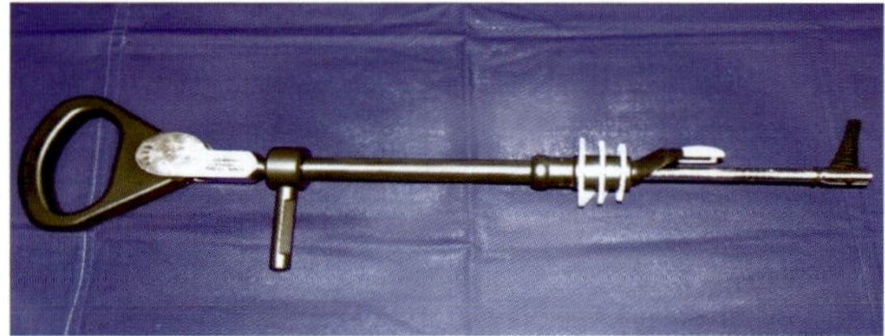

Fig. 2.17: Clermont-Ferrand uterine manipulator

Electronic Tissue Morcellator (Fig. 2.18)

- It is used to morcellate myoma into small bits and remove it piecemeal.

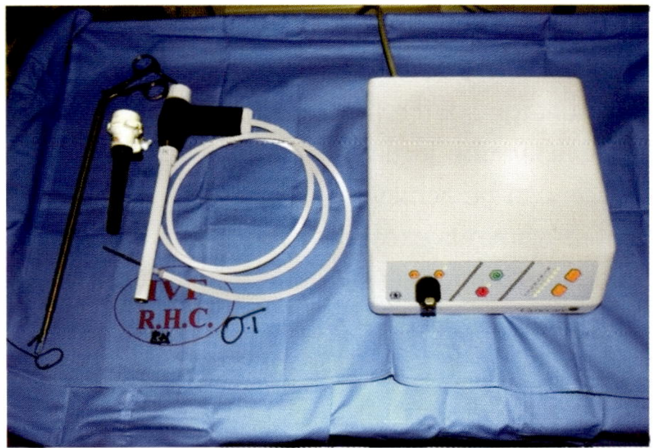

Fig. 2.18: Electronic tissue morcellator

Laparoscopy Specimen Retrieval Bag

It facilitates removal of specimen from the abdominal cavity and avoids contamination of the abdomen with its contents.

TIPS

a. Handle all equipments with utmost care.

b. Maintenance of all equipments is the secret of their longevity.

c. All instruments should be cleaned with a brush and water to remove all clots. Ultrasonic cleaners and enzymes are also available to remove all the clots.

d. Instruments should be dried thoroughly before being replaced in their chambers.

e. When the xenon light source is kept in contact with the skin/ drape, there is burning of that part suggesting that if this aspect is ignored during surgery, the patient may have electrical burns.

f. Light cables are always kept in the larger circular pattern to avoid breakage of the inner fibers.

g. In endoscopic surgery, you cannot look at the foot switches every time before cauterizing. Your left foot senses the foot switches.

> *A set of good quality instruments is better than a cupboard full of standard ones.*

So it is important to have fixed position of monopolar and bipolar foot switches. If you are used to keep the bipolar foot switch medially, always keep it medially only. This will avoid accidental thermal injury especially if accessory instruments carrying both these cautery currents are inside at a time. If one is using the ultrasonic energy source (i.e. harmonic), then hand instrument with hand activation facility should be used.

h. Sterilization can be achieved as follows:
   i.   Metal instruments except the telescopes can be autoclaved.
   ii. Rapid sterilization can be done by placing in cidex solution for 20 minutes.
   iii. Other instruments (tubings/cables) can be placed in formalin chambers.

Most important aspect of endoscopic surgery is to have a proper operation theater setup, instruments and adequate facilities to deal with complications.

> **"It is not the instruments that makes the surgery safe but it is the surgeon who makes the use of instruments safe for the patients"**

(Photographs courtesy: Ruby Hall IVF and Endoscopy Centre/Dr PG Paul)

3 Energy Sources in Endoscopic Surgery

Learning energy sources is of paramount importance in doing endosurgical procedure.

A clear understanding of its physics and its application to surgical procedure is necessary.

It is equally important to maximize safe delivery of these energy sources.

Aim

1. To discuss and understand the fundamental therapeutic modalities of the available energy sources.
2. To discuss the inherent risks and advantages of each.

Types of energy sources available are:

ELECTROSURGERY

Electrosurgery is the generation and delivery of current between active electrode and dispersive electrode in order to elevate the tissue temperature for purposes of fulguration, desiccation and cutting.

How temperature affects tissue therapeutically?
1. Cutting requires a high current, low voltage continuous wave form.
2. Fulguration requires a high voltage low current non continuous wave form designed to coagulate by spraying long electrical sparks best to control capillary oozing.
3. Desiccation is a form of coagulation.

Two types of electrical circuits can be employed in electrosurgery: Unipolar and Bipolar.

Monopolar/Unipolar Current

Principle: The current flows from the electrosurgical unit through the operating electrode through the patient to the dispersing or ground electrode and finally back to the generator. Uses high frequency continuous wave form mainly for cutting.

Range: 20-80 watts

Precautions: Thermal injuries are very common. Faulty contact between the ground electrode and the patient can result in current dispensing through unwanted pathways of lesser resistance, resulting in undesired thermal injury, especially bowel.
- Proper insulation of instruments to be maintained.
- The electrosurgical unit is supposed to stop functioning if contact is faulty.
- Patient plate to be attached.
- Full view of the instrument in the peritoneal cavity. Full view of the surrounding structures as current can jump and cause thermal injury to surrounding structures.

Disadvantages: Lateral and in depth spread of current.

Bipolar Current

Principle: In bipolar current the circuit is closed, by placing the tissue between two electrodes, so that the current goes through the intervening tissue.

This type of current can coagulate, and desiccate but not achieve cutting.

Precautions: Grasper tip should not be touched to surrounding tissue like bowel while in action as current spreads not only within tips of the grasper but laterally as well.

Disadvantages:
- Lateral thermal spread.
- Charring and sticking of instruments with "eschar" disruption.

TIPS

Tips of Electrocautery
- Mainstay of endosurgery. Always invest in a standardized electrosurgical unit.
- Should offer good blend.
- Attach a standard cautery handle to the machine.
- Coagulate bit by bit in small spurts

- To avoid charring and sticking
    - i.   Stop coagulation before bubbles stop
    - ii. Do not cauterize indiscriminately for longer periods
    - iii. Invest in cautery, which stops automatically once tissue is coagulated
    - iv. Bipolar always works best in presence of blood but when cuatery is done in presence of blood charring does occur.
- Spread is always there though less in bipolar than monopolar.
- Use bipolar current often.
- Also bipolar hook is now available.
- Bipolar is most effective as the mechanism of coagulation is by fast tissue spread and its generation.
- Monopolar never works in presence of blood.
- Monopolar should not be activated when not in touch with any tissue (free in the peritoneal cavity) as it will cause jumping of current.
- Monopolar should never be activated under water as current will spread through water. Thorough suction of fluid should be done before activating monopolar current.

LASER

Many media are used to produce laser light in gynecology including CO_2, Argon gases, Nd Yag and KTP crystals for purpose of hemostasis and cutting.

The safety of patients and operating team are of paramount importance, hence trained and experienced assistants are invaluable during the procedure.

Precautions
- Operation rooms should be labelled.
- All the staff in the OT should wear protective goggles.
- Laser plume can cause respiratory damage.
- Increased equipment costs.

ULTRASOUND DISSECTOR/ULTRASONIC SCALPEL/HARMONIC SCALPEL (FIG. 3.1)

Proposed as an alternative energy source—

Parts: The ultrasonic scalpel system consists of: a current generator, a hand piece that houses an ultrasonic transducer, an instrument having an end effector (specific types include blade or shears) used to cut tissue, a foot pedal, and a hand switching adaptor.

Laparoscopic as well as open surgery handles are available.

Principle

- The instrument operates by means of a blade that vibrates longitudinally at a frequency of 55.5 kHz. The end of the device oscillates at about 50,000 cycles/sec which results in precise cutting.
- The scalpel coagulates and cuts by using lower temperatures than those used by electrosurgery or lasers.
- Ultrasonic scalpel technology controls bleeding by coaptive coagulation at low temperatures ranging from 50 to 100°C. Vessels are coapted (tamponaded) and sealed by a protein coagulum.
- Coagulation occurs by means of protein denaturation when the blade couples with protein, denaturing it to form a coagulum that seals small coapted vessels, when the effect is prolonged, secondary heat is produced that seals larger vessels.

Advantages

- Minimal lateral thermal tissue damage.
- Minimal charring and desiccation.
- Fewer instrument exchanges simplify procedure steps as it coagulates and cut.
- No electricity to or through the patient.
- Greater precision near vital structures.
- Minimal smoke for improved visibility in the surgical field.
- Lesser wear and tear.

Disadvantages

- Slower than other energy sources.
- Ultrasonic tip has a limited life span.
- Disposable attachments increase the cost per patient.
- Can not be used as vessel sealing device for vessels with diameter more than 3 mm.

TIPS

Tips of Harmonic

- A sophisticated energy source generates energy through ultrasonic waves.
- A must for advanced laparoscopy.

- No spread of energy.
- Disposable handle, delicate but reusable and durable.

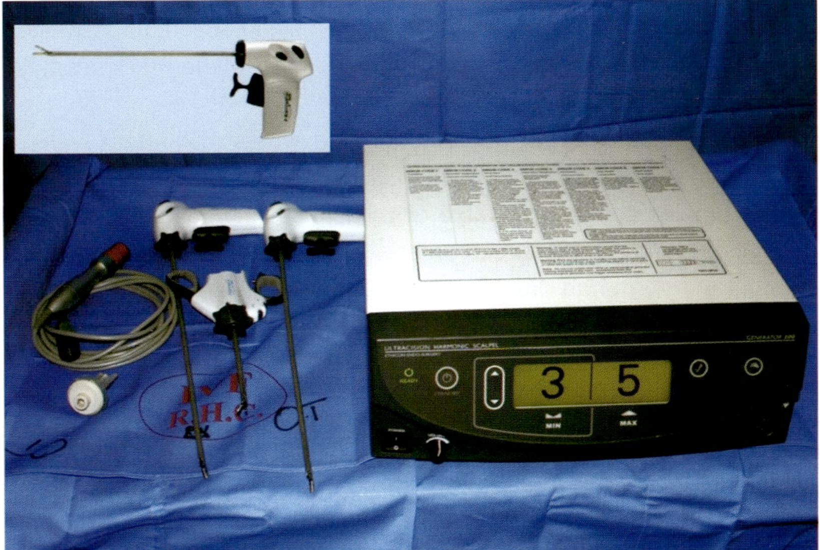

Fig. 3.1: Harmonic scalpel

Argon Beam Coagulator

- Argon Beam Coagulator used in both open procedures and minimally invasive surgery.
- More effective and cost efficient than conventional electrosurgery.
- Delivers current to the tissue in a directed beam of ionized argon gas.
- Flow of gas blows away blood and debris from the surgical field and produces a coagulated surface that is more uniform and shallower than that produced in standard electrosurgical coagulation.
- Coagulates bleeding tissue faster with reduced blood loss and tissue damage.
- Produces less smoke than conventional electrosurgery.

GYRUS PK TISSUE MANAGEMENT SYSTEM

The Gyrus PK Tissue Management System (Gyrus Medical, Inc, Minneapolis, Minnesota) instruments provide a unique technology called—Vapor pulse coagulation (VPC) and plasma kinetic cutting forceps.

Vapor Pulse Coagulation (VPC)

- Produces faster, more uniform results with pulsed energy instantly delivered in a controlled manner.
- VPC's pulse-off periods allow tissue to cool and moisture to return to the targeted area, greatly reducing hot spots and coagulum formation.
- Results in evenly coagulated target tissue; minimal thermal spread, less sticking, and enhanced hemostasis.
- It does require its own generator, which works in tandem with the instruments manufactured by *gyrus pk*.
- This bipolar device is capable of reliably sealing/dividing arteries as large as 6 mm, but it is recommended restricting its use to vessels no larger than 5 mm in diameter to allow a safety margin.
- Thermal spread affects only the area surrounding the divided vessel.

Plasma Kinetic Cutting Forceps

- The second device, the Plasma Kinetic Cutting Forceps (Gyrus Medical, Maple Grove, Minn.) utilizes advanced, solid-state generator software to deliver pulsed energy with continuous feedback control.
- The cycle stops once the device senses that tissue response is complete.
- The cool-down phase ensures that collagen and elastin matrix reforms without tissue fragmentation.

THE LIGASURE SYSTEM (VALLEYLAB, BOULDER, COLORADO): PRINCIPLE

- Uses a unique combination of pressure and energy to create vessel fusion.
- Melting the collagen and elastin in the vessel walls, and reforming it into a permanent, plastic-like seal accomplish is this fusion.
- A feedback-controlled response system automatically discontinues energy delivery when the seal cycle is complete, eliminating guesswork and minimizing thermal spread to approximately 2 mm for most *LigaSure* instruments.

TIPS

Tips of Ligasure
- It does not rely on a proximal thrombus as does classic bipolar electrocautery.

- Results in virtually no sticking or charring, and the seals can withstand 3 times normal systolic blood pressure vessel sealing and a pedicle shearing device.
- Energy is delivered through a sophisticated insulated hand instrument programmed and timed so that safe amount and duration of energy is delivered.
- Laparoscopic as well as open handle available.
- Effective in vessel sealing especially for large pedicles.
- Convenient as coagulates and cuts in a single application one after the other no need of additional scissors and thus change of instruments.

Cautery is the mainstay of endosurgery

(Photograph courtesy: Ruby Hall IVF and Endoscopy Centre)

4 Medicolegal Issues in Endoscopic Surgeries

- Any therapeutic procedure, surgical or medical requires to be offered to the patient within the framework of what is 'ethical'. 'Ethical' implies that the benefits of treatment clearly outweigh the risks of the procedure.
- One has to understand that laparoscopic surgery is a technically driven modality of treatment, which requires training, experience and is typically characterized by a long learning curve till the surgeon establishes skills.
- Evidences in literature have shown that most of the complications occur during the learning curve of the surgeon and therefore, to offer safe technique to patient, it is important to identify your own limitations and capabilities.
- It is imperative that the technique that you use is standardized and the equipment and the instrumentation be of standard quality. This not only offers comfort to the surgeon but also safety and goes a long way in avoiding complications.
- More than 80% of the clinical situations in gynecology today are tackled laparoscopically. The literature unfortunately lacks clear-cut guidelines as to what should and should not be done laparoscopically. These guidelines to be evolved require uniformity of practice, standardization of techniques and modalities. This modality being skill driven also depends upon the competence of the operating surgeon and therefore the need to understand one's own capabilities and limitations. The disease also requires to be properly evaluated and complications, if any, foreseen prior and evaluated.
- It is not only the problem in the court and the public litigation which should be a cause of concern to the surgeon but also the fact that any untoward occurrence or complication receives rejection from the community and therefore one should practice laparoscopy with utmost

responsibility and established standards to allow this modality to evolve, progress and receive acceptability.

- One should be utmost careful while selecting the patient, disciplined while performing the surgery and have an open mind towards the need of conversion to the open approach, if the need so arises in the interest of the patient. The need to convert to the open modality should not be considered as a complication of laparoscopic surgery. At any cost, one should not cause any harm to the patient.

- Laparoscopic surgery has distinct advantages and some very important limitations. These require to be understood by the surgeon while offering this mode of treatment to the patient. The patient should be taken into confidence like any other treatment modality that we offer, so that there are no misunderstandings, false assurances and consequently unpleasantness on the part of the patient.

- It is important that a proper preoperative counseling is offered which will go in the long run to avoid any litigations from the patient arising out of this unpleasantness.

- There are no clear cut guidelines for what is right and what is wrong.But the surgeon should, with responsibility be absolutely thorough in documentation and recording of all the events of the surgical session and its aftermath. There are important directives of the Supreme Court with respect to the informed consent in such situations, which were evolved as a result of a case, related to laparoscopic surgery contested in the Supreme Court in the year 1995 under the CPA 1986 Section 21 of Negligence compensation.

- The Supreme Court of India has come out with very important jugdement in the case of Sameera Kohli vs Dr Mandhanda, case no. CA 1949 of 1004 decided on 16th January 2008.

The story goes as such—

The appellant went to the respondent clinic with her mother. On admission, the appellant's signatures were taken on consent form for diagnostic and operative laparoscopy on 10th May 1995—Appellent was put under GA and was subjected to a laparoscopic examination. When the appellant was still unconscious, assistant doctor came out of the operation theater and took the consent for hysterectomy from the appellant's mother, who was waiting outside. Thereafter, the respondent performed an abdominal hysterectomy and bilateral salpingo-oophorectomy and this case went against the respondent resulting in the Supreme Court summarizing the principles relating to consent as follows:

1. A doctor has to seek and secure the consent of the patient before commencing a treatment (the term treatment includes surgery also). The consent so obtained should be real and valid which means that; the patient should have the capacity and the competence to consent; his consent should be voluntary; and his consent should be on the basis of adequate information concerning the nature of the treatment procedure, so that he knows what he is consenting to.

2. The adequate information to be furnished by the doctor (or a member of his team) who treats the patient, should enable the patient to make balanced jugdement as to whether he should submit himself to the particular treatment or not. This means that the doctor should disclose:
    i. Nature and procedure of the treatment and its purpose, benefits and effect
    ii. Alternatives, if any, available
    iii. An outline of the substantial risks
    iv. Adverse consequences of refusing treatment.

3. But there is no need to explain remote or theoretical risks involved, which may frighten or confuse the patient and result in refusal of consent for the necessary treatment. Similarly, there is no need to persuade a patient to undergo a fanciful or unnecessary treatment. A balanced should be achieved between the need for disclosing necessary and adequate information and at the same time, avoid the possibility of the patient being deterred from agreeing to a necessary treatment or offering to undergo an unnecessary treatment.

4. Consent given only for a diagnostic procedure, cannot be considered as consent for the theraupetic treatment.Consent given for a specific treatment procedure will not be valid for conducting some other treatment procedure. The fact that the unauthorized additional surgery is beneficial to the patient, or that it would save considerable time and expense to the patient or would relieve the patient from pain and suffering in future, are not grounds of defence in action in tort for negligence or assault and battery. The only exception to the rule is where the additional procedure though unauthorized, is necessary in order to save the life or preserve the health of the patient and it would be unreasonable to delay such unauthorized procedure until patient regains consciousness and takes a decision.

5. There can be common consent for diagnostic and operative procedures where they are contemplated. There can also be a common

consent for a particular procedure and an additional or further procedure that may become necessary during the course of surgery.

6. The nature and extent of information to be furnished by the doctor to the patient to secure the consent need not be of the stringent and high degree mentioned in Cantebury, but should be of the extent which is accepted as normal and proper by a body of medical men skilled and experienced in the particular field. It will depend upon the physical and mental condition of the patient, the nature of treatment, the risk and the consequences attached to the treatment.

7. In view of our finding, that there was no consent by the appellent for performing hysterectomy and salpingo-oophorectomy, performance of such a surgery was an unauthorized invasion and interference with appellent's body, which amounted to a tortuous act of assault and battery and therefore a deficiency of service. But as noticed above, there are several mitigating circumstances. The respondent did it in the interest of the appellent. As the appellant was already 44 years old, and was having serious menstrual problems, the respondent thought that by surgical removal of the uterus and ovaries, she was providing permanent relief. It is also possible that the respondent thought that the appellant may approve the additional surgical procedure when she regained consciousness and the consent by appellant's mother gave her the authority to do the same.

8. This is a case of respondent acting in excess of consent but in good faith and for the benefit of the appellant. Though the appellant has alleged that she had to undergo hormone therapy, no other repercussions is made out as a result of the removal. The appellant was already fast approaching the age of menopause, and in all probability required such hormone therapy. Even assuming that AH-BSO surgery was not immediately required, there was a reasonable certainty that she would have ultimately required the said treatment for a complete cure.

9. On the facts and circumstances, we consider that interests of justice would be served if the respondent is denied the entire fee charged for the surgery and in addition, directed to pay Rs. 25,000 as compensation for the unauthorized AH-BSO surgery to the appellant.

10. This particular Supreme Court ruling along with the elaborate case has been on purpose included for each one of us to be able to device a proper consent under the guidelines laid down by the Supreme Court of India.

11. Proper equipment has to be available.
12. Careful case selection is important.
13. Detailed communication complications and develop a standardized system and a habit to remain within the ethical framework.

TIPS

- The surgeon should be adequately trained as regards the procedure and informed consent is vital.
- Standard techniques should be followed.
- The procedure and specially the precautions taken should be documented.
- Possibility of complications, specially in a high risk patient, should be counseled well in advance.
- Postoperative instructions and follow up should not be neglected.

5   Prevention of Complications in Endoscopic Surgeries

Complications are inherent in any surgical procedure and laparoscopy is no exception. Since complications can occur even with a relatively easy procedure, it is imperative that all surgeons must learn to recognize the complications expeditiously and manage the events.

The risks increase exponentially with the complexity of procedures, the inexperience of the surgeon and with any deviation from the standard techniques.

The learning curve for laparoscopic procedures is lengthy and the risk of complications is greatest in the early period of the surgeon's learning.

Preoperative complications can be at different stages, such as

During Anesthesia

- Proper preoperative workup of the patient with cardio-respiratory assessment.
- Sensitivity of the drugs to be checked.
- Monitoring of the patient with pulseoxymetry, cardiogram and ET CO_2 to prevent complications.
- Prolonged ventilation with difficult intubation may fill the stomach with air and make it prone for injury with Veress needle or trocar hence Ryle's tube instillation is necessary to decompress the stomach just prior to veress insertion.
- Ryle's tube instillation to prevent Mendelson's syndrome.
- General anesthesia combined with epidural in long cases helps to keep bowel collapsed and decrease oozing.

During Positioning of Patient

Prevention of nerve injuries especially those involving the brachial plexus, ulnar, femoral and common peroneal nerves.

- Padded Allen stirrups provide good support and allow proper positioning which can be changed in a draped position during surgery.

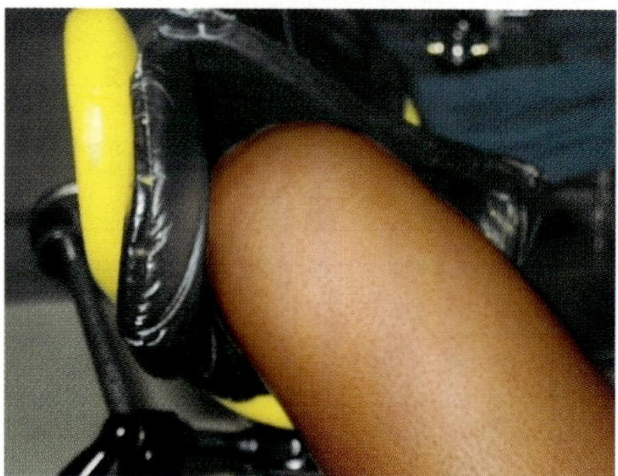

Fig. 5.1

- In lithotomy position, good cushion support prevents injury to common peroneal nerve (Fig. 5.1).
- Shoulder rest should be placed laterally on acromio-clavicular joint to prevent injury of brachial plexus (Fig. 5.2).

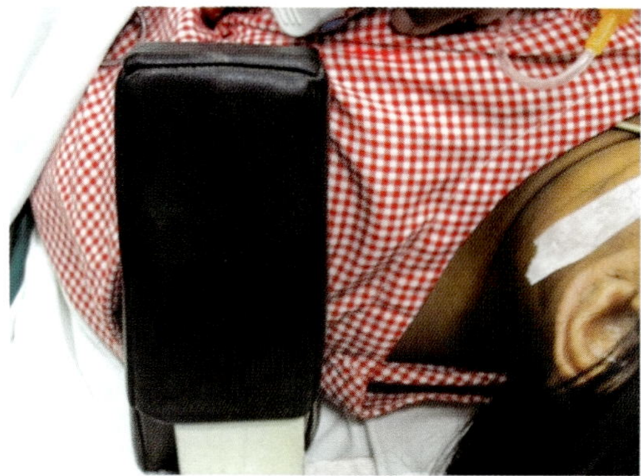

Fig. 5.2

- Placing the left arm extended at the elbow joint, pronated and tucked loosely by the side of the body and the right arm flexed and kept on the chest as if on a sling can prevent both ulnar and brachial plexus injuries (Figs 5.3A and B).

> ***Every surgery open or endoscopic has its own share of complications. The greatest hazard to the patient is not the surgery but the 'Surgeon'***

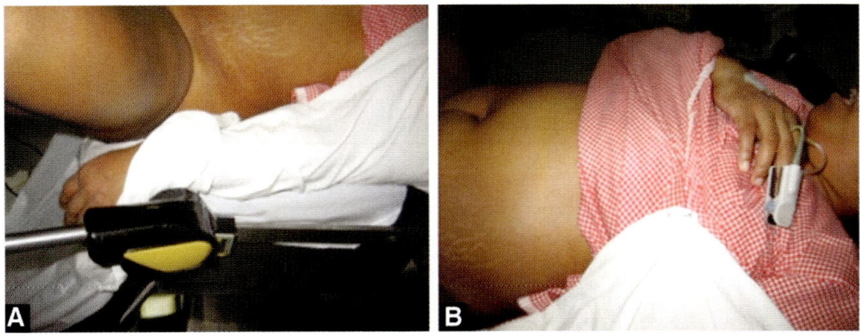

Figs 5.3A and B

During the Technique

Prevention of Complications due to Pneumoperitoneum

- Pneumoperitoneum pressure should not exceed more than 15 mm of Hg to avoid cardio-respiratory embarrassment and injuries to major vessels.
- Entry of veress needle or trocar in peritoneal cavity should be confirmed before starting inflow of CO_2 to prevent complications due to extra peritoneal insufflation.
- Embolization can be prevented by use of CO_2 for pneumoperitoneum than air.

Prevention of Trocar or Veress Needle Injuries

Most of the vessel injuries are mainly due to technical errors and hence these need to be corrected by —
- Proper stabilization of abdominal wall during trocar insertion.
- Avoid forceful and jerky trocar insertion, guard trocar with index finger tip to prevent sudden and wrong entry of trocar. Screwing motion gives better control than direct trusting.
- Visualization of inferior epigastric vessels before insertion of ancillary trocars.
- Direction of entry of trocar should be towards the tip of coccyx (Fig. 5.4).
- All accessory trocars should be placed under vision.
- In cases of previous scarred surgery, (laparoscopic/laprotomy) it is preferable to use Palmer's point for primary trocar insertion.
- Don't give head low position unless primary port is taken.

> *Every surgeon should pick up the right surgical technique for the right patient, understating his/her limitations and mastery over the technique.*

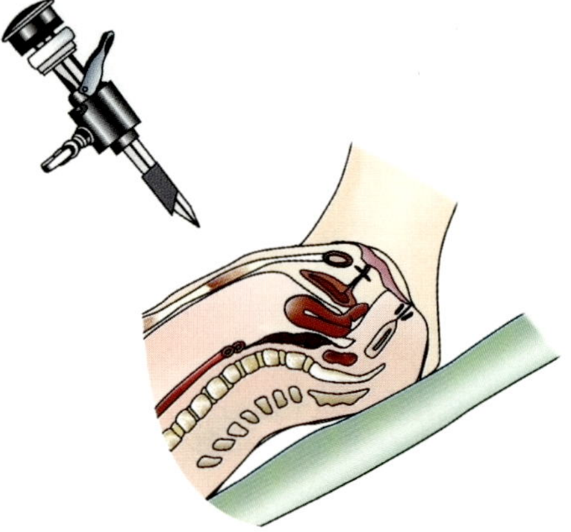

Fig. 5.4: Correct direction of entry of trocar

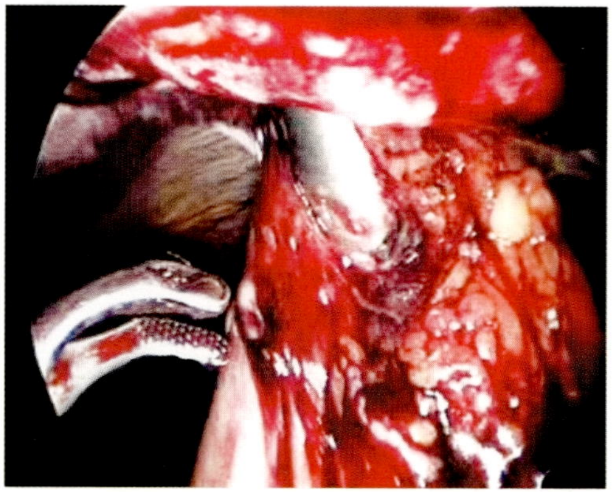

Fig. 5.5: Entry of primary trocar directly in bowel

Prevention of Bowel Injuries

- Good bowel preparation is must prior to any laparoscopic surgery.
- Open trocar entry by Hasson's technique or Palmer's point entry in cases of previous scarred surgery.
- Instruments with defective insulation should be discarded and not repaired.
- Avoid dangling of instruments specially monopolar and bipolar forceps at a time inside the peritoneal cavity at the beginning and learning curve.

> **Endoscopic surgery should not be 'in competition' but should be 'complimentary'.**

- Use of plastic abdominal wall grips with metal cannula should be avoided to prevent bowel injury by direct coupling.

Prevention of Urinary Tract Injuries

- Bladder should be emptied adequately before veress or primary trocar insertion.
- Good tissue planes and proper dissection of bladder during the procedure prevents bladder injuries.
- While performing hysterectomy – tips to prevent bladder and ureteric injuries (refer to respective chapters).
- Ureteric stenting in case of extensive adhesions, e.g. Endometriosis, prevents injury to the ureter.

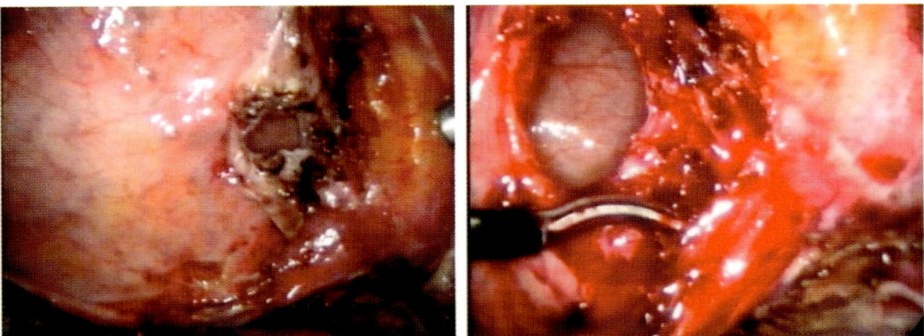

Fig. 5.6: Inadvertent opening of bladder

Prevention of Electrosurgical Injuries

- Periodic check of instruments is must to find out any break or breach in insulation.
- Whole length of the cautery pad should be in contact with the broad skin surface of the buttock or legs to prevent skin burns.
- All instruments carrying monopolar current should be inspected regularly for insulation. Monopolar cautery can not be used under water or free in air as current spreads or jumps to near by organs.

Morcellator Related Injuries

- The rotating blade of the morcellator should be visible throughout the procedure and it should be retracted when not in use.
- The specimen should be completely separated from surrounding structures and vessels before the morcellation.

Prevention of Postoperative Complications

- Early ambulation.
- Coverage of antibiotics-intraoperative and postoperative period.
- Deep breathing exercises.
- Ensure adequate hydration on previous day especially for patients who are on bowel preparation to prevent postoperative electrolyte imbalance in extensive cases.
- Early suspicion in case of abnormal signs and symptoms.

TIPS

- Use of stockings and or anticoagulants to prevent deep vein thrombosis.
- Keeping operating time to a minimum by improving surgical skills and standard equipments.
- Suturing rectus sheath whenever incision more than 7 mm is taken and using 'Z' technique for primary trocar insertion can prevent herniation.
- Exposure, identification of anatomic landmarks and careful dissection will reduce the risk of ureteric injury.
- The presence of gas and/or blood in the urinary drainage bag allows early recognition of bladder injury. Cystoscopy is confirmatory.

PREVENTION OF COMPLICATIONS DURING HYSTEROSCOPY

Preoperative Prevention

1. By using an ideal distending media, in right quantity, water intoxication and hyponatremia can be prevented.
2. Uterine perforation is the commonest complication that can be encountered during septum resection, adhesiolysis of Ashermann's syndrome and myomectomy, which can be prevented by —
   - Gentle cervical dilatation.
   - Introduction of hysteroscope under vision.
   - Using energy setting appropriate for the procedure.
   - Making all cutting strokes from fundus towards cervix or lateral alternating technique in case of broader septum.

- By recognizing thinness of cornual opening and obeying 1st law of holes, i.e. stop digging once inside the holes.
- By performing simultaneous laparoscopy.
- During septum resection in its final phase by stopping the resection till small area of bleeding is seen indicating myometrium is reached.
- Should get reorientation of cavity from time to time by withdrawing telescope till internal os and taking panaromic view.

3. Over abduction of the thighs to be avoided.
4. Keeping operating time to a minimum.
5. Detection of fluid overload by signs and symptoms like transient hypertension followed by hypotension.
6. Keep fluid pressures below 80 mmHg.
7. Meticulous accountancy of fluid balance.
8. The procedure must be abandoned if the deficit rises to 2 liters or there is evidence of venous congestion.
9. In case of suspected electric injury after uterine perforation, laparoscopy may be performed to examine bowel, pelvic blood vessels and aorta.

TIPS

- Every surgery open or endoscopic has its own share of complications. The greatest hazard to the patient is not the surgery but the 'Surgeon'.
- Every surgeon should pick up the right surgical technique for the right patient, understating his/her limitations and mastery over the technique."

> *The flexible surgeon is familiar with all available techniques so that the best approach is selected for the individual patient*

(Photographs courtesy: Dr PG Paul)

6   Port Placement

Usually in gynecologic endoscopic surgeries, all ports are at and below umbilicus level but position of the ports either in lower or upper abdomen depends upon the size and pathology of uterus and if any previous lower abdominal surgeries.

ROUTINE PORT PLACEMENTS

Usually 3 to 4 ports are taken.

Primary Port

1. Taken either infraumbilical or intra-umbilical-
   - Verres needle for pneumoperitoneum followed by 10 mm trocar insertion or
   - Direct 10 mm trocar insertion

Ancillary Ports

1. Two 5 mm ports on surgeon's side, 10 cm apart
   a. Lower port in iliac fossa, approximately 2 fingers medial and one finger above anterior superior iliac spine.
   b. Upper port 10 cm up and little medial to lower port.
2. Third 5 mm port is on the contralateral side usually in line with the primary trocar (A) or can also be taken in similar manner as lower port of ipsilateral side (B) as in Figure 6.1.

TIPS

1. Left-sided (surgeon's side) lower 5 mm port should be valve-less to carry suture material. Right-sided 5 mm port should have outlet to remove the smoke intermittently.

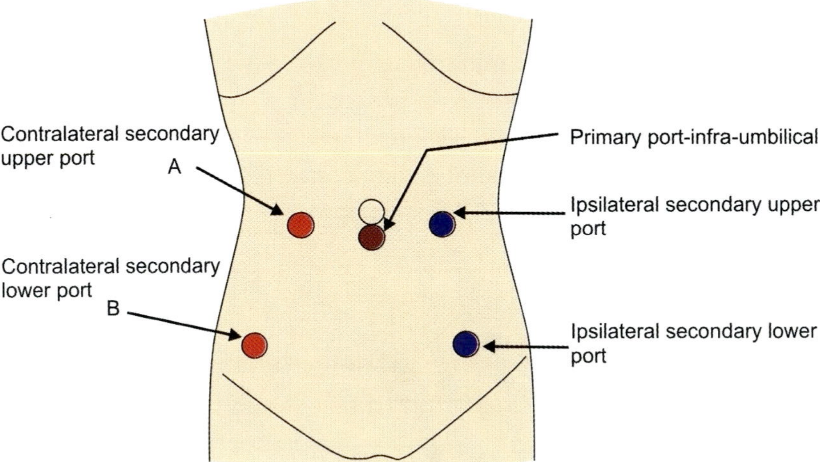

Fig. 6.1

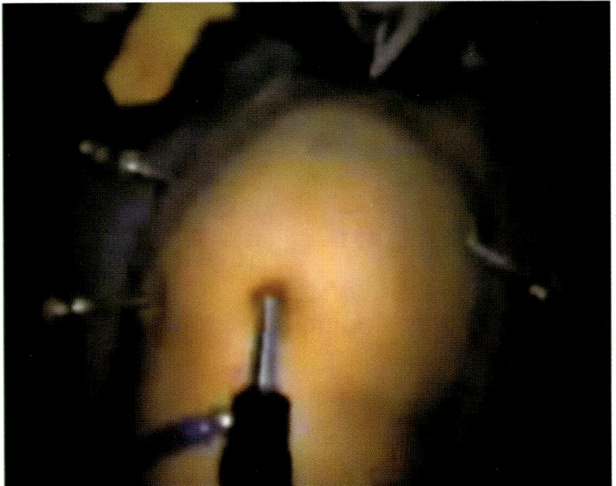

Fig. 6.2

2. Ancillary ports are introduced always under vision.
3. Site of ancillary ports is the individual's choice as per the suturing techniques and height of surgeon. For e.g. one can take one port on each side and third in the suprapubic area.

IN DIFFICULT SITUATIONS, LIKE

a. Previous lower abdominal surgeries
b. Large myomas
c. Large adenexal masses

Primary Port

1. At Palmer's point with 5 mm trocar
   Under vision, 10 mm trocar is passed at epigastric region (below xiphisternum) or supra-umbilical region.
   5 mm trocar at Palmer's point is then converted into ancillary port.
2. At supra-umbilical region 2-3 fingers above umbilicus.

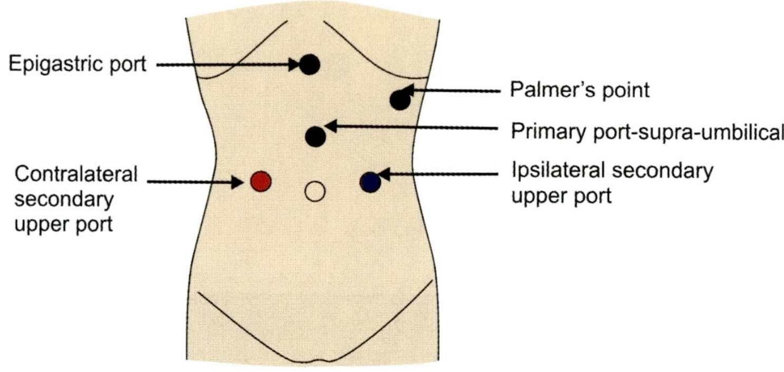

Fig. 6.3

TIPS

- While entering Palmer's point, 3 resistances are encountered
  - Anterior rectus sheath
  - Posterior rectus sheath
  - Parietal peritoneum
- Before selection of Palmer's point ensure
  - Deflation of stomach with Ryle's tube
  - Absence of splenomegaly
- Care has to be taken when primary supra-umbilical port is taken, as bifurcation of aorta and inferior vena cava will come directly under the entry of the trocar.

HASSON'S TECHNIQUE OF OPEN TROCAR INSERTION

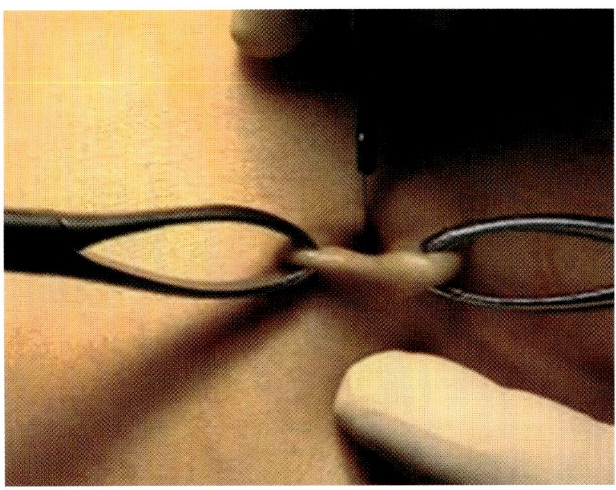

Fig. 6.4: Intraumbilical incision

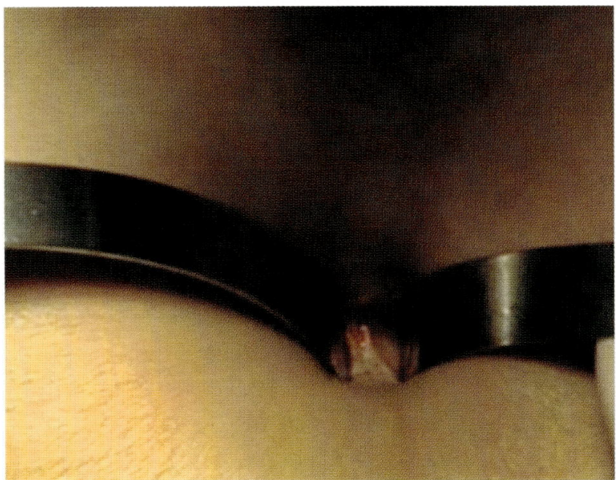

Fig. 6.5: Rectus sheath exposed

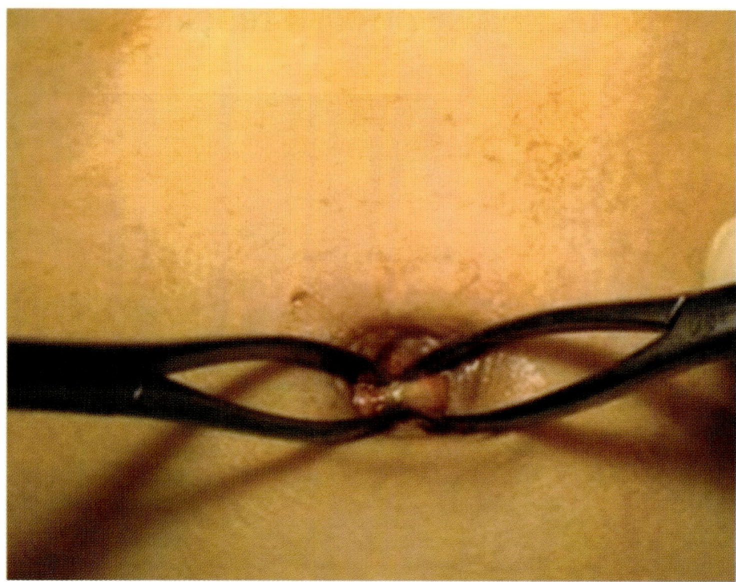

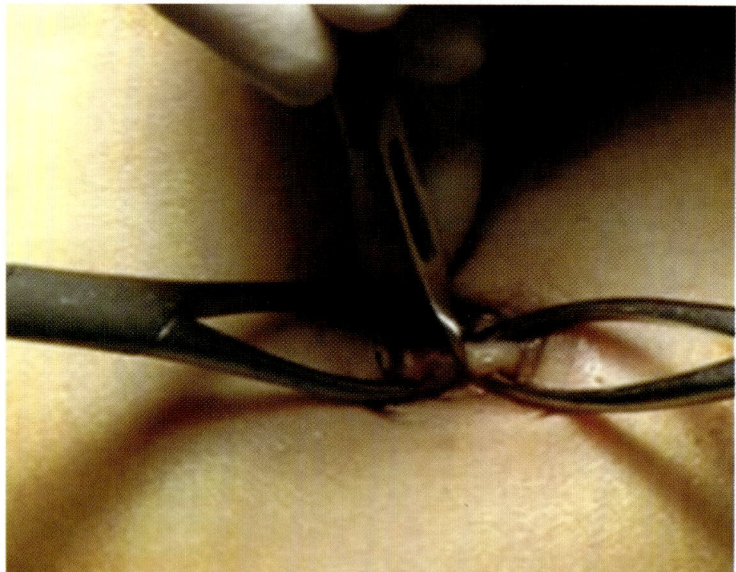

Figs 6.6A and B: Rectus sheath hold and cut

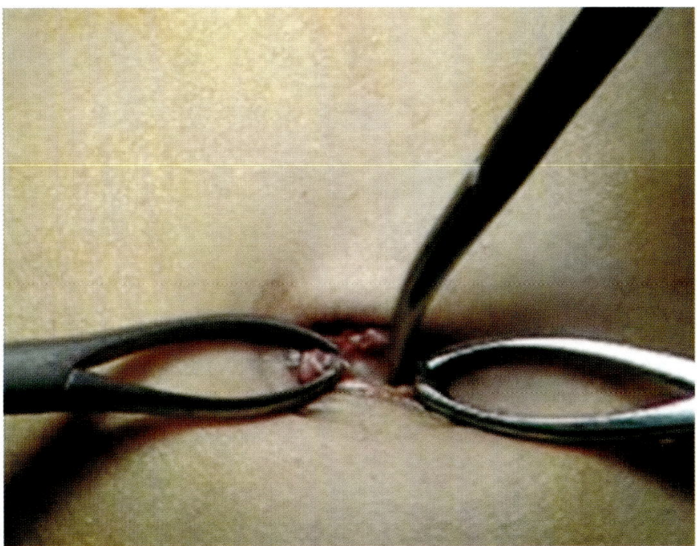

Fig. 6.7: Peritoneum dissected

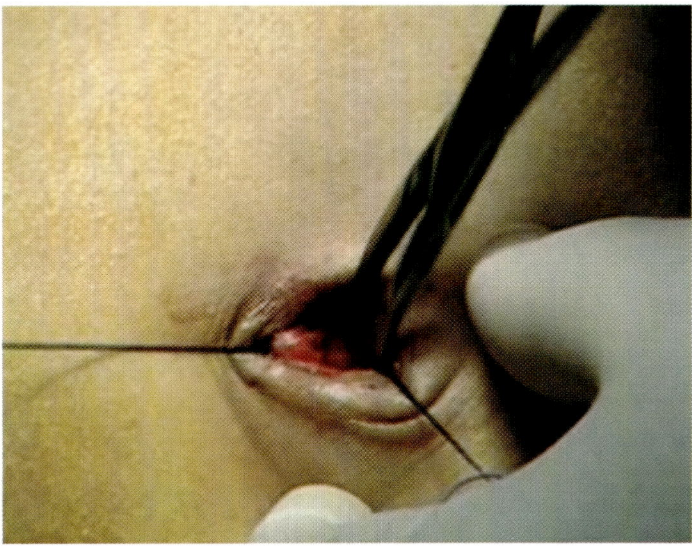

Fig. 6.8: Peritoneum opened after taking stitches at rectus, one on each side

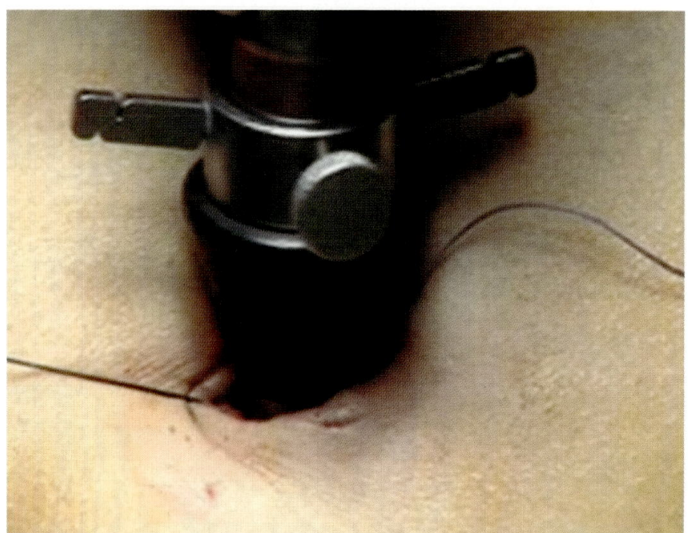

Fig. 6.9: Hasson's trocar in place

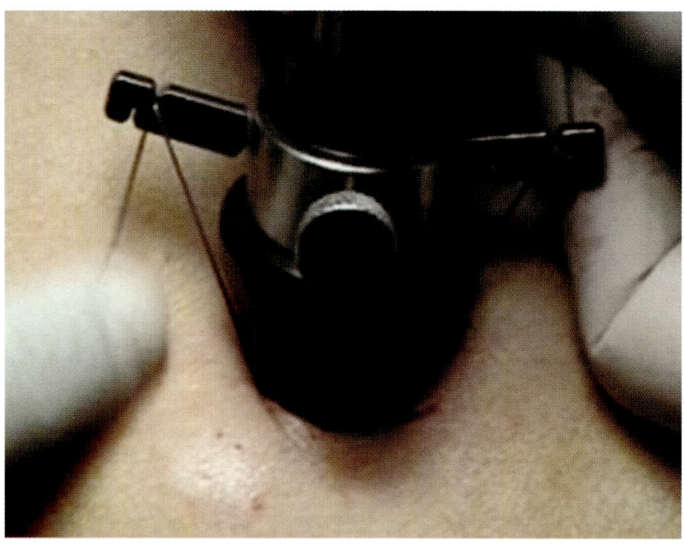

Fig. 6.10: Hasson's trocar fixed with stitches taken at rectus

(Photographs courtesy: Ruby Hall IVF and Endoscopy Centre)

Section Two

Hysteroscopy

7   **Diagnostic Hysteroscopy**

PREOPERATIVE PREPARATION

Diagnostic hysteroscopy does not need any other preoperative preparation. It is usually performed in immediate postmenstrual period.

ANESTHESIA

Under short General Anesthesia.

IMPORTANT EQUIPMENTS

Hysteroscope (4 mm) with diagnostic sheath.

TECHNIQUE

- 2 Allis forceps are placed on the anterior lip of the cervix to straighten the cervix and the uterus.
- Cervix is dilated manually with serial dilators to the one size more than the outer diameter of the outer sheath of hysteroscope so as to avoid forceful entry of hysteroscope.
- Hysteroscope is gently inserted under vision to limit the risk of uterine perforation. The insertion of the scope into uterine cavity is done with inflow on. This inflow of fluid also helps to wash up any blood clots coming in contact with lens tip.
- The outflow is partially on to make the vision clear. The movement of scope follows the anatomy of cervix.
- Once inside the cavity, scope is positioned in the center with the distal tip being kept at the distance of 1.5 to 2 mm from the fundus.
- Fixing the position of the camera in the left hand and holding the light cable in the right hand, scope is rotated by 90° clockwise and 180° anticlockwise, to see right and left cornu respectively. Hysteroscope is

withdrawn slowly till internal os. A panoramic view is taken. Hysteroscope is further withdrawn to view and examine the entire cervical canal since better view of cervical canal can be obtained during removal than during insertion.

TIPS

- In case of slight isthmic stenosis, atraumatic dilator i.e. plastic dilator can be used initially, as it is difficult to create wrong passage with plastic dilator.
- Also, paracervical block can be given with 2% xylocaine.
- Insertion of the scope into uterine cavity is done with inflow on. This inflow of fluid also helps to wash up any blood clots coming in contact with lens tip

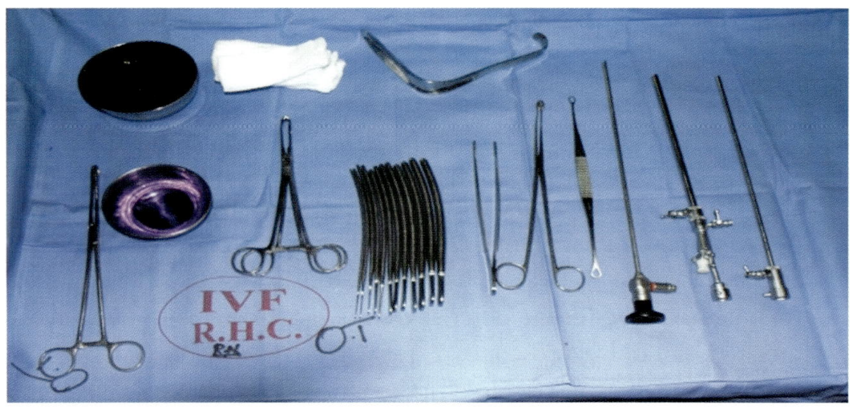

Fig. 7.1: Trolley of diagnostic hysteroscopy

Right cornu

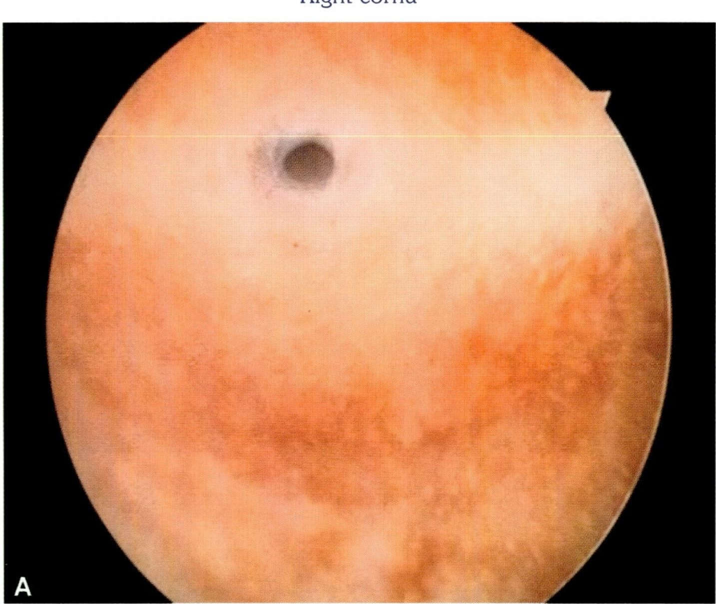

Left cornu

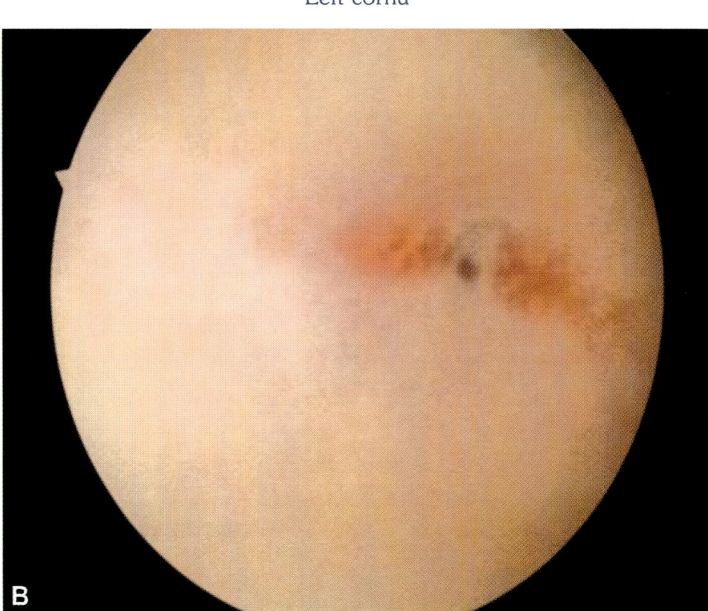

Figs 7.2A and B: Rotation of telescope allows visualization of tubal orifice

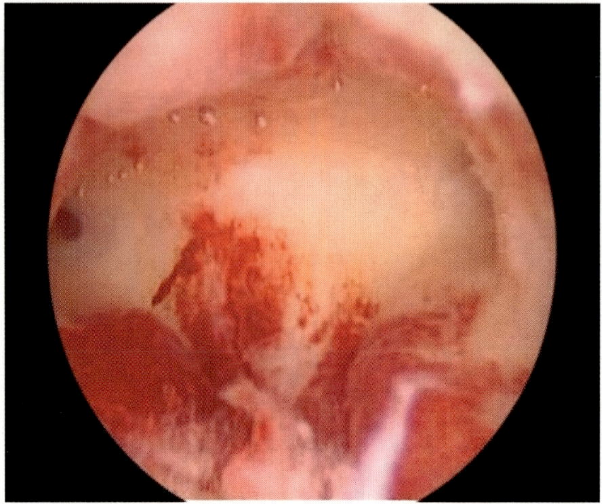

Fig. 7.3: Panoramic view from internal Os

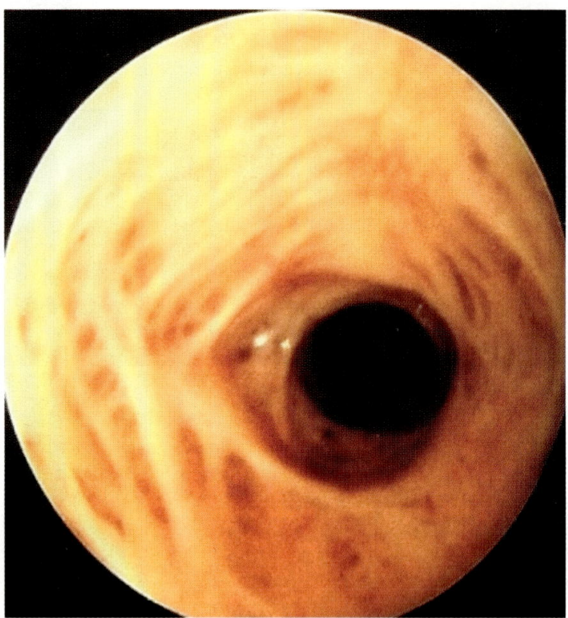

Fig. 7.4: Mild stenosis of cervical canal

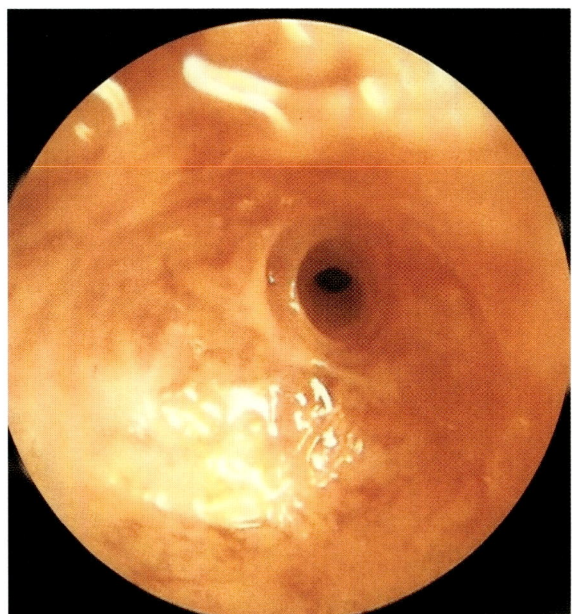

Fig. 7.5: Extensive stenosis of cervical canal

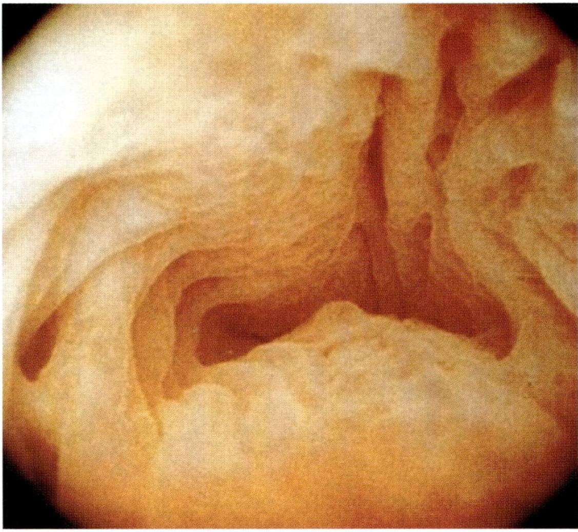

Fig. 7.6: Normal cervical canal

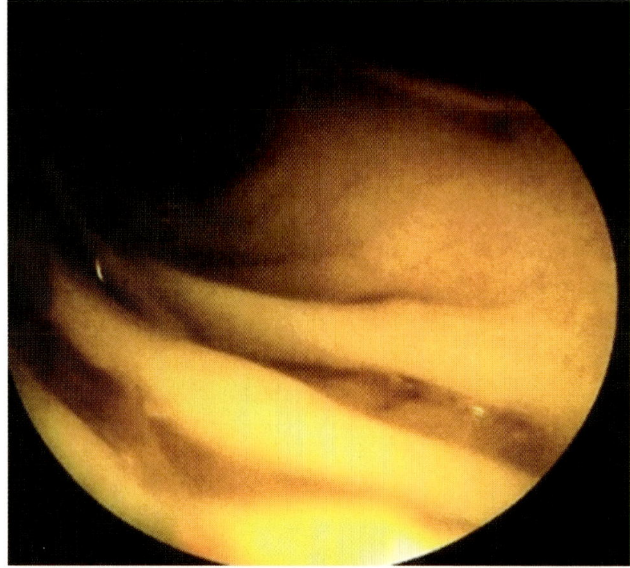

Fig. 7.7: Palmate folds of cervical canal

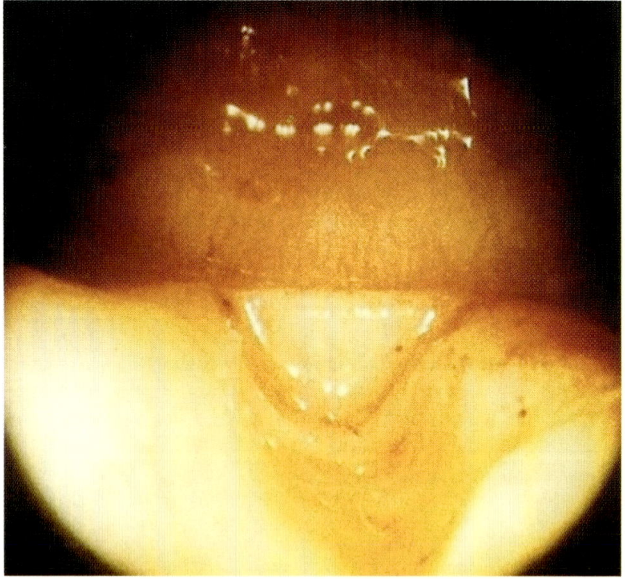

Fig. 7.8: Measurement of endometrial thickness

VARIOUS PATHOLOGIES DIAGNOSED
DURING HYSTEROSCOPY

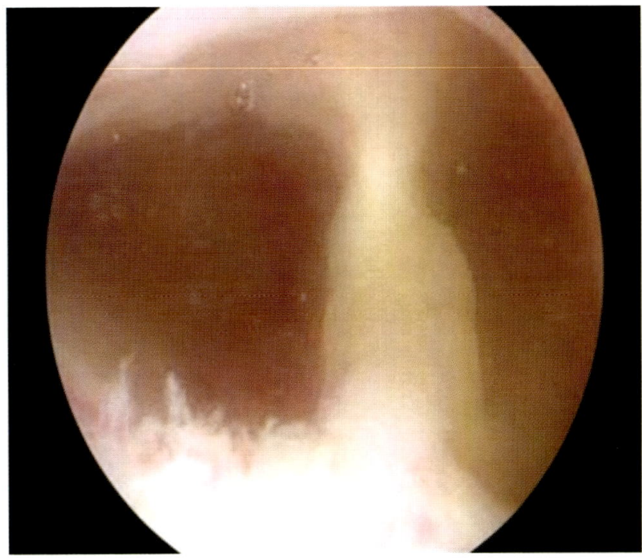

Fig. 7.9: Uterine septum

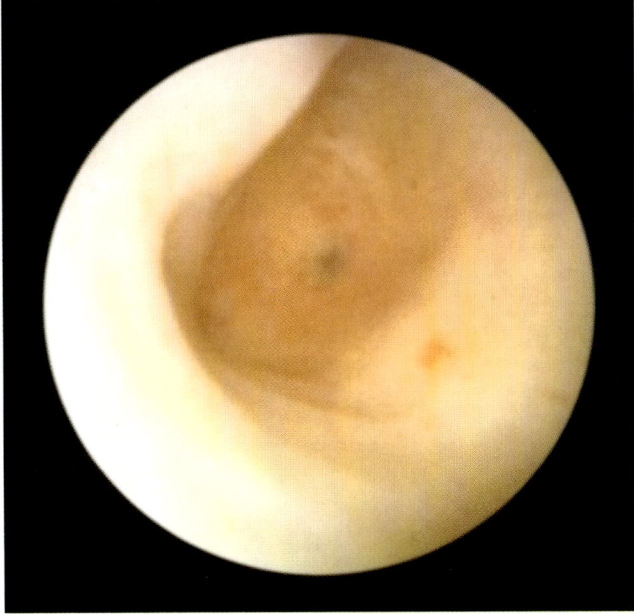

Fig. 7.10: Unicornuate uterus

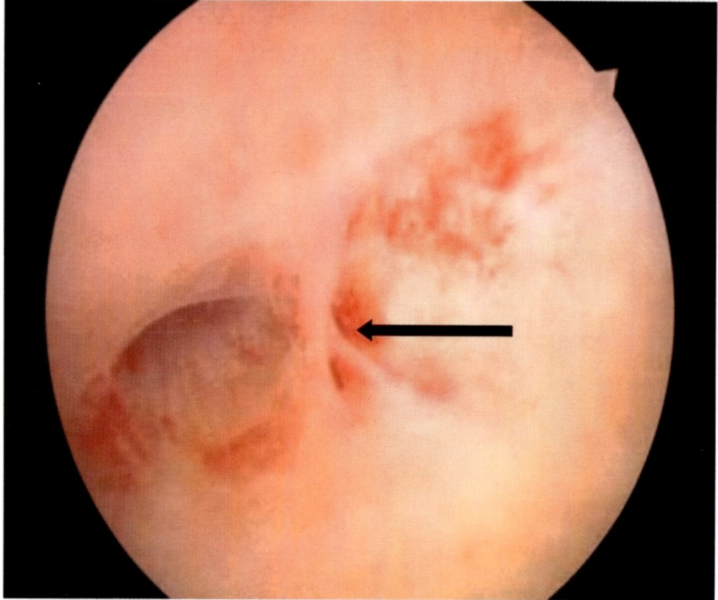

Fig. 7.11: Flimsy adhesions at cornu

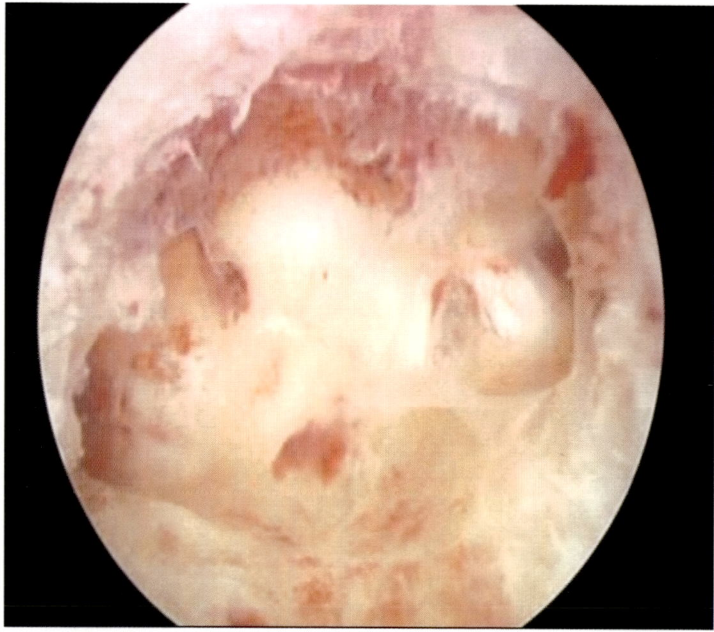

Fig. 7.12: Flimsy adhesions in cavity

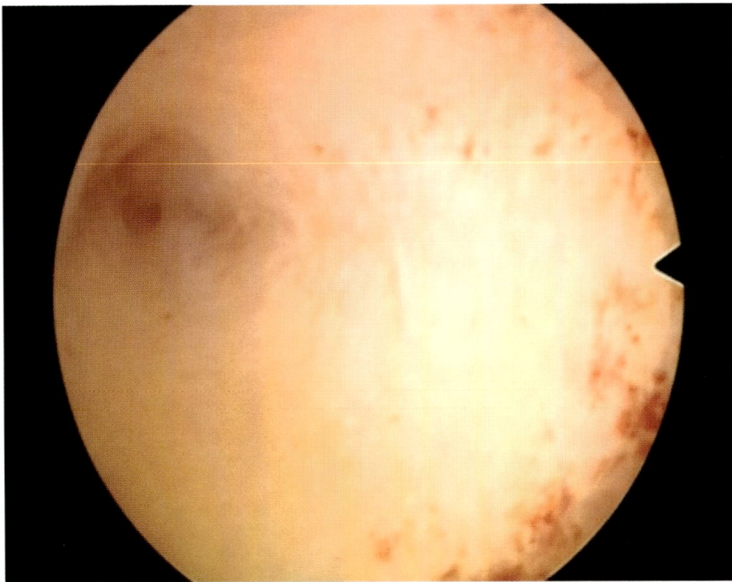

Fig. 7.13: Right cornual block

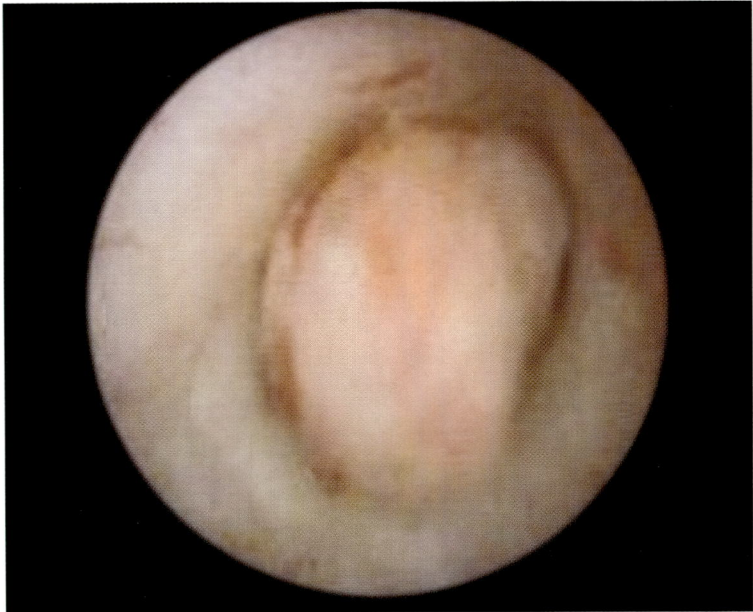

Fig. 7.14: Benign endometrial polyp at cornu

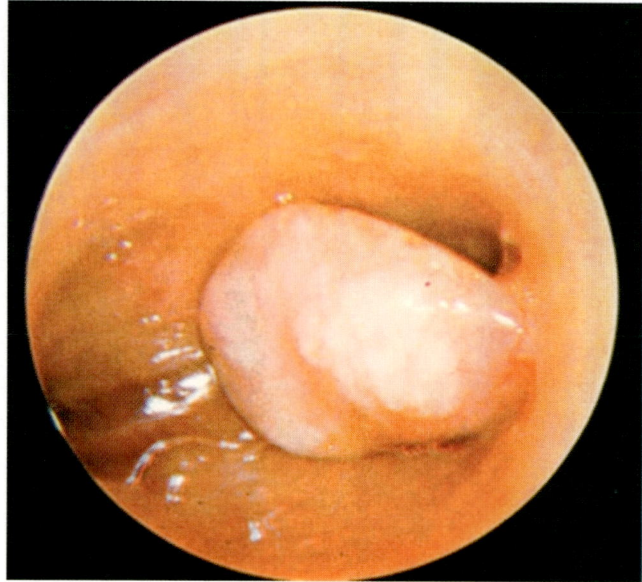

Fig. 7.15: Polyp at left lateral wall

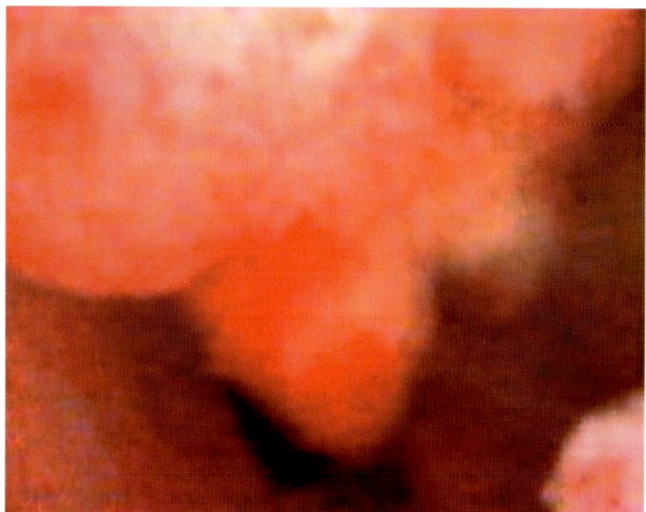

Fig. 7.16: Multiple polyps

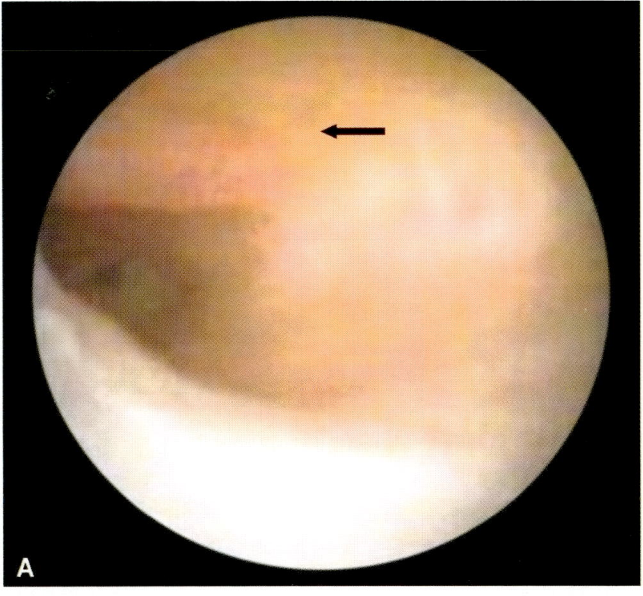

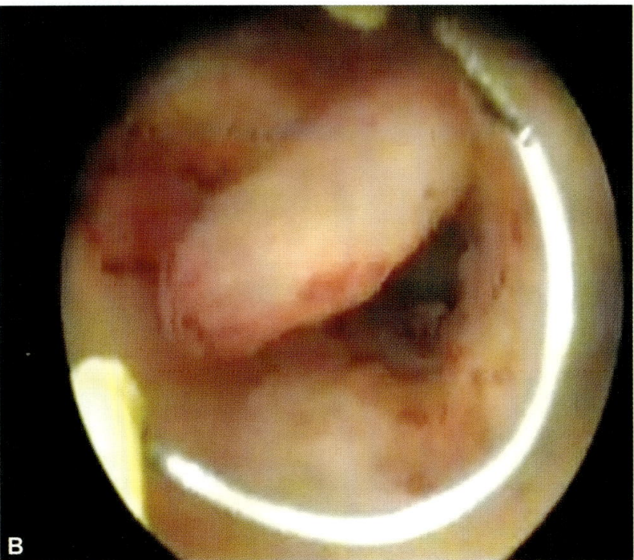

Figs 7.17A and B: In benign polyps (single or multiple) we recommend resection with resectoscope without using energy source. This avoids damage to basal endometrium

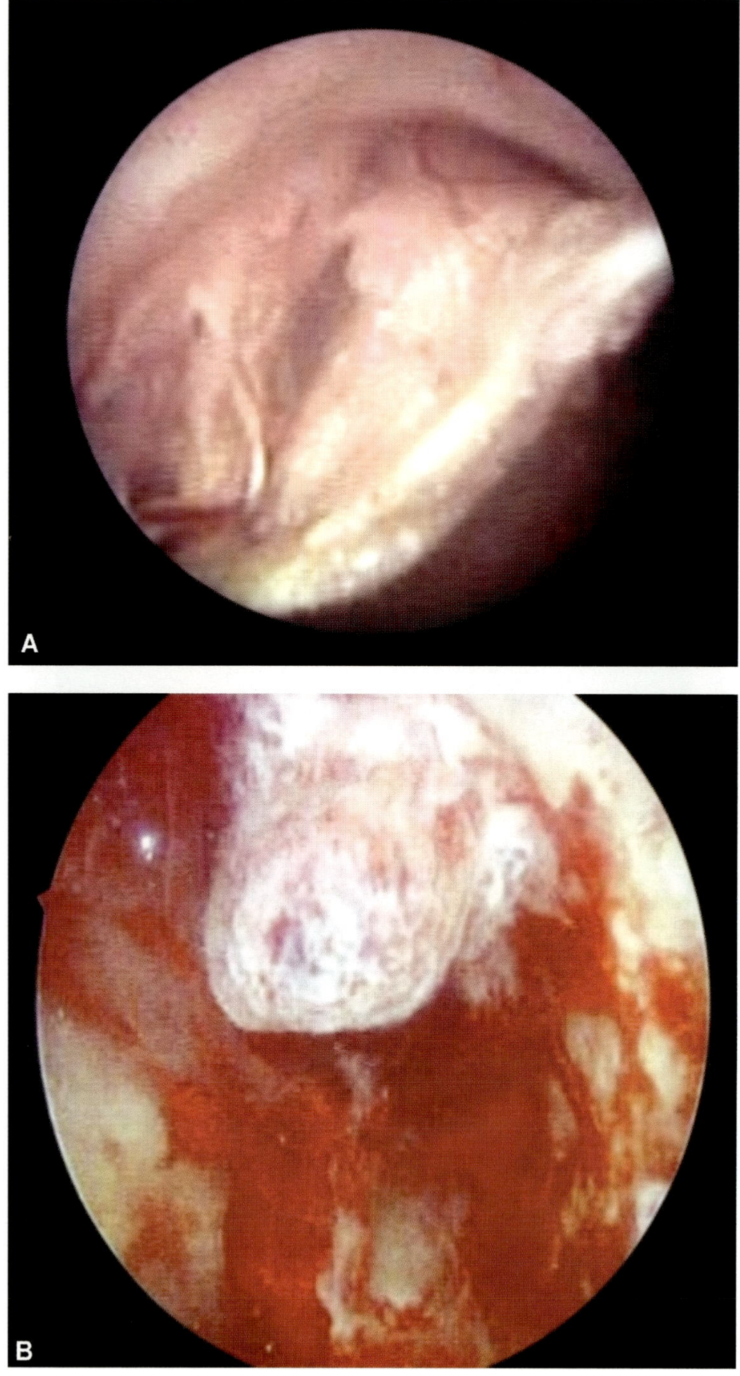

Figs 7.18A and B: Malignant endometrial polyps

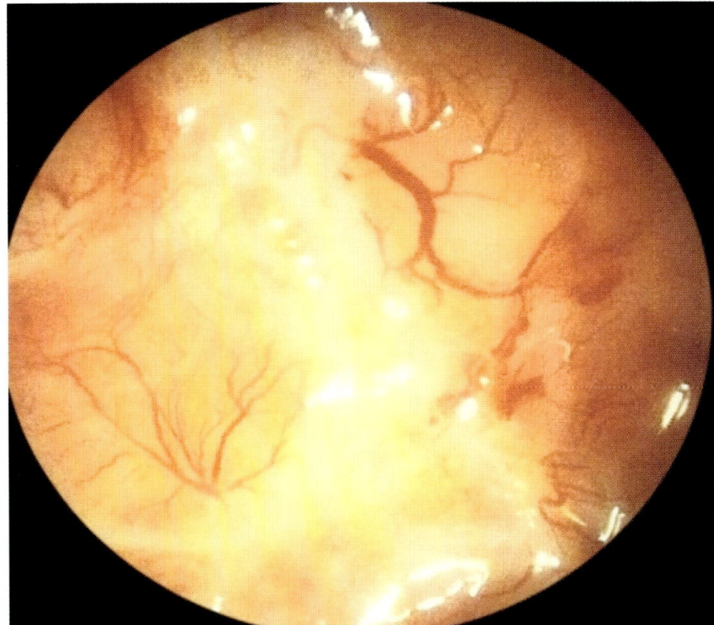

Fig. 7.19: Vascular endometrium in endometrial hyperplasia

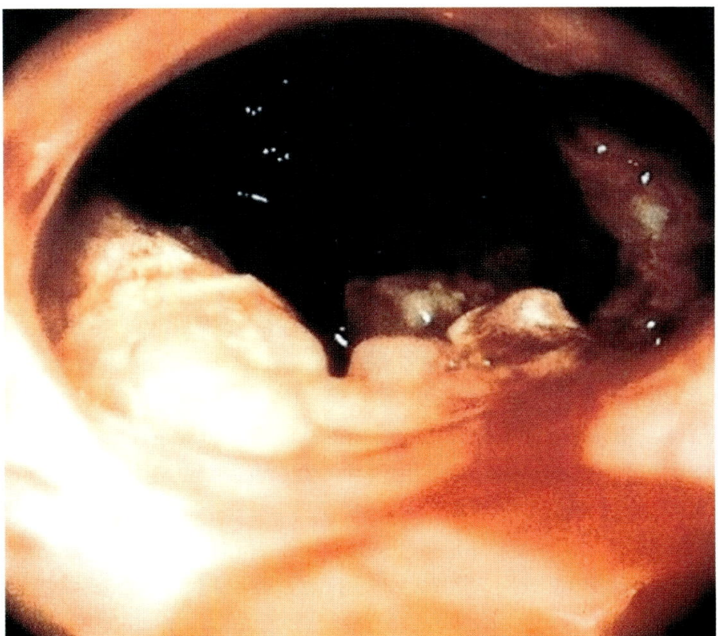

Fig. 7.20: Ca endometrium

(Photographs courtesy: Ruby Hall IVF and Endoscopy Centre)

8 Office Hysteroscopy

PREOPERATIVE EVALUATION

History and general examination of patient.

PREOPERATIVE PREPARATION

It is done in the immediate postmenstrual period when endometrial thickness is thin.

Office hysteroscopy does not need any other preoperative preparation.

IMPORTANT EQUIPMENT

- Versa scope with disposable sheath, or
- Betochhi office hysteroscope.

TECHNIQUE

- Bimanual examination of uterus to know direction of uterus
- Holding of cervix is not required
- Hysteroscope with the inflow channel ON is passed through the introitus. Fluid distends the vagina and cervix is identified **(vaginoscopy)**
- Once the external os is seen, the hysteroscope is negotiated through the external os into the canal, the influx of the fluid keeps on distending the further passage allowing the smooth entry of hysteroscope in uterine cavity under vision.
- Smaller lesions like polyp or a band of intrauterine synechie can be released with the use of Versa Point in same sitting.

TIPS

1. In case of patulous introitus, external compression on both sides over labia is given so as to allow sufficient vaginal distension and to minimize fluid wastage.
2. In acutely anteverted or retroverted uterus countertraction by applying Allis forceps or vulsellum on the cervix helps to negotiate internal os.

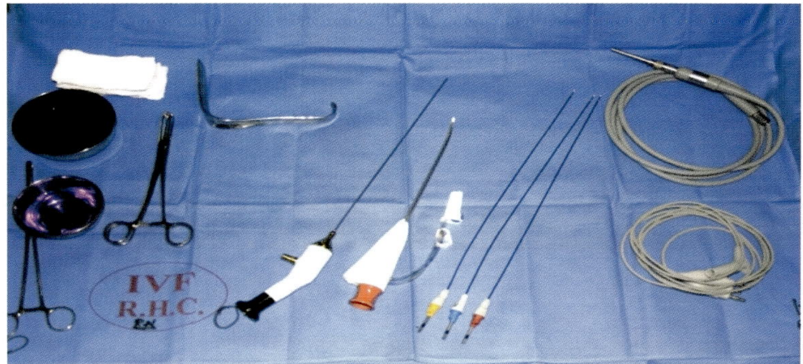

Fig. 8.1: Trolley of office hysteroscopy

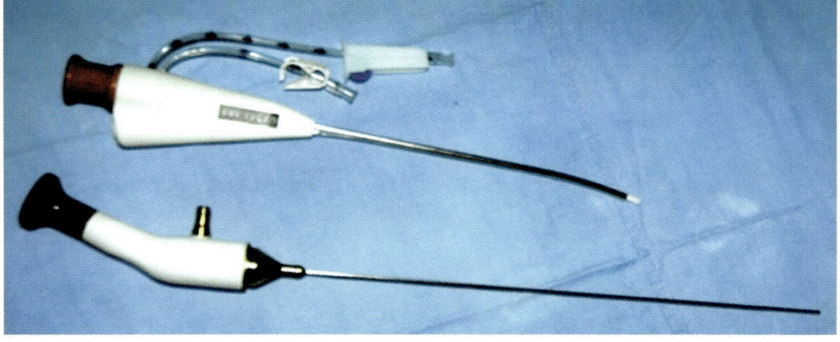

Fig. 8.2: Versa scope with operative sheath

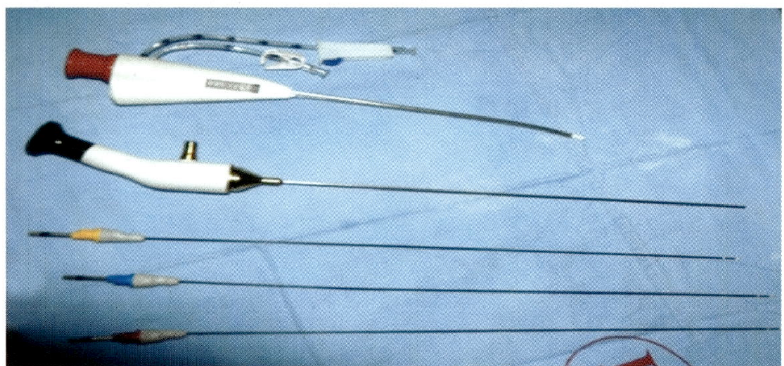

Fig. 8.3: Versa scope with operative sheath with electrodes

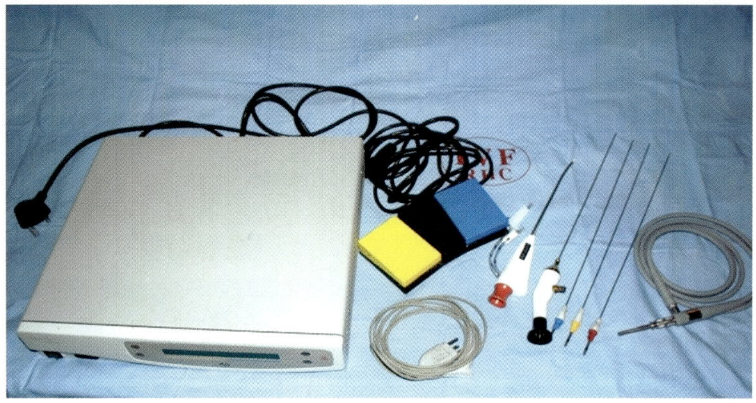

Fig. 8.4: Versa scope with versapoint and operative sheath

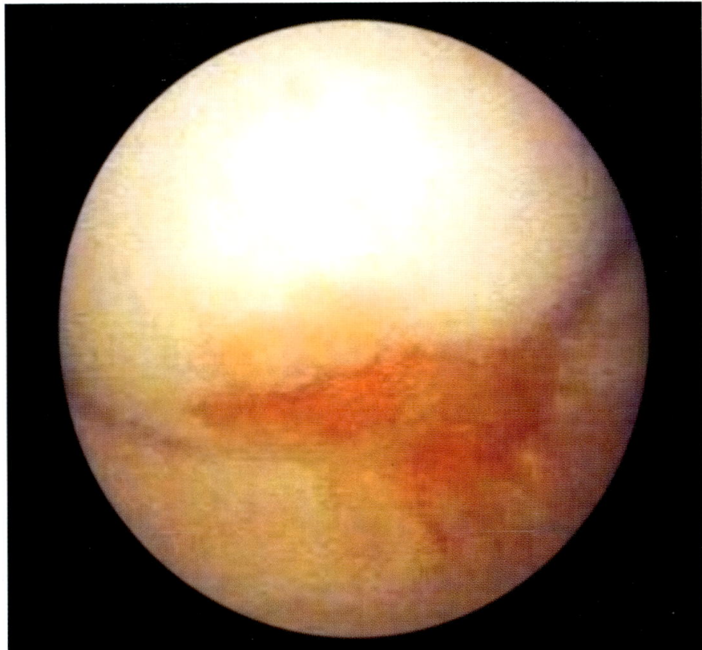

Fig. 8.5: View of external os on vaginoscopy

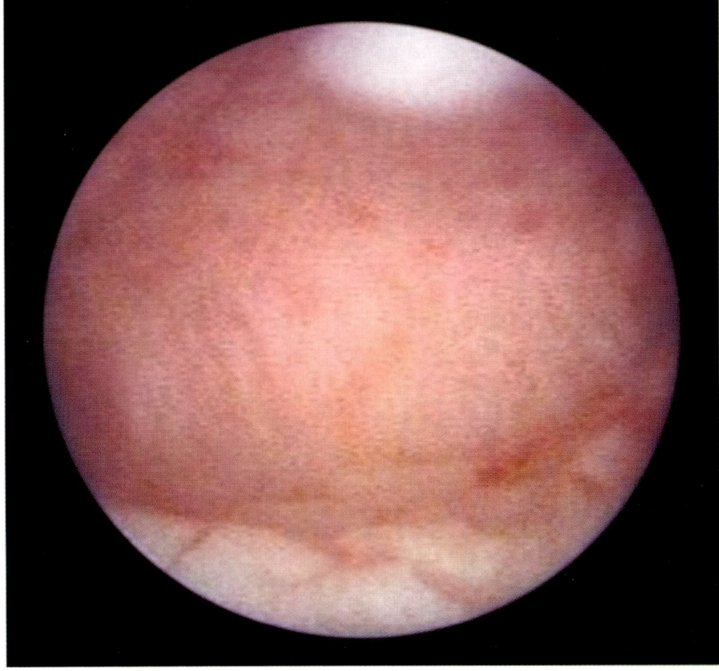

Fig. 8.6: Panaromic view of cavity

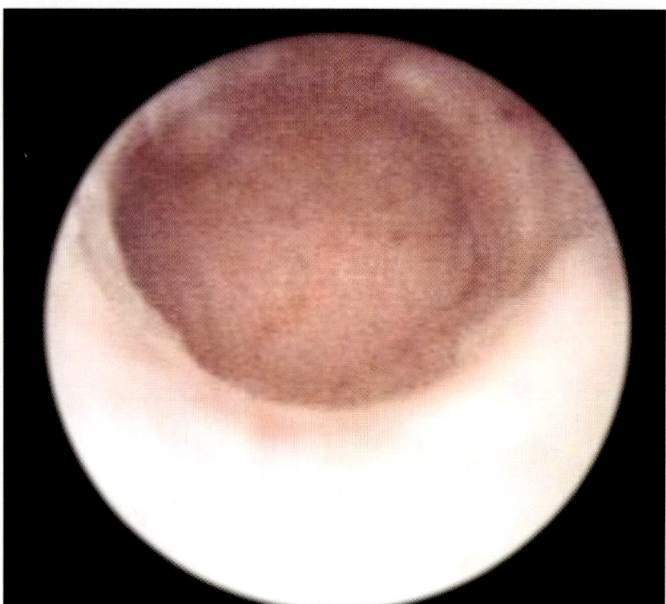

Fig. 8.7: Visualization of cavity while withdrawing the scope

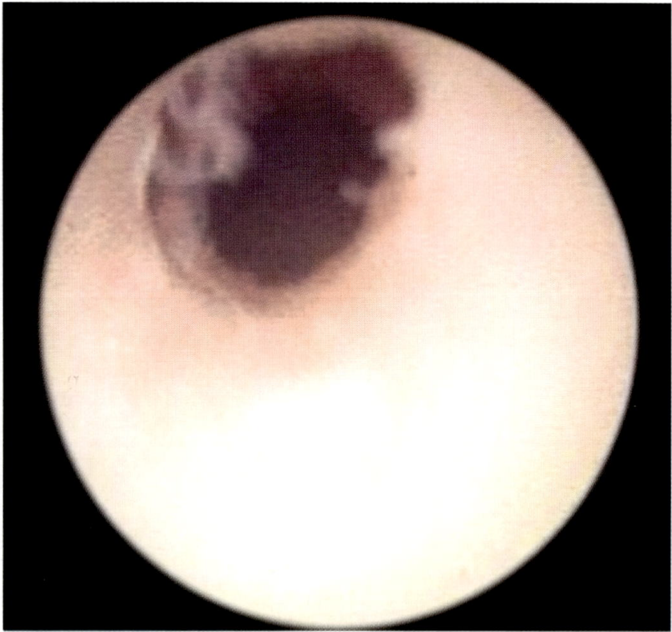

Fig. 8.8: View of internal os while withdrawing the scope

(Photographs courtesy : Ruby Hall IVF and Endoscopy Centre)

9 Hysteroscopic Myomectomy

PREOPERATIVE EVALUATION

- Transvaginal ultrasound (TVS) should be performed to confirm the diagnosis and to assess number, size and location of the myomas.
- It must indicate the extent of myomal intra-mural extension.

PREOPERATIVE PREPARATION

- It is preferred to do the procedure in immediate post-menstrual period.
- It does not require any particular preparation of the patient.

IMPORTANT EQUIPMENTS

- Resectoscope with forward bend loop
- Hysteromat/pressure bag
- Glycine 1.5%

CLASSIFICATION OF SUB-MUCOSAL FIBROID

It is divided into 3 sub-types:

Type 0 Pedunculated fibroid without intra-mural extension

Type I Sessile with intra-mural extension of fibroid of <50%

Type II Sessile with intra-mural extension of fibroid of >50%

The degree of intra-mural extension can be assessed by transvaginal ultrasonography or by hysteroscopy by observing the angle between fibroid and the endometrium at the attachment to the uterine wall.

TECHNIQUE

1. Diagnostic hysteroscopy is performed to confirm the ultrasonographic findings.

2. Cervix is further dilated to accommodate the resectoscope. Ensure the free movement of resectoscope.
3. For leiomyoma resection, a 26 fr resectoscope is normally used with 30° telescope. After cervical dilatation, the resectoscope with the electro-surgical working element (90° cutting loop) is introduced.
4. Distension of the uterine cavity is obtained with glycine.
5. Irrigation is controlled with an electronic suction and irrigation pump, which automatically controls both intra-uterine pressure and flow rate. The system also ensures constant suction and allows us to calculate the precise amount of fluid loss.
6. Intra-uterine pressure should be adjusted such that it gives adequate distension and clear vision.
7. Following settings are generally used: Flow rate of approximately 250 ml/min, pressure of 80-100 mmHg, monopolar electricity generator at 60-100 watts and suction pressure of 0.25 bar. Fluid balance is recorded by measuring the infused and drained fluid from continuous flow resectoscope.
8. Resection is performed by placing the electrical loop behind the myoma to be resected and retracting it towards the distal lens of hysteroscope. Myoma is shaved down with slicing technique.
9. Type 0: It is systematically shaved off with the resectoscope loop until the pedicle is reached. There is no need for hydrostatic massage. In case of large fibroids, too much crowding of pieces can be tackled by removing them with ovum forceps intermittently.
10. Type I and Type II:
    - Resection is done by placing the loop behind the myoma and retracting it towards the scope. Myoma is shaved down with slicing technique with cutting loop to the level of myometrium till myoma becomes flat. After having dissected the portion of myoma protruding into the cavity, an attempt is made to remove the part nested deep in the myometrial wall.
    This can be achieved by 2 techniques:
    i. By giving hydromassage by controlled variation of endo-cavitary pressure (opening and closing the endo-uterine aspiration system) myoma will start protruding in the cavity which can be sliced off. Like this we may be able to remove myoma completely in the same sitting. Usually we are able to see pink capsule on myometrium as end result.

   ii. Cold knife technique which consists of simple, mechanical passage of the resectoscope loop along the capsule lining of the myoma, detaching if from the fibrous bridges that anchors it to the uterine wall, without any electro-coagulation.

11. The operation can be considered complete when only myometrium can be seen throughout the entire surgical area. Utmost care should be taken to prevent damaging the smooth muscle fiber bundles. If it is impossible to totally remove the intra-mural fibroid in one sitting, in spite of trying the above techniques, because of it is too deep location and/or technical difficulties, the remaining myoma can be coagulated until dry. This effect is achieved by placing the loop in direct contact with remaining wall of the myoma and applying a high coagulation current for approximately 30 seconds. The fibroid can then be treated at a later date (2-3 months later) as over the period intra-mural component of myoma migrates into the uterine cavity.

TIPS

1. Meticulous attention to intraoperative fluid balance is imperative, if fluid deficit more than 1 to 1.5 liters is detected, serum sodium is measured and hyponatremia, if present, should be treated. For every liter of electrolyte free fluid that is absorbed the sodium will go down approximately 10 mEq /lit. This helps surgeon to determine when to stop a case. If deficit is approximately 1500cc it is advisable to put in a Foley's catheter and give diuretic.

2. Absorption of large volumes of electrolyte free, low viscosity fluid especially with large myoma is the trigger of some systemic changes during the operation. Myomectomy of large myomas is liable to hyponatremia, hypo-osmolality, increased CVP, increased PT and aPTT and increased most of the cardio dynamic parameters. These changes deserve performing the procedure by an experienced hysteroscopic surgeon using a quick technique with least possible Glycine volume and minimal intrauterine pressure to achieve the goal of a safe minimal access surgery.

3. It is advisable not to remove big anterior and posterior fibroids in the same sitting to avoid intra-uterine adhesions/ synechie formations.

4. Type 0 myoma should never be dislodged at the base first, which is the most tempting thing to do. One should avoid this as removal of floating myoma from uterine cavity creates a great problem.
5. While resecting Type I and Type II myoma particular care is taken regarding the intra-uterine pressure. If pressure is very high, fibroids will be pushed deep into the wall making resection difficult and also it may increase the intravasation of fluid. To prevent this, minimal least pressure is kept that gives adequate distension and clear vision.

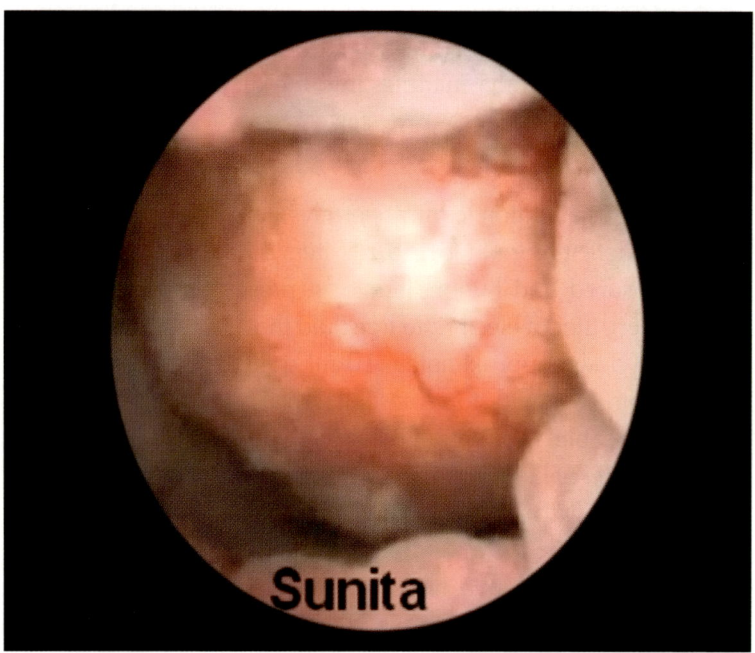

Fig. 9.1: Type 0 myoma
(intracavitatory-completely in the cavity)

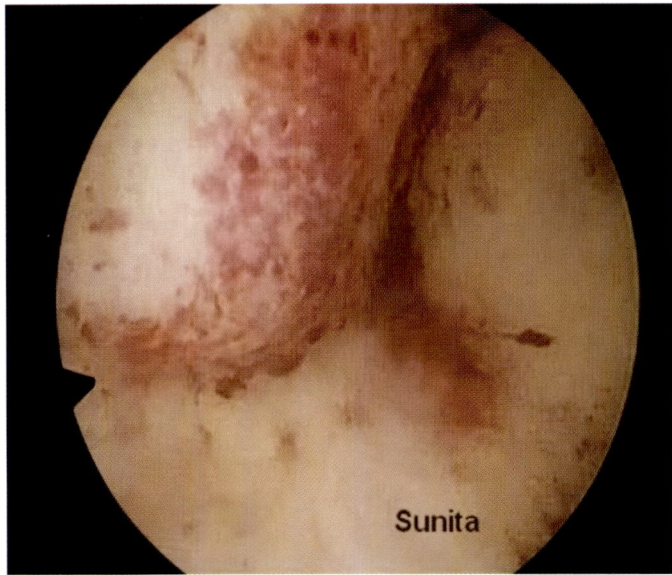

Fig. 9.2: Type I myoma
(>50% in cavity)

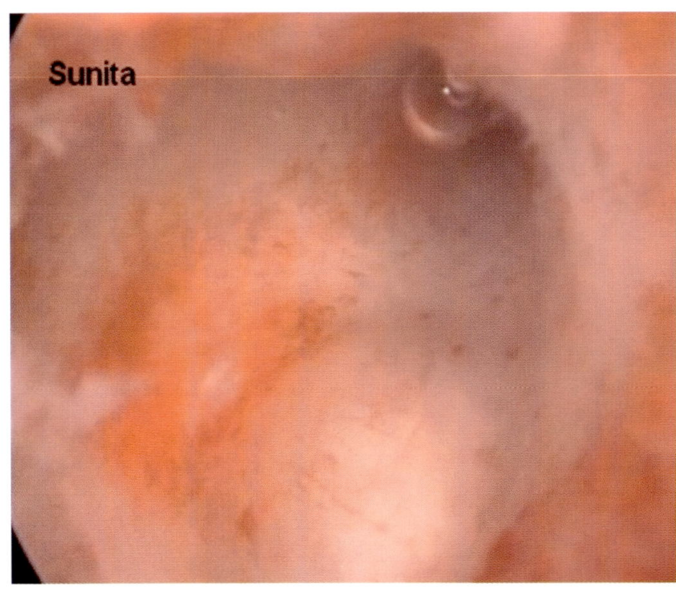

Fig. 9.3: Type II myoma
(<50% in cavity)

RESECTION OF TYPE 0 MYOMA

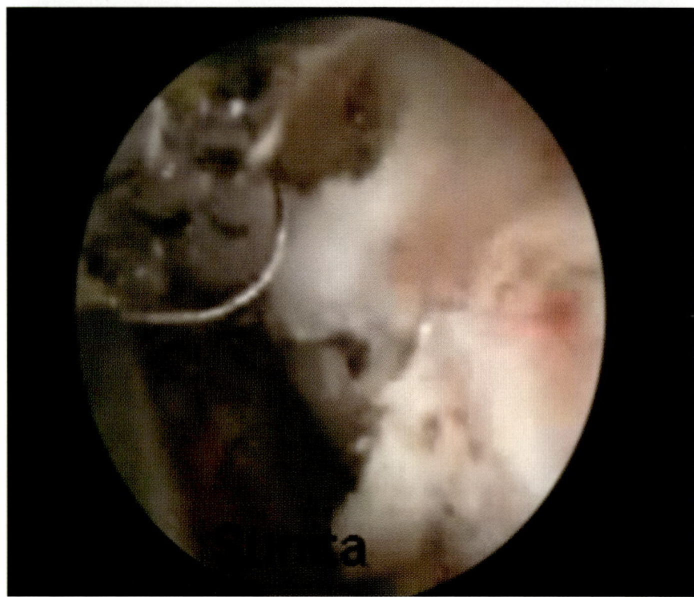

Fig. 9.4: Resection of myoma

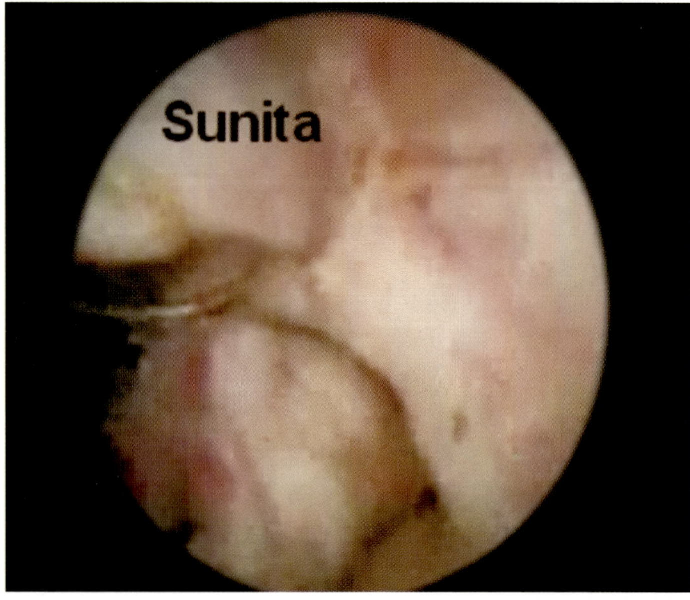

Fig. 9.5: Resection till pedicle base

RESECTION OF TYPE II MYOMA

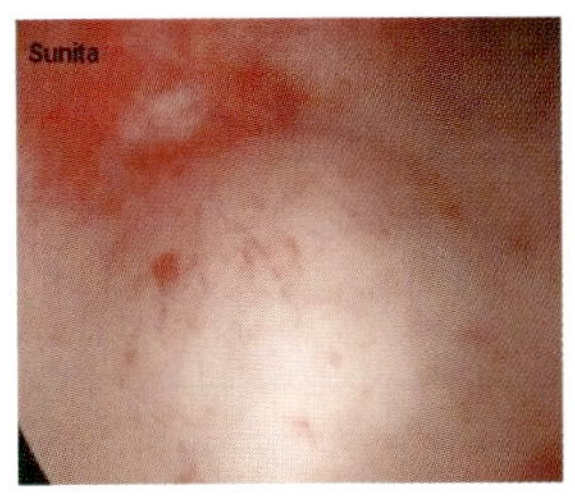

Myoma

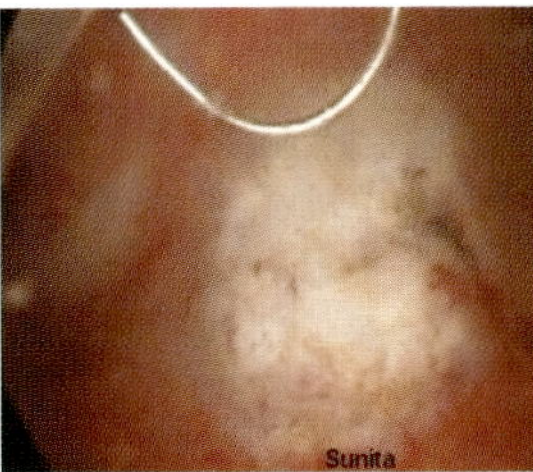

Resection with loop

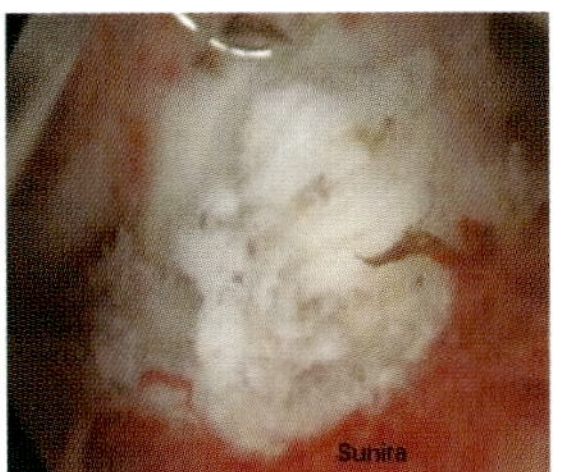

Resection till myoma
becomes flat

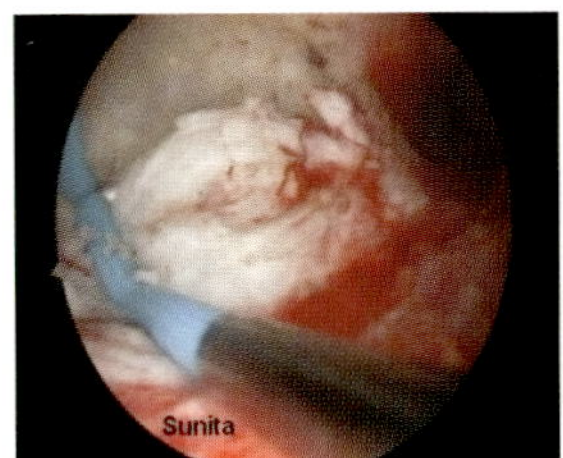

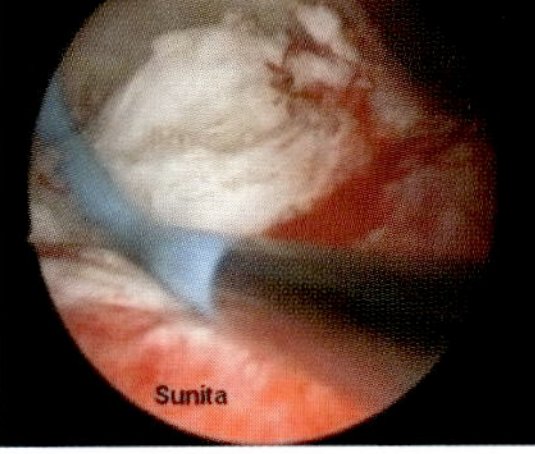

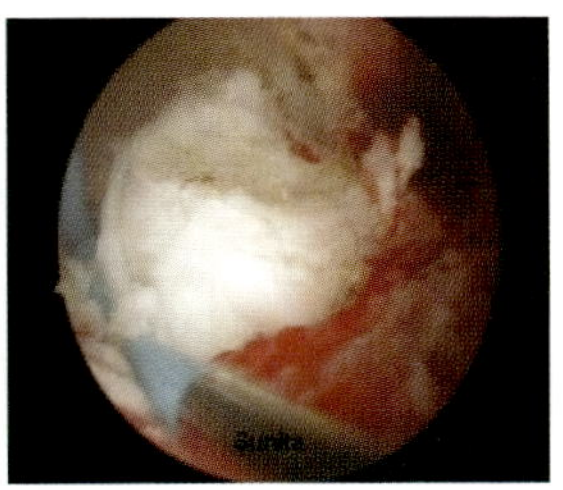

Cold knife enucleation

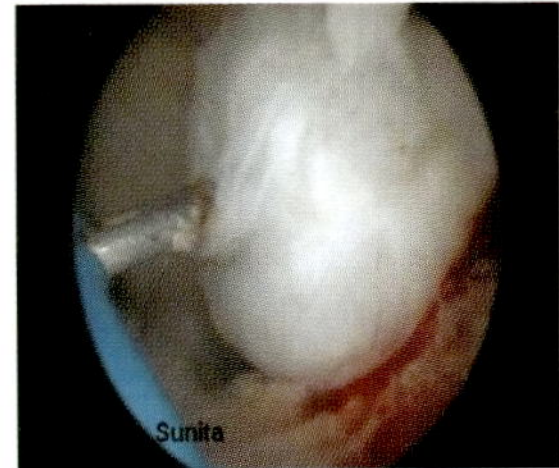

Completely enucleated ….encapsule

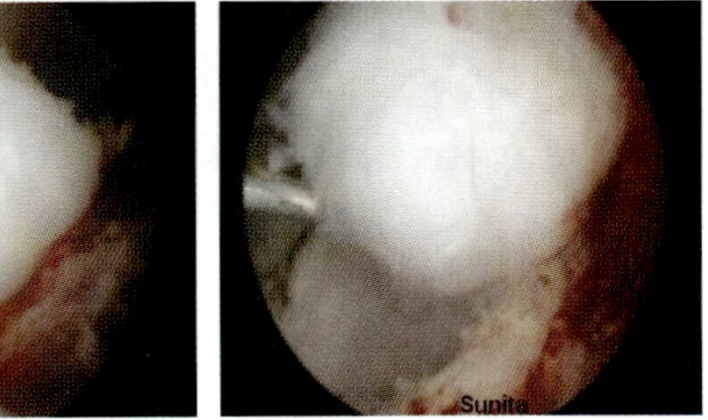

Completely enucleated
with crater in background

Fig. 9.6

(Photographs courtesy: Ruby Hall IVF and Endoscopy centre)

10 Hysteroscopic Management of Intrauterine Adhesions

PREOPERATIVE EVALUATION

- History of oligomenorrhea/amenorrhea following dilatation and curettage or suction and evacuation.
- Hysterosalpingography - may help to outline the extent of uterine cavity occlusion.
- Transvaginal sonography

PREOPERATIVE PREPARATION

Usually done immediate postmenstrually, but in patients who have amenorrhea, it can be planned anytime.

INSTRUMENTATION

- Therapeutic hysteroscope with
  Scissors
  Versa point
  Monopolar/bipolar needle
  Resectoscope with Collin's knife
- Hysteromat/ Pressure bag
- Glycine 1.5% w/v or normal saline depending on the energy source to be used.

TECHNIQUE

1. Bimanual palpation should be done to evaluate the position of uterus.
2. Gradual gentle dilatation of the internal os is done.
3. Diagnostic hysteroscopy should be done by using therapeutic sheath to confirm the diagnosis.

4. The set pressure of hysteromat should be between 180-200 mm of Hg with a minimum amount of pure cutting current between 60-80 watts.
5. Either monopolar needle/scissors/versa point is passed through therapeutic sheath to release adhesions.
6. If one wishes to use Collin's knife, further dilatation is needed to accommodate resectoscope with the Collin's knife.
7. 1.5% glycine is required whenever cautery current is used (for monopolar/bipolar needle or Collin's knife).
8. One should withdraw the scope till internal os from time to time, to have a panoramic view of cavity for orientation and to avoid going in the wrong plane.
9. Adhesiolysis should be stopped once the pink myometrium is reached.

POSTOPERATIVE CARE

- Estrogen and progesterone treatment– Premarin 0.625 mg, 6 weeks + Duphaston 20 mg for latter 4 weeks.
- Second look hysteroscopy if adhesions are moderate to severe and patient is for IVF

TIPS

1. Care should be taken not to damage the basal endometrium that may interfere with rapid re-epithelialization of the area.
2. In case of severe adhesions, simultaneous laparoscopy is helpful and more than one sitting may be needed.
3. Good intra-uterine pressure should be maintained.

> ***The only criterion for success is a subsequent
> pregnancy resulting in a viable birth.***

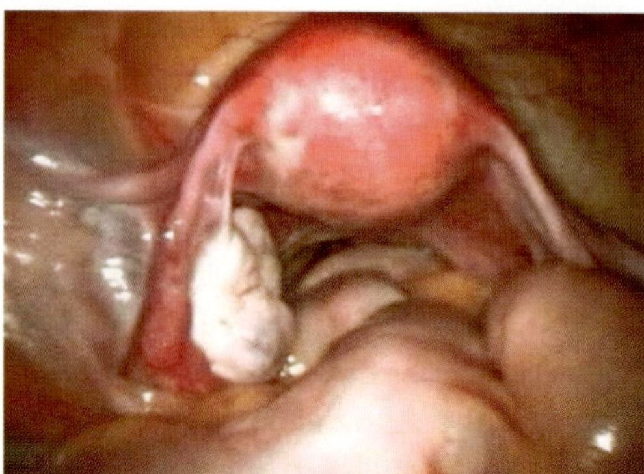

Fig. 10.1: Laparoscopy showing normal uterus
(Hysteroscopy was showing cavity like unicornuate uterus as shown below)

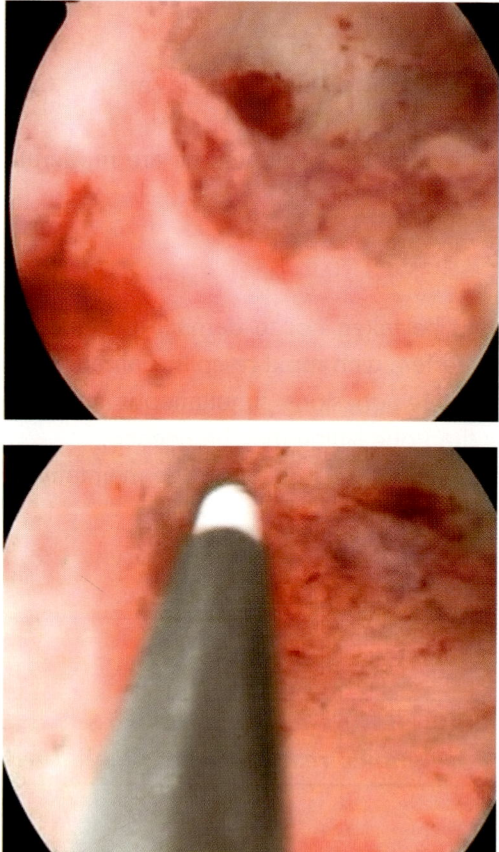

Fig. 10.2: Hysteroscopy showing intrauterine adhesions on right half of the cavity. With versa-point upper right point is fixed in correspondence with left cornu, no dissection will go in cranial direction from this point, this step avoids fundal perforation

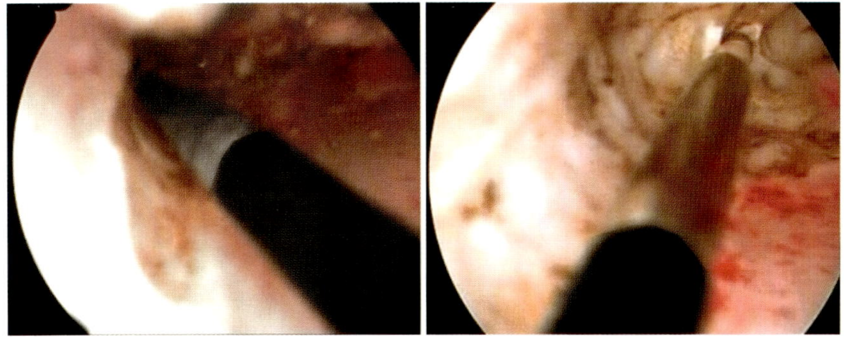

Fig. 10.3: With versascope lateral and vertical strokes taken so as to release adhesions

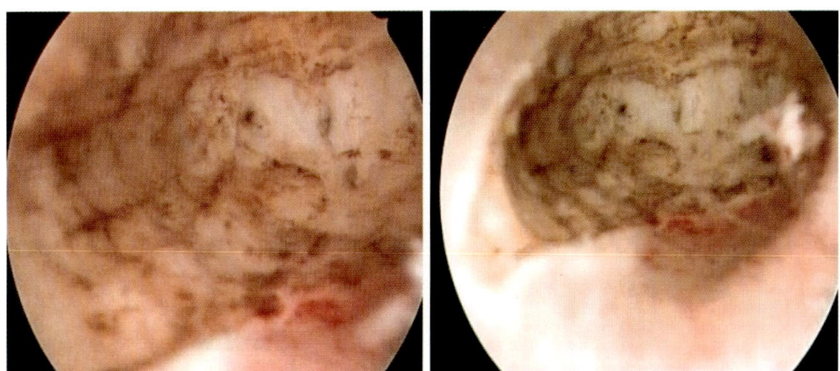

Fig. 10.4: Towards end

Fig. 10.5: End result (Nearly normal cavity)

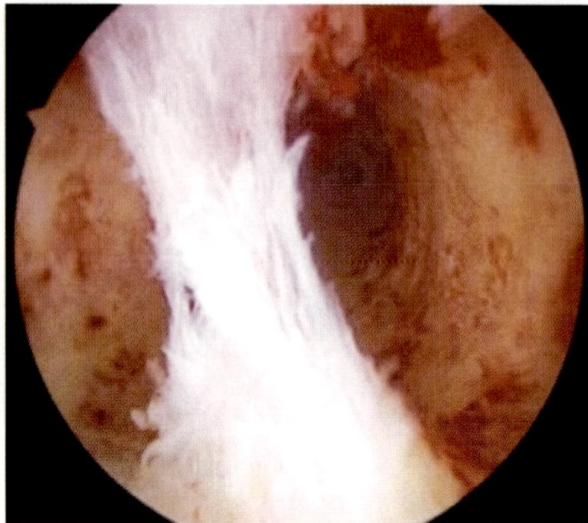

Band of intrauterine adhesion at isthmus

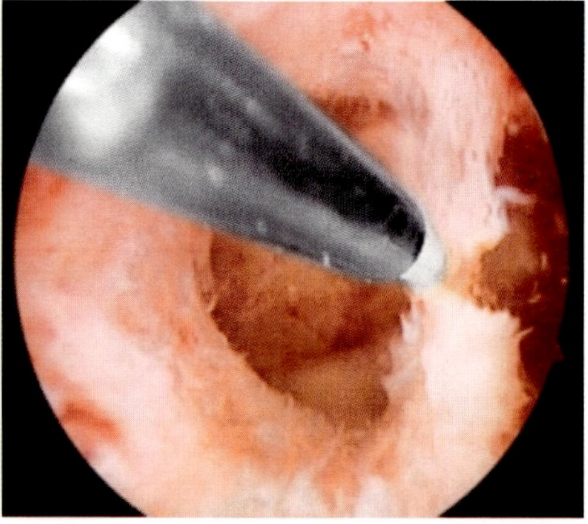

Adhesion released with versa point

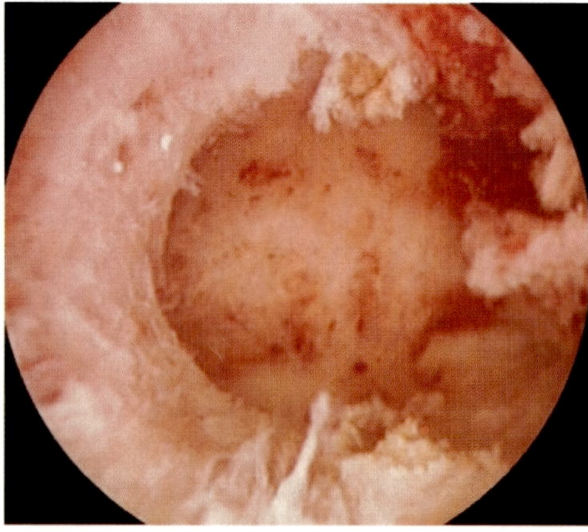

End result

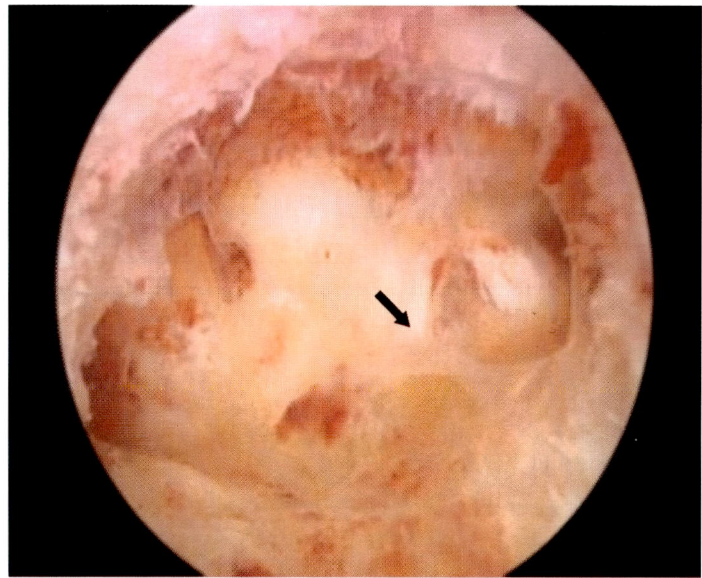

Flimsy adhesions in cavity

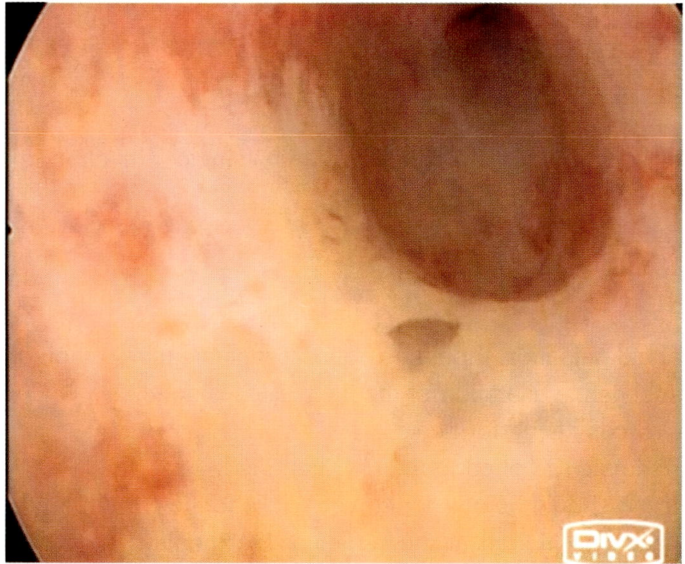

Flimsy adhesions near cornu

(Photographs courtesy: Ruby Hall IVF and Endoscopy Centre)

11 Hysteroscopic Cannulation for Proximal Tubal Block

PREOPERATIVE EVALUATION

- History of infertility
- Hysterosalpingography can give a false positive diagnosis of cornual block.

PREOPERATIVE PREPARATION

- Cannulation does not need any other preoperative preparation.
- It is performed in the immediate postmenstrual period.

IMPORTANT EQUIPMENTS

- Hysteroscope with therapeutic sheath (single 7 fr channel is also sufficient).
- Cannulation set with guide wire.

TECHNIQUE

- Bimanual palpation should be done to evaluate the position of uterus.
- Gradual gentle dilatation of the internal os is done.
- Hysteroscopy is performed.
- Approximate site of cornu can be identified.
- Telescope should be positioned very close to the cornu and the cornu should be positioned at the center of the monitor (so automatically when the guide wire comes out it will enter the cornu).
- Once this position is achieved, guide wire and cannula are passed through the operative sheath and is pushed so as to be seen in the field of vision.
- Guide wire negotiates the cornu and the cannula is guided over it.
- Cannula is pushed just 2-4 mm beyond the cornu and guide wire is removed.

- Methylene blue is injected through the distal end of cannula; dye is seen coming out from the fimbrial end of cornu simultaneously by laparoscopy
- If cornual block is rigid, cannulation will not be successful.

TIPS

- Presence of 2 separated monitors, camera and light source for laparoscopy and hysteroscopy each, makes surgery simple and hastlefree.
- The aim of surgery is opening the cornual end of fallopian tube, so never pass guide wire through full length of fallopian tube. It will damage the ciliary and endothelial layer.

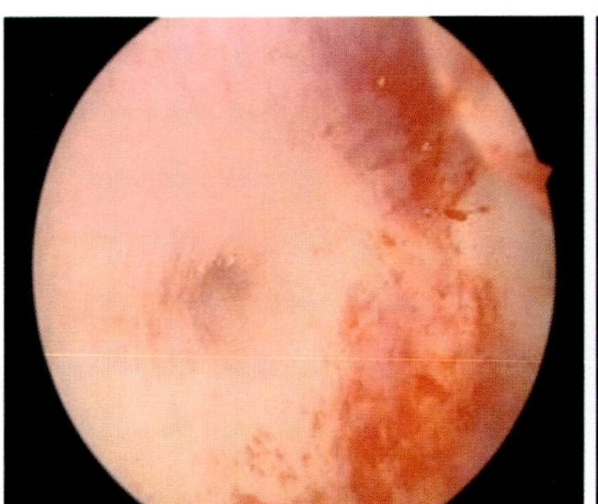

Right cornual block

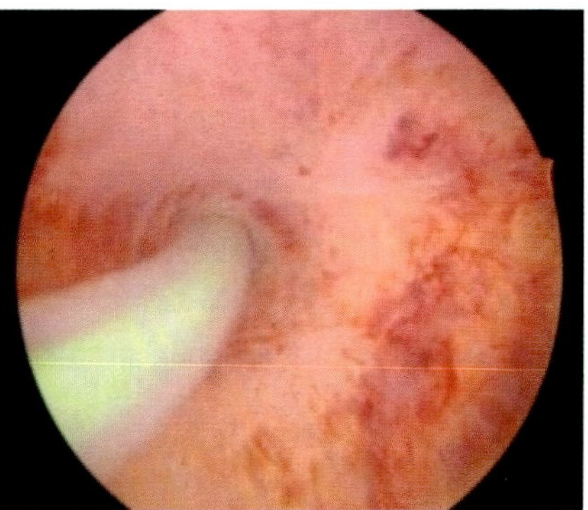

Guide wire passed

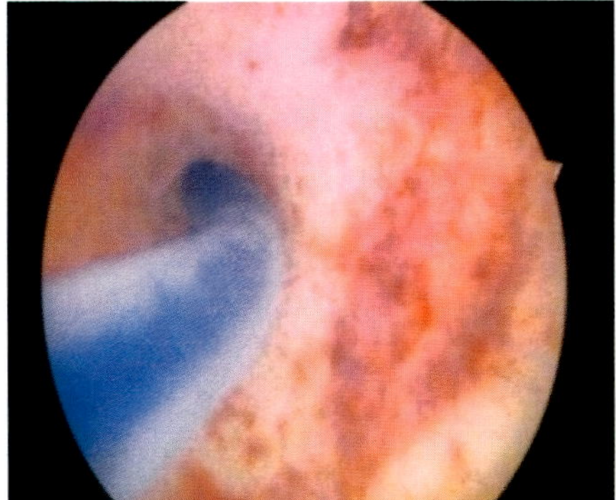

Dye injected

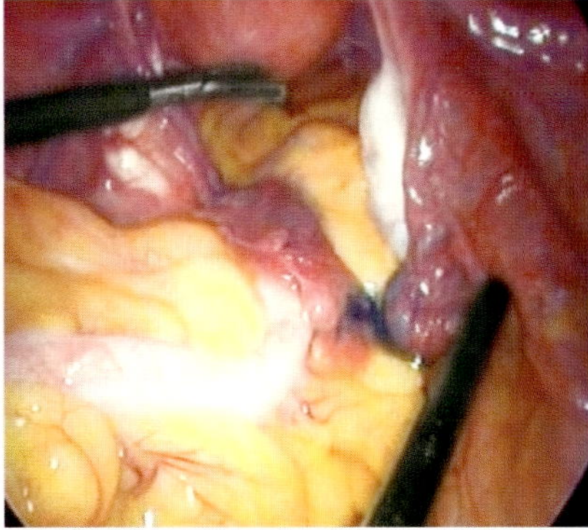

Free spillage seen through laparoscopy

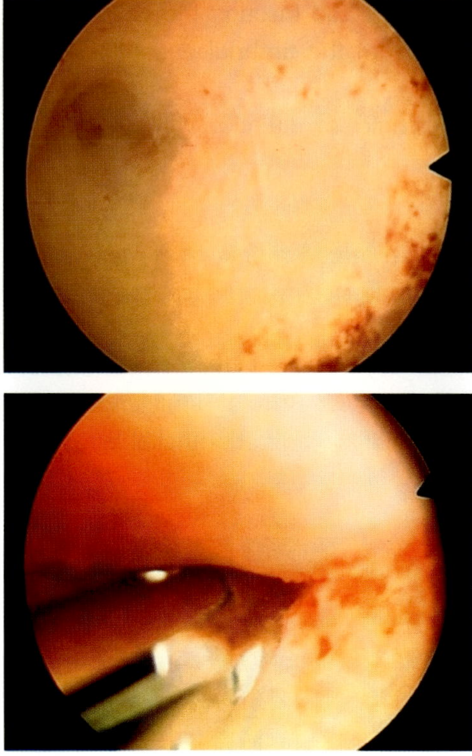

Occasionally flimsy fibers at cornu can be released with scissors or blunt forceps

(Photographs courtesy : Ruby Hall IVF and Endoscopy Centre)

12 **Hysteroscopic Resection of Septum**

PREOPERATIVE EVALUATION

- Bad obstetric history/ infertility
- 3-D transvaginal sonography

PREOPERATIVE PREPARATION

Preferably done in postmenstrual period.

SPECIAL INSTRUMENTS

- Therapeutic hysteroscope with
  Scissors
  Versa point
  Monopolar/bipolar needle
  Resectoscope with Collin's knife
- Hysteromat/ Pressure bag
- Glycine 1.5% w/v or normal saline depending on the energy source to be used.

TECHNIQUE

First, a diagnostic hysteroscopy is performed to confirm the diagnosis of the septum. (Laparoscopy is needed in case of complete broad septum to differentiate from bicornuate uterus).

1. Bimanual palpation should be done to evaluate the position of uterus.
2. Gradual gentle dilatation of the internal os is done.
3. Diagnostic hysteroscopy should be done by using therapeutic sheath to confirm the diagnosis.
4. The set pressure of hysteromat should be between 180-200 mm of Hg with a minimum amount of pure cutting current between 60-80 watts.

5. Both the ostia are visualized before the resection of the septum.
6. The septum is visualized.
7. Either monopolar needle/scissors/versa point is passed through therapeutic sheath to release adhesions.
8. Incision is taken from the distal to the cephalic end.
9. When it is thin septum, incise it from distal to cephalic which causes fibroelastic band to retract.
10. In case of broader septum, 1st step is a lateral alternating technique of side-to-side resection up to 0.5 cm from fundus. Then the remainder is removed sweeping from cornu to cornu to avoid damage to this area.
11. Panaromic view is obtained from time-to-time by withdrawing the telescope till the internal os for getting judgement in cases of broad septum.
12. End result is visualizing both ostia in one line.

TIPS

- Always see both ostia before starting for resection of septum.
- While resection, always stay in the midline of the septum.
- Care should be taken not to damage the basal endometrium that may interfere with rapid re-epithelialization of the area.
- Good intra-uterine pressure should be maintained.
- It is better to have 2-3 cm space remaining than overdoing the resection, as it may cause thinning of fundal myometrium and chances of rupture in subsequent pregnancy.

RESECTION OF COMPLETE SEPTUM

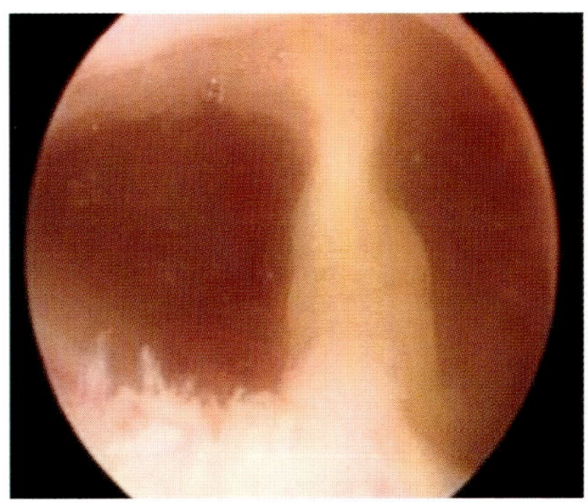

Complete septum upto internal Os

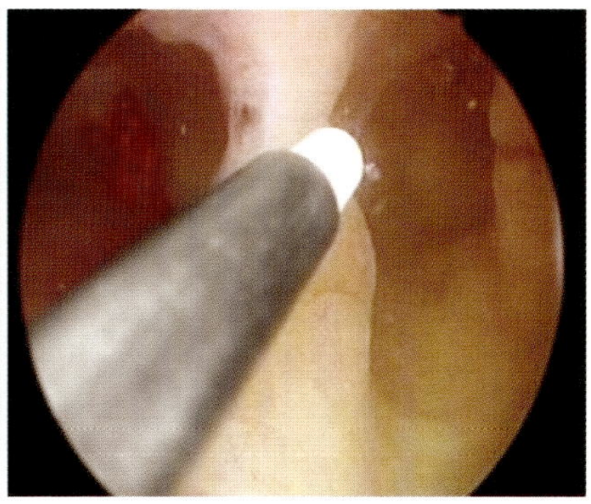

Resection with versapoint

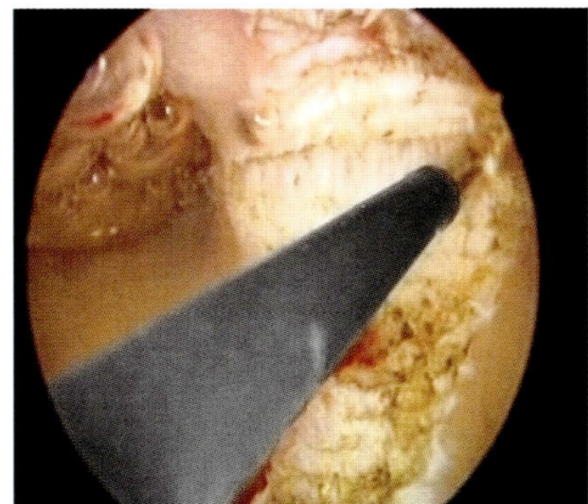

Resection in process

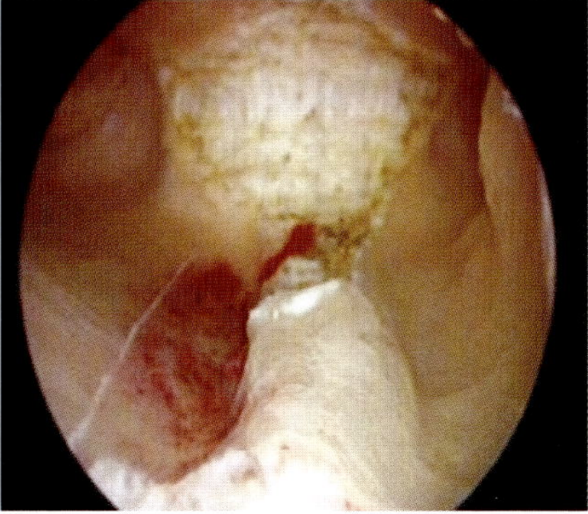

Resection towards end

RESECTION OF PARTIAL BROAD BASE SEPTUM WITH COLLIN'S KNIFE

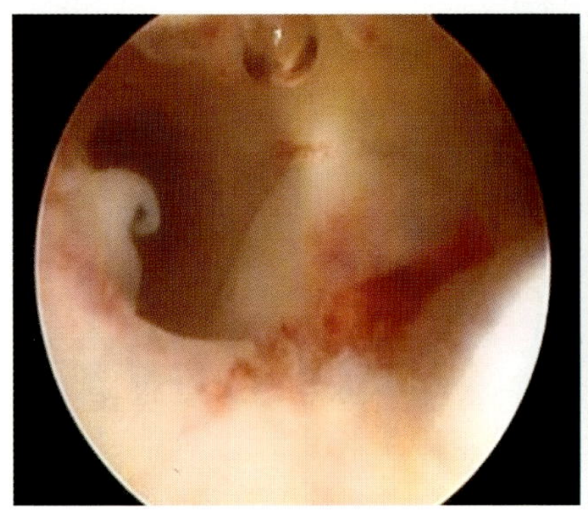

Partial broad septum

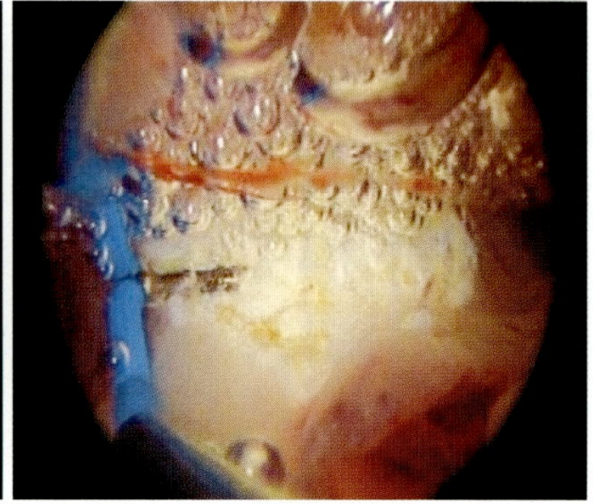

Side-to-side resection in process using Collin's knife

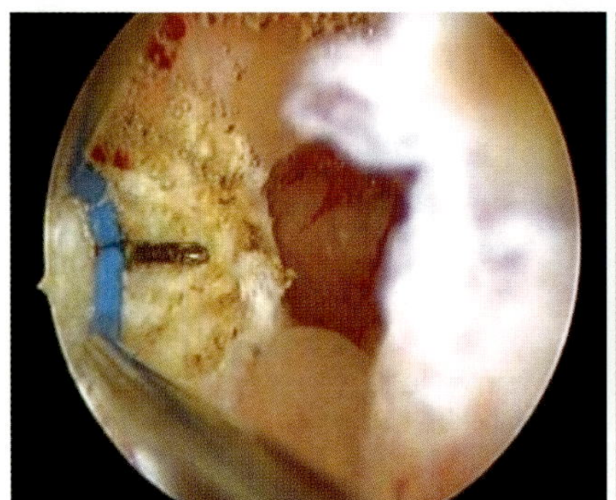

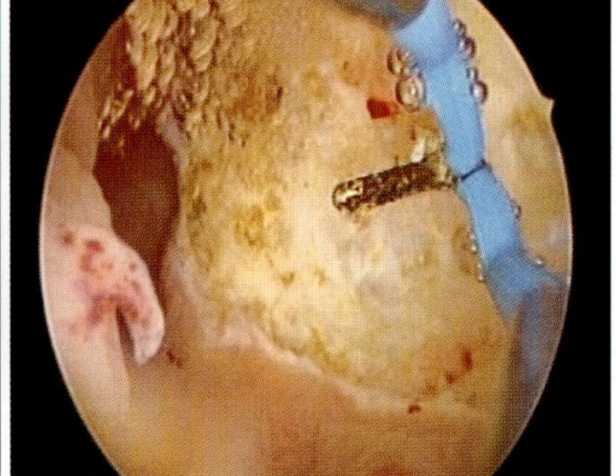

Resection towards end

RESECTION OF PARTIAL BROAD BASED SUBSEPTATE UTERUS WITH VERSAPOINT

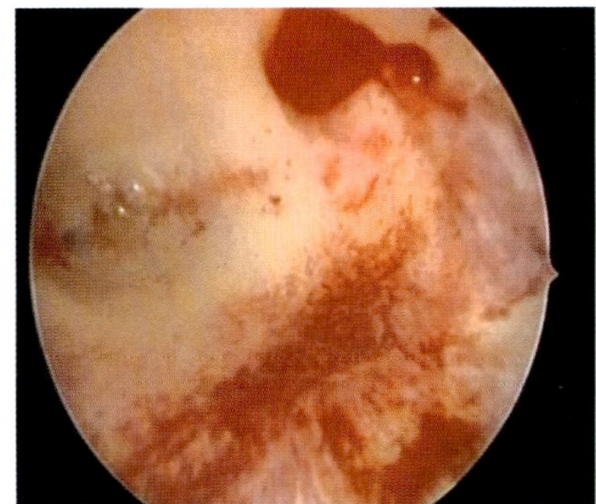

Subseptate uterus

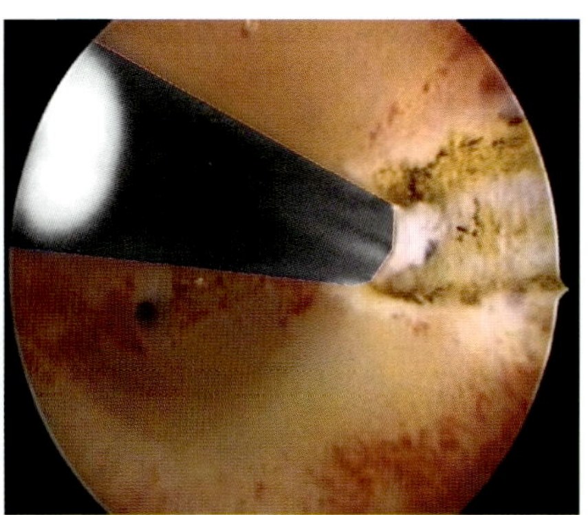

Resection with versapoint

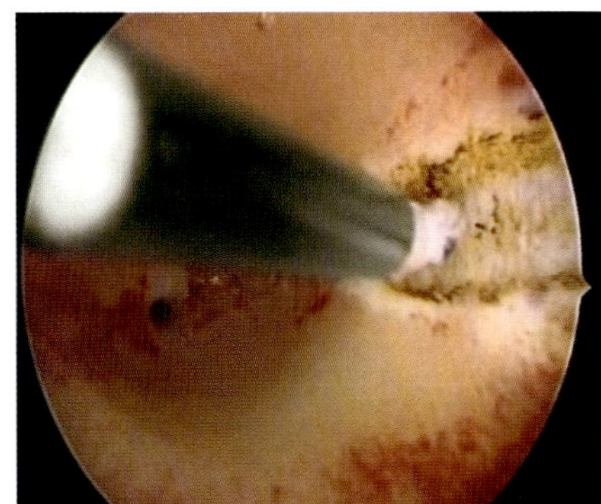

Resection in process

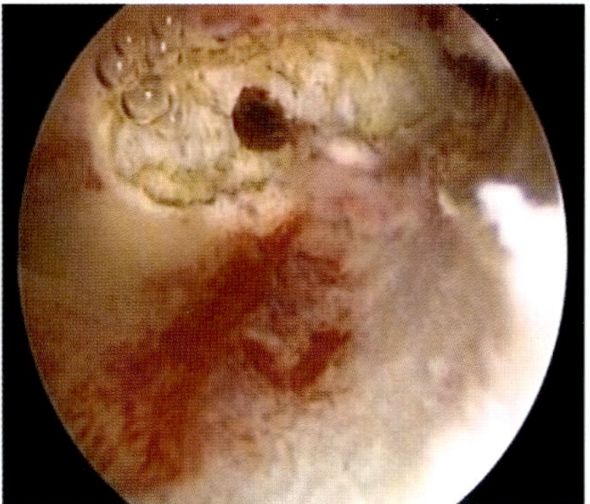

End result

(Photographs courtesy : Ruby Hall IVF and Endoscopy Centre)

Section Three

Laparoscopy

13 Laparoscopic Hysterectomy

PREOPERATIVE EVALUATION

Proper case selection is necessary (depending on the skills and laparoscopic surgeon).

PREOPERATIVE PREPARATION

Bowel Preparation

- *Diet*—One day prior to surgery soft diet till afternoon followed by clear liquid diet (about 8-10 glasses) and then, nil by mouth for 8 hrs prior to surgery.
- *Peglec powder*—dissolve the pack in 2 liters of water to be given over 2-3 hrs on previous evening.

  or
- Exelyte solution 90 ml to be added in 300 ml of limca / fruit juice to be given on previous evening.

  No need for admission for the above preparation. Patient can be admitted 6 hours prior to surgery. (High-risk cases need prior admission, evaluation and fitness).

Position of Patient

Patient is placed in a low modified lithotomy position (Fig. 13.1) on the Allen's stirrups with adjustable and padded leg rest.

- If Allen stirrup are not available then standard lithotomy bars with padded rest for the knee joint is suitable, kept at 45° downwards.

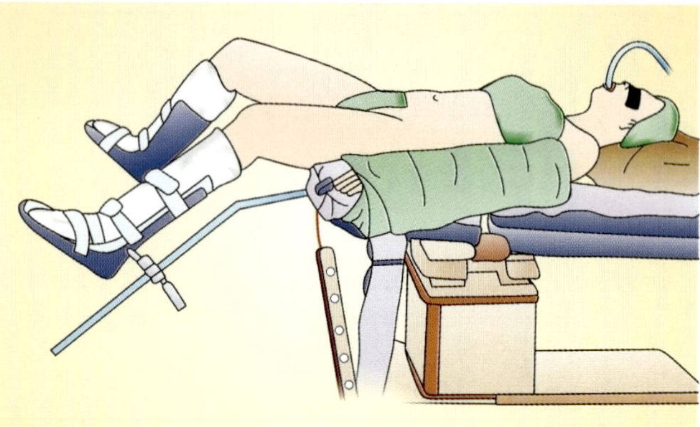

Fig. 13.1: Patient's position – modified lithotomy position
(extended hips and legs at 135° to the horizontal)

IMPORTANT EQUIPMENTS

- One or two 10 mm trocars
- Three or four 5 mm trocars
- 2 non traumatic graspers
- 1 claw forceps
- 2 scissors (tissue cutting and suture cutting)
- 1 bipolar forceps (and one stand by)
- Monopolar spatula or hook
- Uterine manipulator or myoma screw (for manipulation of uterus)
- Pair of needle holders
- Respective grasper if other energy source is to be used.

TECHNIQUE

Manipulator

Uterine manipulator [self designed – refer to instrument session (*See* Fig. 2.11)] is inserted to facilitate better mobilization of the uterus.

Port Placement

1. Position of the ports either in lower abdomen or upper abdomen depends upon the size and pathology of uterus and previous lower abdomen surgeries, if any.
2. Head low only after primary trocar insertion.

3. Secondary trocars can be:
   A. Two 5 mm ports on surgeon's side usually 10 cm apart and upper port a little medially. Third 5 mm port is on the contralateral side usually in line with the primary trocar. Left-sided lower 5 mm port should be valve-less to carry suture material. Right-sided 5 mm port should have outlet to remove the smoke intermittently.
   B. One on surgeon's side, one in the midline and one on the contra-lateral side. (Individual choice as per the suturing techniques and height of surgeon) (For details, refer to chapter on Port placement).
4. A 10 mm 0° laparoscope or occasionally 30° laparoscope is introduced through primary port. CO_2 is used for pneumoperitoneum at a rate of 3-9 liters/min with a pressure cut off at 15 mmHg. Then Trendelenberg's position is given.

STEPS OF LAPAROSCOPIC HYSTERECTOMY

1. Thorough inspection of pelvis (Fig. 13.2) (i.e. examination of uterus, adenexa, anterior and posterior pouch) should be performed first. Correction of anatomy should be done if adhesions are present (Fig. 13.3). Tracing of ureter through its full course from pelvic brim till entry underneath the uterines is must before proceeding for hysterectomy (Figs 13.4 and 13.5).
2. Uterus should be pushed in and to the opposite side when the contra-lateral ligaments are taken. This causes apparent lengthening of the ligament, which then can be easily cauterized by keeping sufficient length from lateral pelvic wall (Fig. 13.6).
3. Procedure is started with division of infundibulopelvic ligaments (IPL), by using bipolar forceps and dedicated generator. Pull the adnexa on the medial side so that maximum length of IPL can be obtained. Always cauterize its lateral most point first (remember not to cross this point further to avoid injury to ureter). Then cauterization should be done medially. Cautery and cutting should be performed serially so as to involve whole bulk of IPL till one reaches the round ligament (Fig. 13.7).
4. Round ligaments are then coagulated and safely divided by scissors with monopolar cautery or Harmonic scalpel (Figs 13.8 and 13.9).
   * Recommend taking IPL first followed by round ligament, (so that both the ligaments can be cauterized and cut in one line) but they can also be taken vice versa.

5. Anterior and posterior lips of broad ligament are separated and cut as much as possible just lateral to uterine wall (Figs 13.10 to 13.12).
6. Maintaining cranial displacement of the uterus with the help of uterine manipulator, uterus is kept in center, midposed and pushed completely in so as to visualize the anterior pouch and bladder margin.
7. Uterovesical fold of peritoneum is then lifted and held in the midline using a Maryland forceps introduced through the right port and cut close to the uterus using a spatula or hook introduced through left upper port (Fig. 13.13). It may be cauterized before cutting to avoid capillary oozing. Usually pneumoperitoneum helps to further create plane. Incision is further extended laterally to the anterior lip of broad ligament to meet the previous cut.
8. Maintaining the position of the uterus, little retroverted, pubo-cervical ligament can be identified and severed with blunt forceps or cauterized and cut. This allows the bladder to push down easily, exposing 1-2 cms of upper vagina. This step of pushing the bladder completely down and laterally causes lateral displacement of the ureters. We always advocate this step before tackling the uterines (Fig. 13.14).
9. After this uterus is completely anteverted, so as to visualize the posterior lip of broad ligament which is cut next to uterus up to uterosacral ligament, after blunt separation from the uterine.
10. Once posterior lip of peritoneum is cut, loose areolar tissue is displaced laterally. This step further pushes ureters laterally and since there is breach in continuity of the peritoneum, current will not pass laterally to ureters while cauterizing the uterine artery.
11. Uterine artery is skeletonized for effective dessication. To identify the right uterine artery, the uterus is displaced upwards and to the left side. This will also cause apparent lengthening of the uterines, so that the ureter will be further away from the point of dessication (Figs 13.15 and 13.16).
12. A substantial segment of the skeletonized uterine artery (1-2 cm) is coagulated or sutured (Figs 13.17A to D) and then the pedicle is divided.

    * Vessel sealing device (Gyrus), if available negates the need for suturing the uterine artery.
13. Keeping the uterine position same, (completely pushed in and to opposite side) transverse cervical ligament is cauterized and cut medial to the uterine stump till the angle of the vault (Figs 13.18 and 13.19).

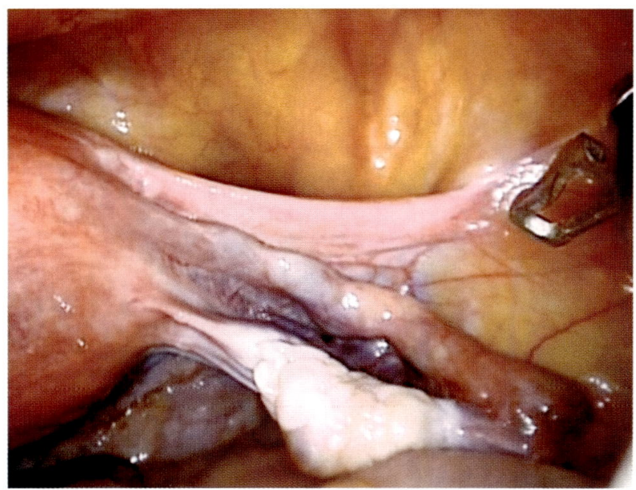

Fig. 13.2: Thorough visualization of right adnexa

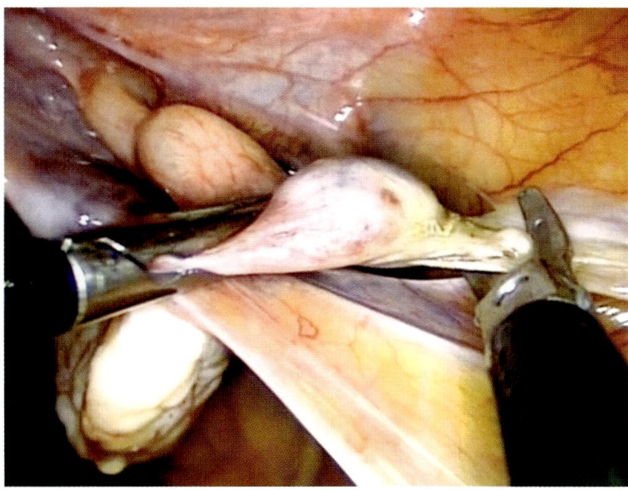

Fig. 13.3: Release of adhesions of fallopian tube from lateral pelvic wall

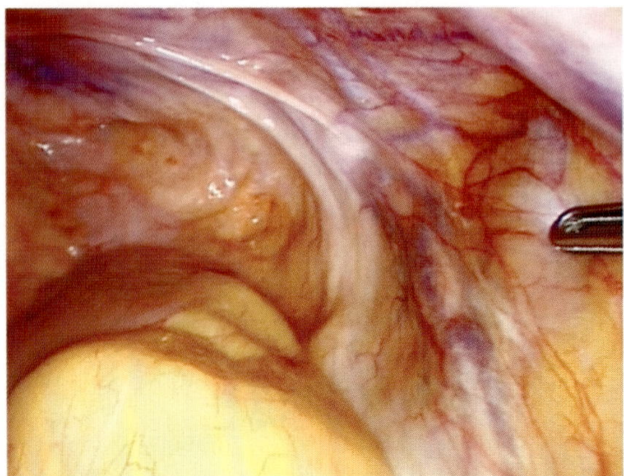

Fig. 13.4: Tracing course of right ureter

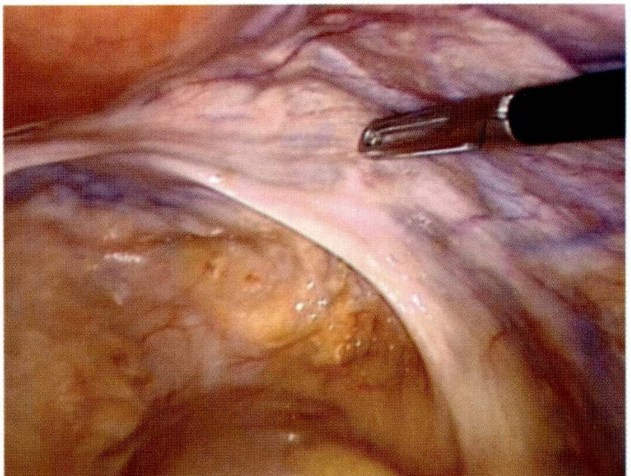

Fig. 13.5: Tracing of ureter till its entry beneath uterines

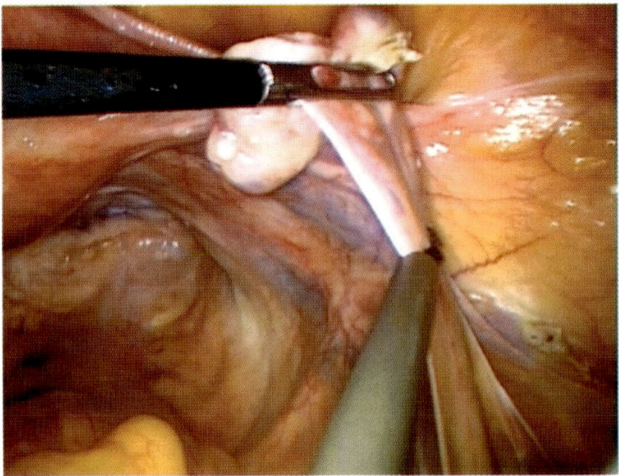

Fig. 13.6: Cauterization of infundibulopelvic ligament

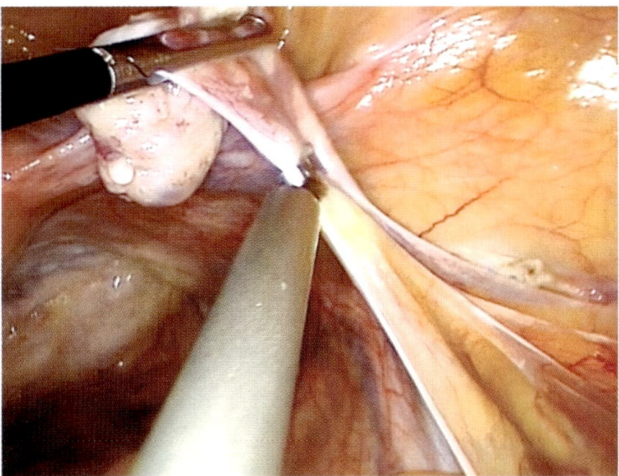

Fig. 13.7: Serial cauterization and cutting of infundibulopelvic ligament

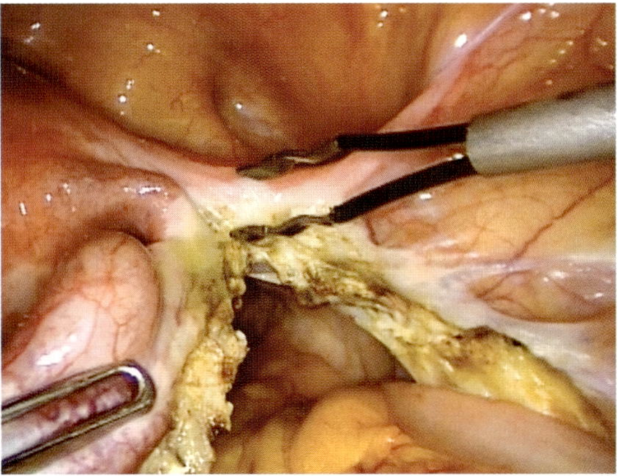

Fig. 13.8: Cauterization of round ligament

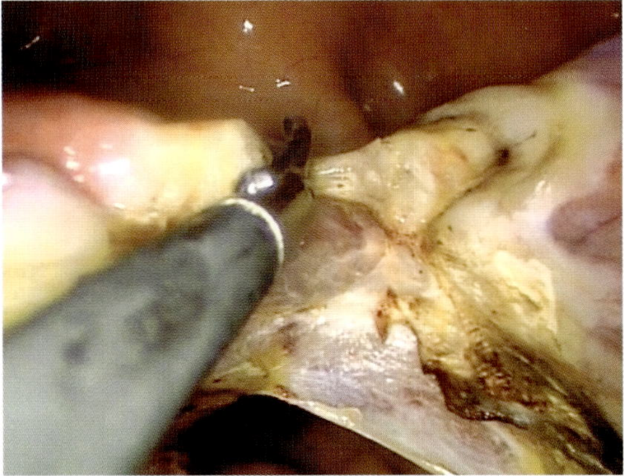

Fig. 13.9: Cutting of round ligament

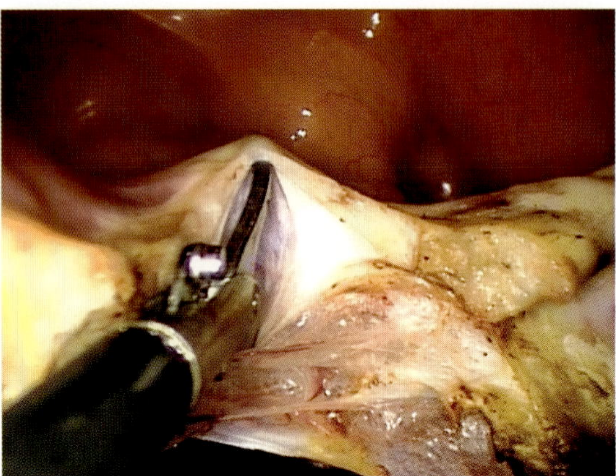

Fig. 13.10: Opening of two lips of broad ligament

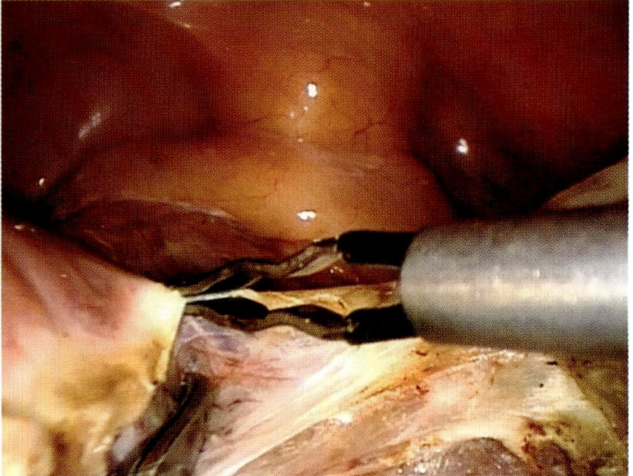

Fig. 13.11: Anterior lip of broad ligament being separated

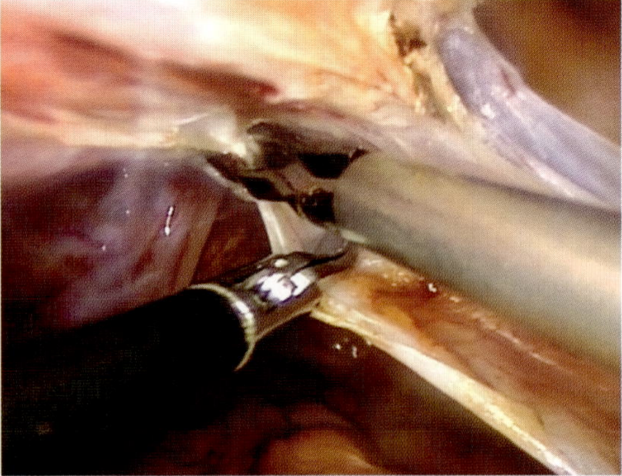

Fig. 13.12: Posterior lip of broad ligament being separated and cut lateral to uterine wall

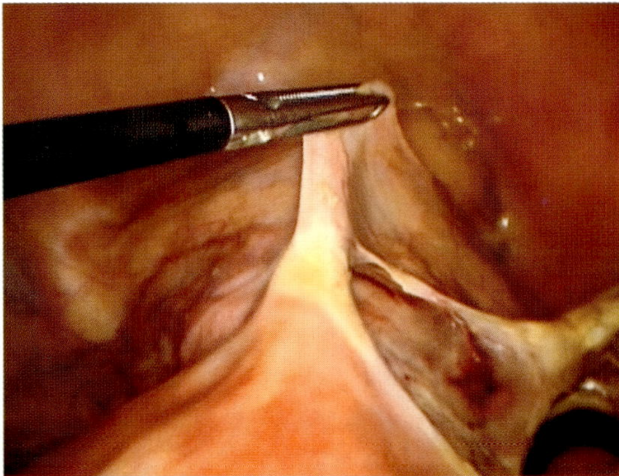

Fig. 13.13: Uterovesical fold of peritoneum lifted and cauterized at isthmic level close to uterus

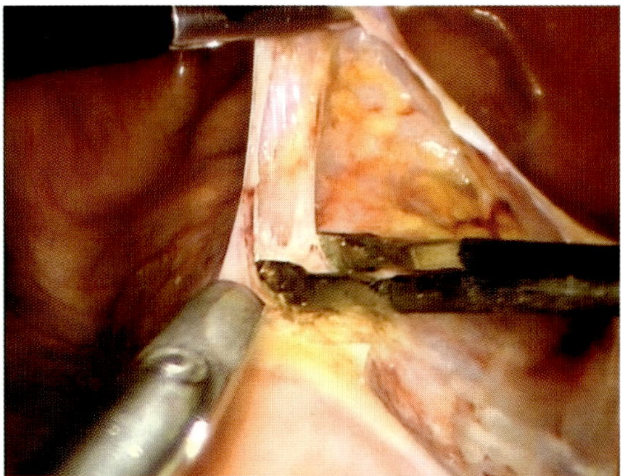

Fig. 13.14: Dissection of pubo-cervical ligament and anterior pouch, pushing bladder down

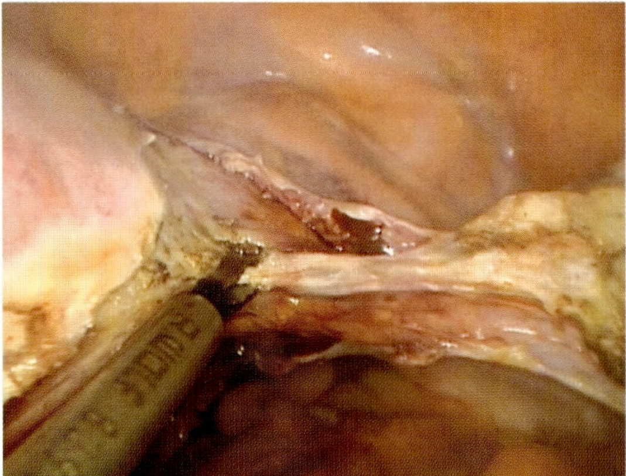

Fig. 13.15: Skeletonization of right uterine artery followed by cauterization

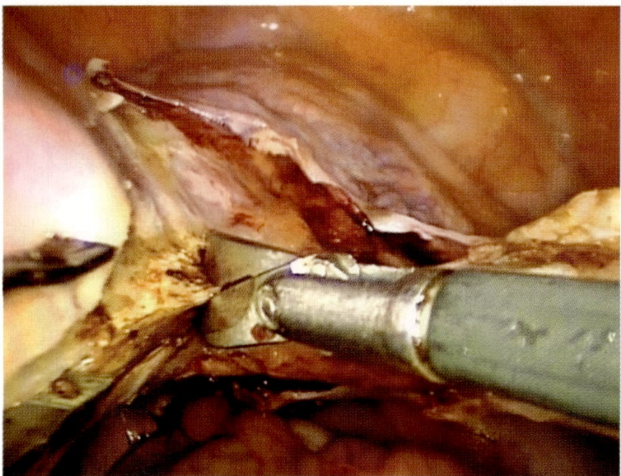

Fig. 13.16: Cutting of right uterine artery

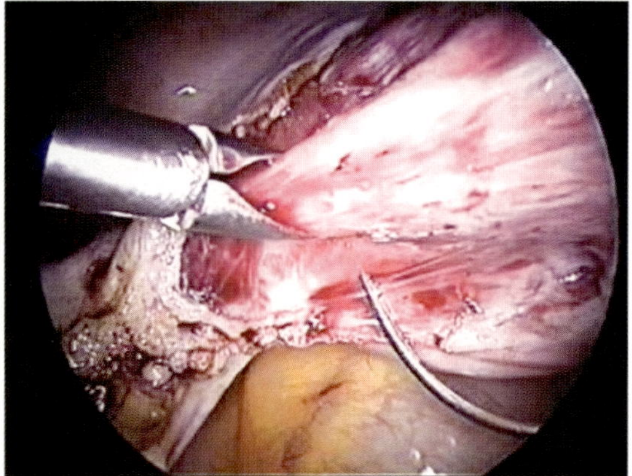

Fig. 13.17A

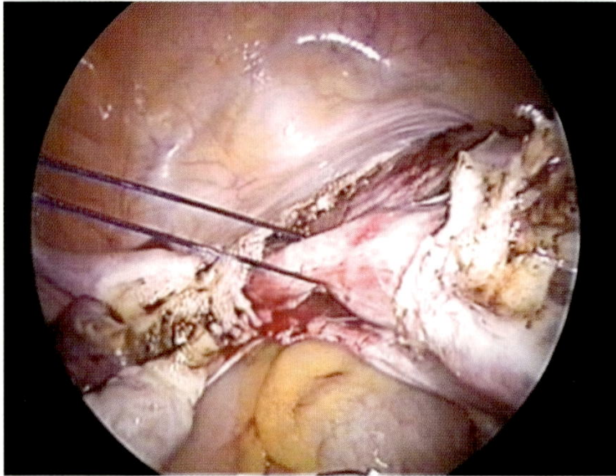

Figs 13.17A and B: Left uterine artery ligation

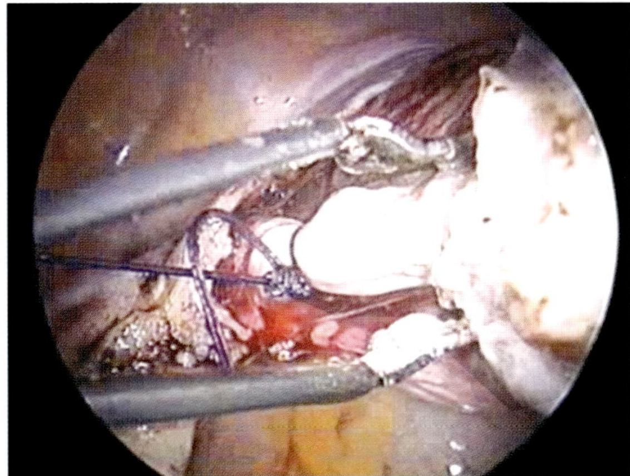

Fig. 13.17C

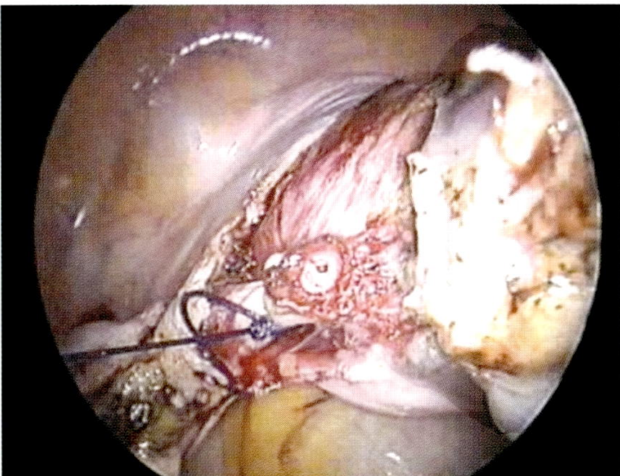

Fig. 13.17D

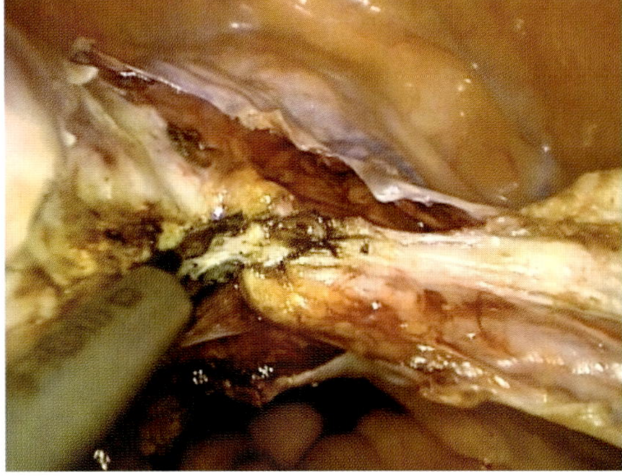

Fig. 13.18: Cauterization of Mackenrodt's ligament

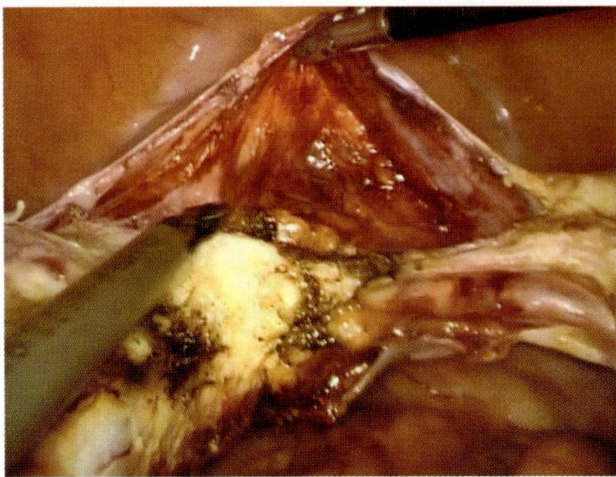

Fig. 13.19: Mackenrodt's ligament cut and angle of vault reached on right side

Before cauterizing it, one should ensure sufficient bladder dissection to avoid thermal spread to the bladder. This anterior displacement and shaving of bladder pillar, transverse cervical ligament and utero-sacral ligament from their attachments maintains the integrity of endopelvic fascia and vascularity.

14. All the steps are done bilaterally.
15. Once you reach the angle of the vault, manipulator is changed to Clermont Ferrand manipulator. (Few endosurgeons use this manipulator from the beginning)
16. Maintaining cranial displacement of uterus, blade of the manipulator is thrusted into the anterior fornix in such a way so as to lift the vaginal wall and displace the bladder downwards. Using the monopolar hook, the vault is cut circumferentially over the blade of the vaginal manipulator. The vaginal assistant tactfully rotates the blade so that the surgeon is able to cut the vault over the blade circumferentially. Here, instead of cutting current, if one uses coagulation current, spurters of vault will not bleed. But one should keep sufficient stretch on tissue to be cut, for the coagulation current to work (Figs 13.20 to 13.23).
17. After completing the circumferential incision, the uterus is gently drawn in the vagina and kept in place, which prevents CO_2 gas leak.
    - Instead of monopolar spatula, harmonic scalpel with open blade on level 5 setting can be used, without any risks of electro-surgical burns.

18. The angles of vaginal vault along with pubocervical and uterosacral ligaments are closed by endoligature on both sides, re-creating the ring of fascia. One or two more interrupted sutures can be taken over vaginal vault (Figs 13.24 and 13.25). After ensuring hemostasis, a complete peritoneum lavage is done (Figs 13.26 and 13.27).

    • As it is not possible to take uterosacral angle and pubocervical fascia vaginally, (the way it can be taken laparoscopically), vault closure from vagina is never recommended.
    • Continuous locking sutures is not recommended for the vault.
    • In case of laxity of uterosacral ligament, plication stitches are taken on both the uterosacral ligaments, taking care of the ureters.
    • Reconstruction of the vault ring is the most important step to avoid vault prolapse.

Post Hysterectomy Inspection

After closing the vault, saline wash is given and the pedicles are inspected. Bladder, ureters and bowel are also thoroughly inspected.

Postoperative Management

1. No need to keep Foley's catheter postoperatively, unless excessive bladder handling and dissection is done. Patient is encouraged to walk to the toilet within 2 hrs.
2. After 6 hours, clear liquids are given and if tolerated soft diet can be given in the evening.
3. Patient can be discharged after 24 to 48 hrs and can resume her normal activities, within a weeks time.

Problems Anticipated and How to Avoid Them?

Opening of the Vaginal Vault

Division of the lateral part of the cervix is technically difficult as the ascending vaginal vessels may cause troublesome hemorrhage if not coagulated completely. This difficulty can be easily overcome by synchronous movements by the surgeon and the vaginal assistant who pushes the colpotomizer in a proper direction according to the surgeon's choice.

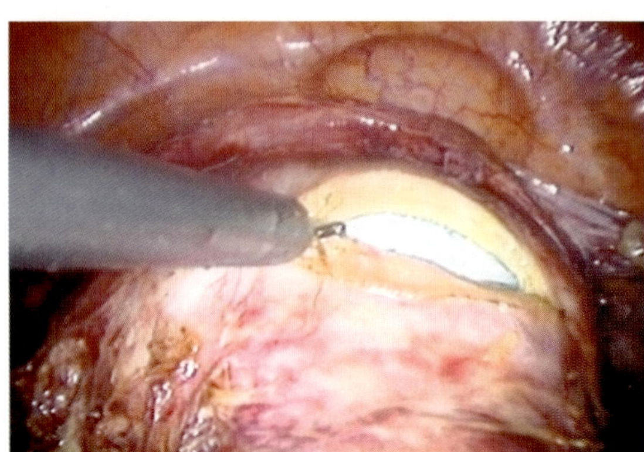

Fig. 13.20: Cutting vault with monopolar hook over uterine manipulator

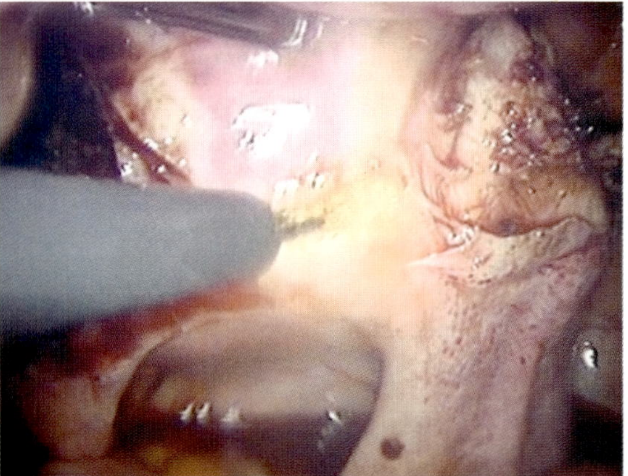

Fig. 13.21: Cutting vault in between uterosacrals

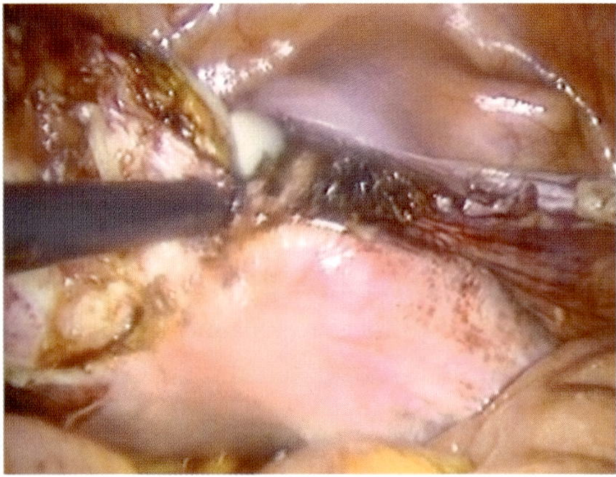

Fig. 13.22: Cutting vault circumferentially

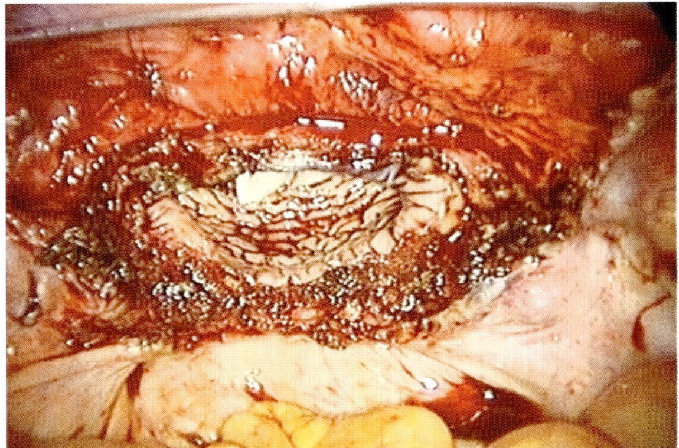

Fig. 13.23: Ring of vault after cutting

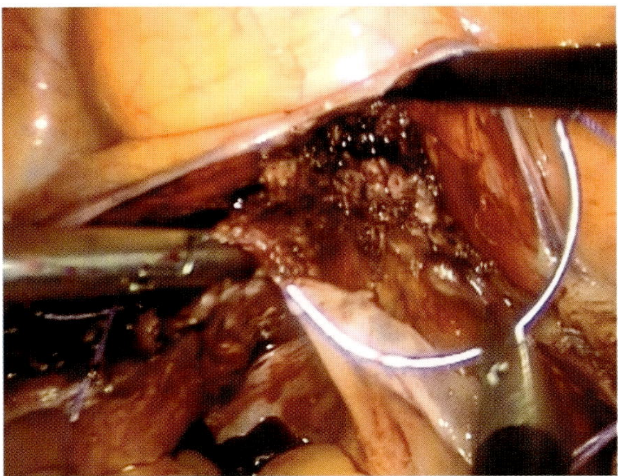

Fig. 13.24: Suturing uterosacral ligaments, vaginal angle, and pubocervical fascia separately on both sides

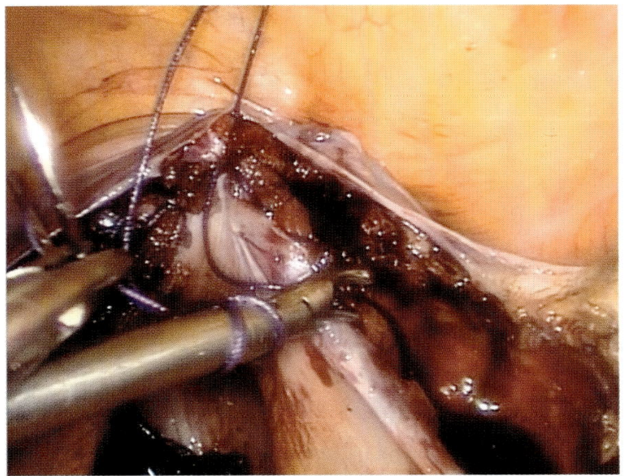

Fig. 13.25: Interrupted suture over vaginal vault

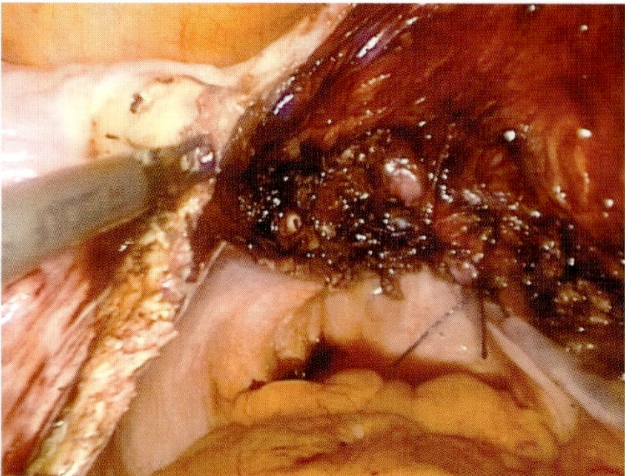

Fig. 13.26: Confirming hemostasis of pedicles.

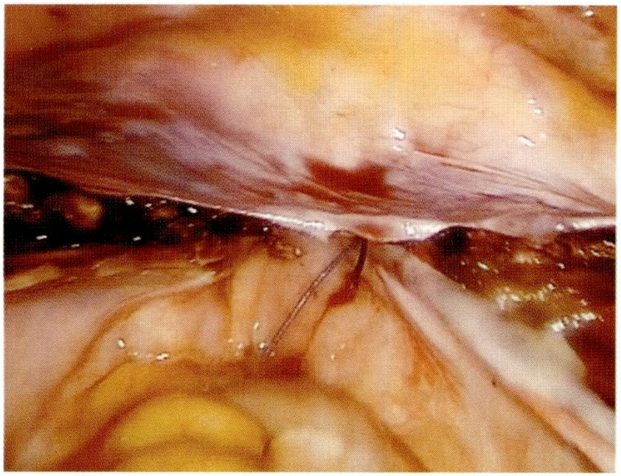

Fig. 13.27: End Result: Clean pelvis. Need not suture visceral peritoneum

Removal of Large Masses/Leiomyoma > 18 weeks

Preferred methods are:

a. All ports in upper abdomen, providing room for vision and surgery.
b. Debulking after uterine ligation (Figs 13.28 to 13.30).
c. Myomectomy before hysterectomy.
d. Securing uterine vessels properly ensuring a bloodless operative field.
e. Use of a 30° 10 mm laparoscope aids good anterior and posterior dissection.
f. In previous CS cases with large uterus, morcellation reduces lacerations of the vagina during specimen removal.

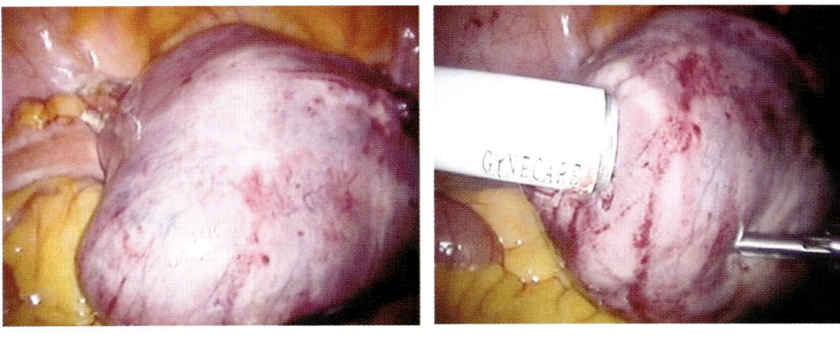

Fig. 13.28   **Fig. 13.29**

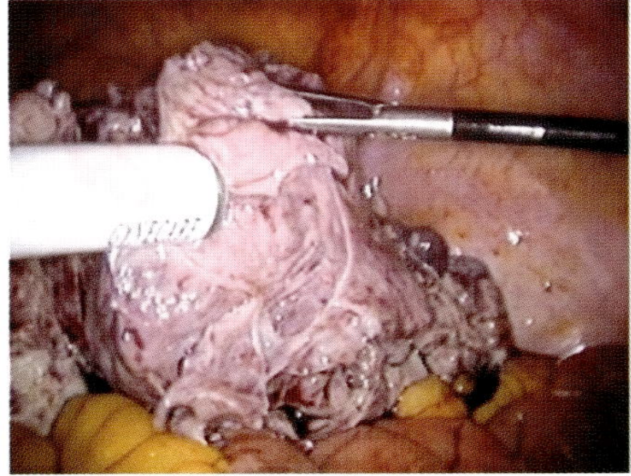

Fig. 13.30

Figs 13.28 and 13.30: In situ morcellation of large uterus after uterine ligation

(Photographs courtesy: Ruby Hall IVF and Endoscopy Centre)

g. Bladder adhesions at isthmus should always be released with sharp dissection by scissors without using energy source or with harmonic scalpel. Throughout the dissection, uterus should be pushed in and is kept midposed, which ensures proper vision and keeps bladder mucosa away from the line of incision.

14 Laparoscopic Radical Hysterectomy

Preoperative Preparation

- FIGO staging
- Mechanical bowel preparation
- Preoperative antibiotics

Instruments and Equipments

- Myoma screw
- Two non-traumatic graspers
- One needle holder
- One Maryland dissector
- Harmonic scalpel
- Bipolar forceps
- Allis' forceps
- Suction cannula
- 0 degree telescope

Technique

1. Regional anesthesia, either spinal or epidural preferred in combination with general anesthesia.
2. Patient is placed in modified Lloyd Davis position at approximately 30- to 45-degree angle.
3. The ports taken are as follows:
    - A total of 5 ports are used.
    - A 10 mm camera port at the umbilicus.
    - A 10 mm working port at the McBurney's point on the right side
    - A 5 mm port pararectally at the midclavicular line
    - A set of 5 mm ports in the mirror image on the left side

The surgeon is on the right side, the assistant and camera surgeon on the left side. The surgeon need not change the position during the contra-lateral dissection.

Procedure

A Myoma screw is introduced from the upper left port and inserted into the fundus for uterine manipulation.

The following standardized steps are followed:

- Step 1: **Anterior U Cut**

The dissection is begun by taking an anterior U cut, cutting the round ligament on the right side with Harmonic Shears.

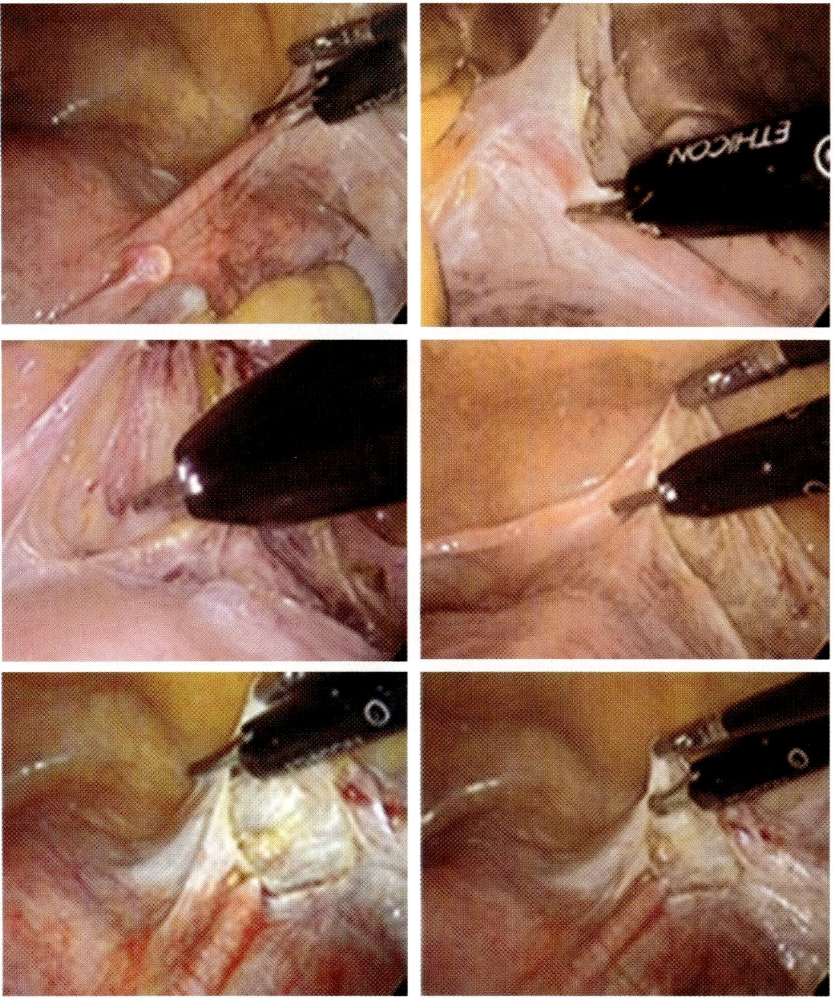

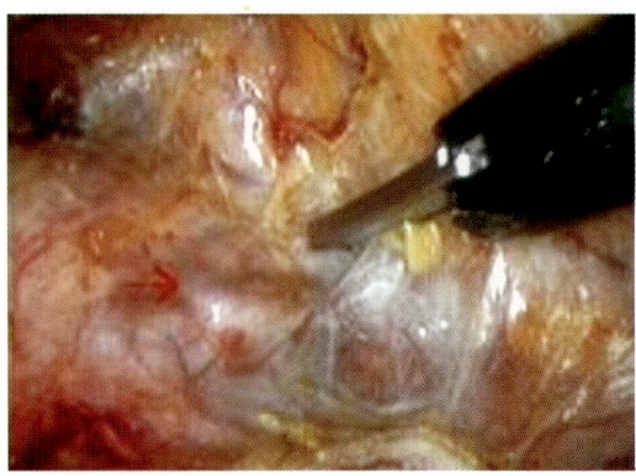

This cut is then extended into the uterovesical fold and is carried downwards up to the urinary bladder. The uterus is pulled cranially and the assistant lifted the bladder. The peritoneum is then incised and the fascial plane between the bladder and the uterus is developed. The bladder when dissected with harmonic shears and then blunt dissection is done with gauze. This dissection is carried downwards to achieve a good vaginal cuff and is facilitated by carbon dioxide insufflations. The peritoneal cut then extended on the left side up to the round ligament. This ligament is cut with the harmonic shears.

- Step 2: **Posterior U Cut**

The peritoneal cut is further extended up to the left infundibulopelvic ligament. The uterus is anteverted and the assistant pushes the rectum to the right side. This stretched the peritoneum medial to the left infundibulopelvic ligament. The ureter is then visualized underneath the peritoneum at the level of sacral promontory.

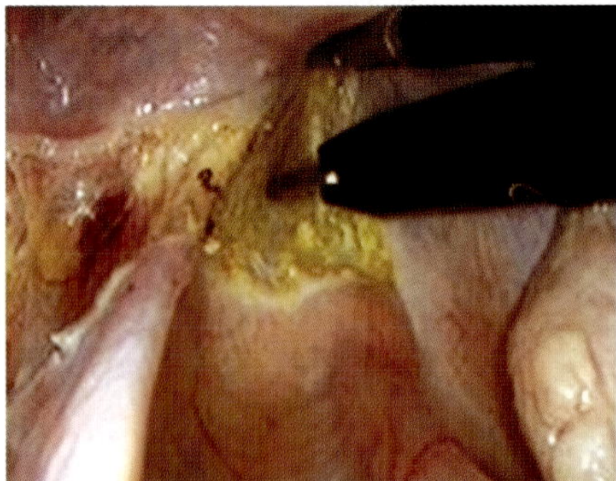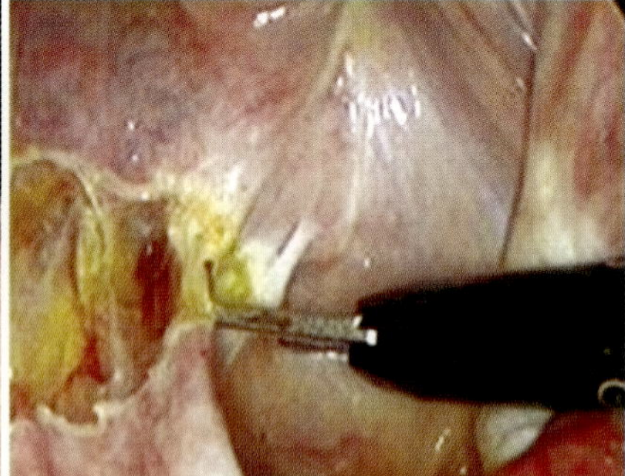

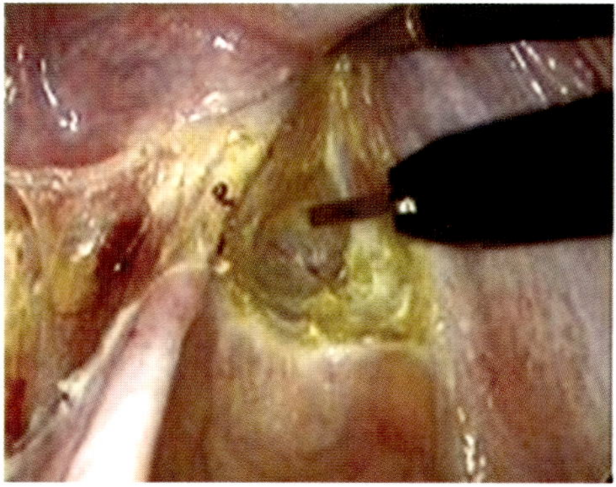

The peritoneum medial to the infundibulopelvic ligament is incised with the harmonic shears to expose the ureter, which is then pushed laterally. The peritoneal cut (Posterior U cut) is extended down into the pouch of Douglas keeping the ureter constantly under vision. The same step is repeated on the right side and the right ureter is pushed laterally. The ureteric dissection is always done parallel to the ureter.

- Step 3: **Dissection of Rectovaginal Space**

The assistant pulls the rectum cranially so as to stretch the peritoneum in the pouch of Douglas. This peritoneum is incised with harmonic shears. The insufflation of carbon dioxide gas opens the loose areolar planes between the two layers of Denonvilliers fascia.

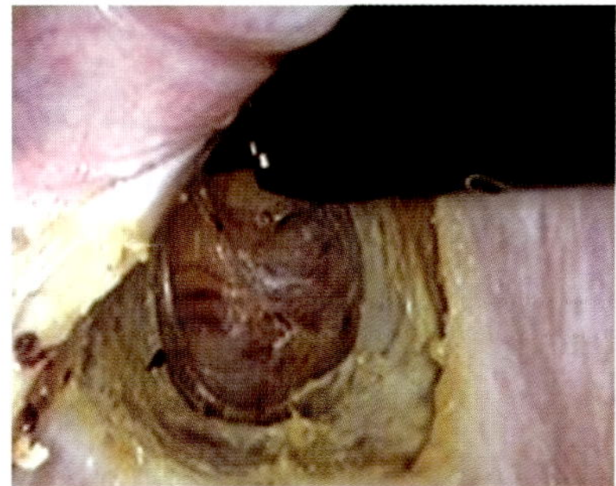
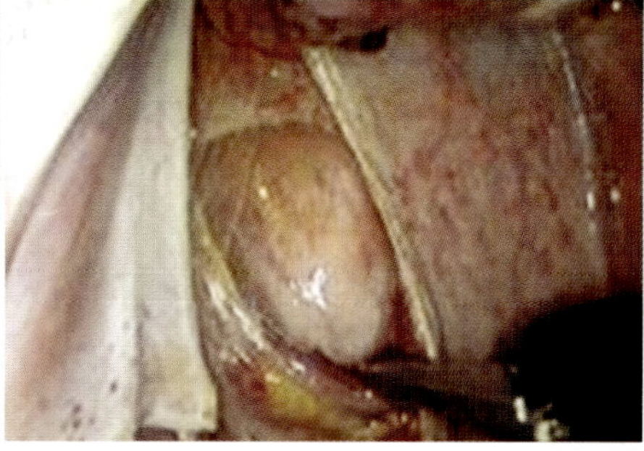

The rectum is dissected off the posterior vaginal wall up to the levator ani. The trick of the trade is to retain the fat on the rectum. One has to remember that the fat belongs to rectum and so the dissection should be between this fat and the posterior vaginal wall. No rectal wall fibers should be visualized.

- Step 4: **Dissection of Pararectal Space**

The left ureter is retracted medially and the posterior leaf of broad ligament above the ureter is cut. This cut is extended downwards towards the bladder so that a window in the broad ligament is created. The ureter is again retracted medially and the Harmonic is swept parallel to the ureter to open the pararectal space. The internal iliac artery which forms the lateral boundary of this space is immediately seen. The only structure which crosses the pararectal space transversely is the uterine artery.

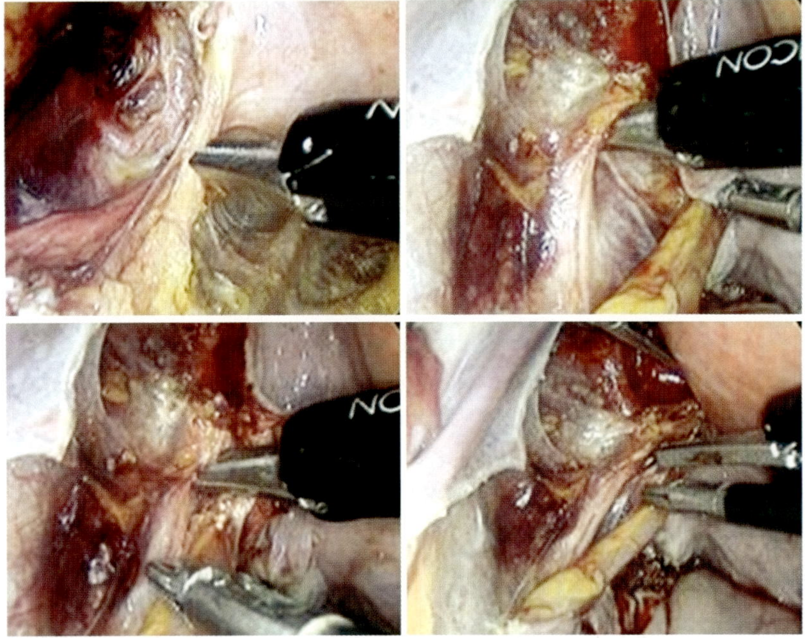

This can be traced to its origin from the internal iliac artery. This artery is then clipped or ligated and cut. The pararectal space dissection is extended caudally up to the leavator ani muscle.

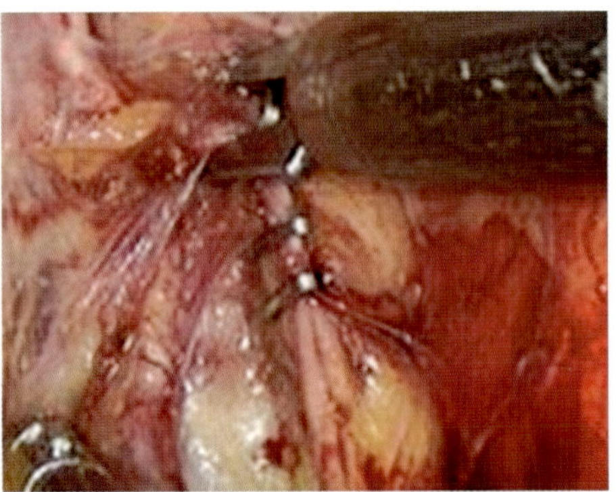

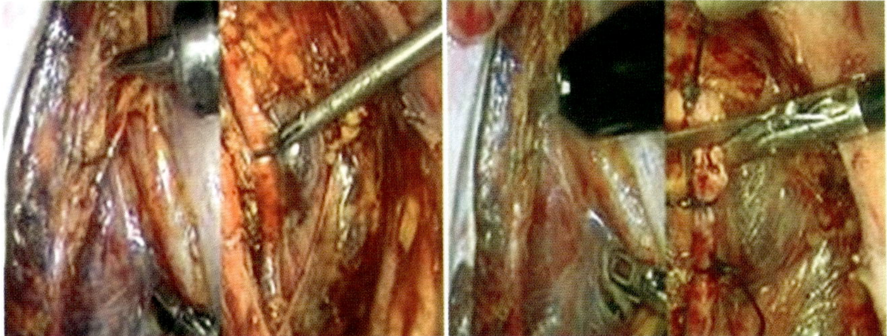

The uteroscaral and Mackenrodts ligaments were thus seen as a single fan-shaped structure. These ligaments were cut with ligature. This cut is extended up to the levator ani.

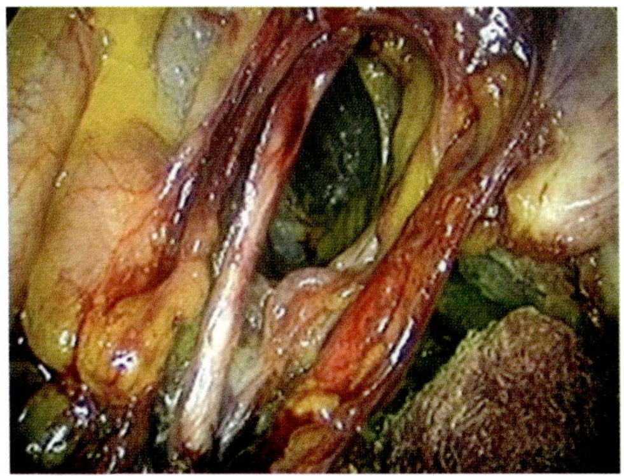

- Step 5: **Lateralisation of Ureter**

The ureter is then retracted laterally and the uterine vein is seen coming from below the ureter. This vein is either clipped or ligated or cut with harmonic shears or with ligature similar steps were taken on the right side. The uterus is pulled cranially and then to the right. This exposes the ureter from the top. The ureter is then traced along its course towards the urinary bladder. At this point, the bladder is held stretched upwards by the assistant surgeon. Thus, the ureteric tunnel could be then visualized along with small veins.

This tunnel was either dissected with Maryland forceps or with harmonic shears. This helped in pushing the ureter further laterally. The ureter could be seen as it enters the bladder at the uterovesical junction. The bladder is then pushed further down to achieve a good vaginal cuff. The ureteric dissection exposed the paracolpos, which is then cut as laterally as possible.

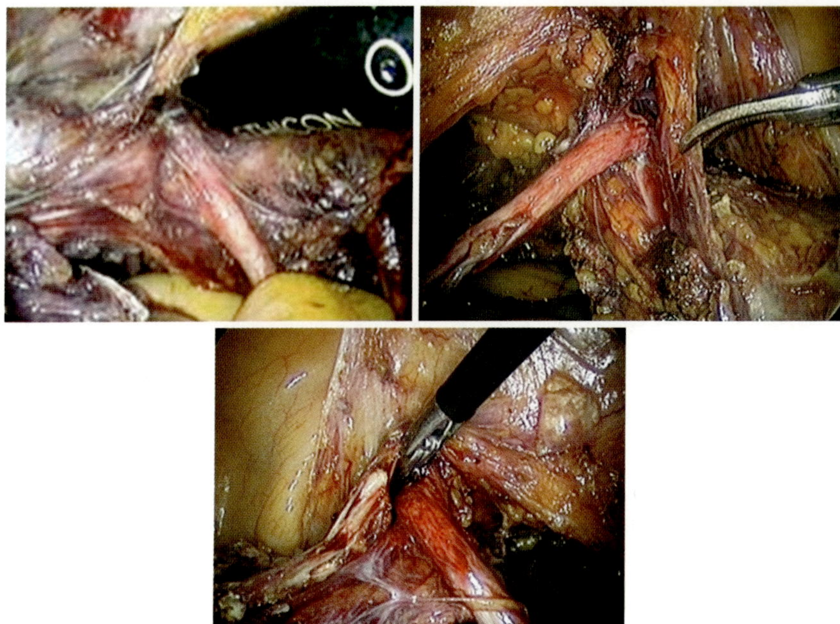

The same steps were repeated on the right side. Finally a good length of vagina below the growth is exposed. The vagina is opened with harmonic shears.

This kind of dissection usually achieves about 2.5 to 3 cm of vaginal cuff. Lastly, the infundibulopelvic ligaments were cut and the entire specimen is separated.

This is then removed through the vagina and the vagina was again packed to prevent carbon dioxide leak. The length of the parametrium and vaginal margin of the specimen is measured.

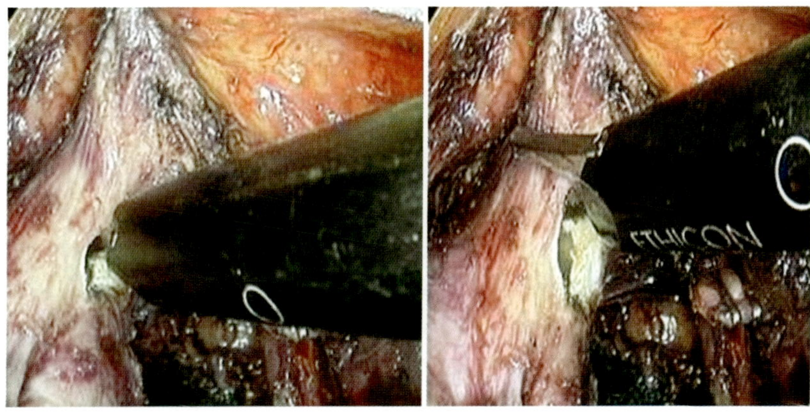

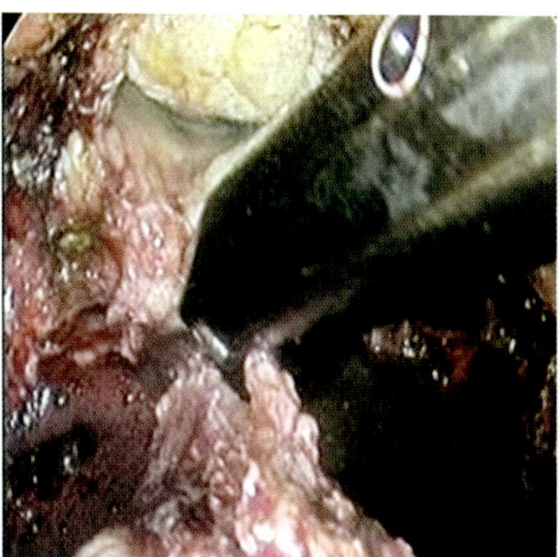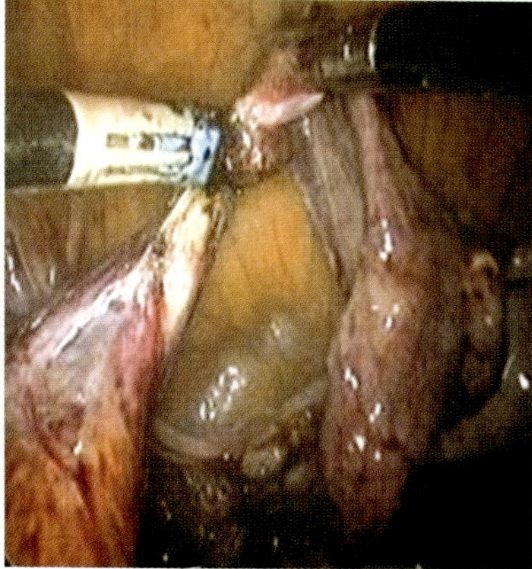

- Step 6: **Lymph Node Dissection**

The lymph node dissection started at the bifurcation of common iliac artery. The suction cannula is the preferred instrument for dissection. The loose areolar tissue along the external iliac artery is swept till the inguinal ligament. All the fibrofatty tissue along the external iliac vein is dissected. At this point the iliac bone is exposed which is the lateral limit of dissection. The nodes in the obturator fossa were visualized by stretching the peritoneum by the assistant. The nodes were swept from the pubic bone cranially. The obturator nerve is exposed and all the nodes above the nerve were cleared. This dissection is done right up to the bifurcation of the iliac vein. The entire fibrofatty tissue is then dissected medially till the internal iliac artery is exposed and cleared off the fibrofatty tissue. This is the medial limit of dissection. At the end of dissection, the external iliac

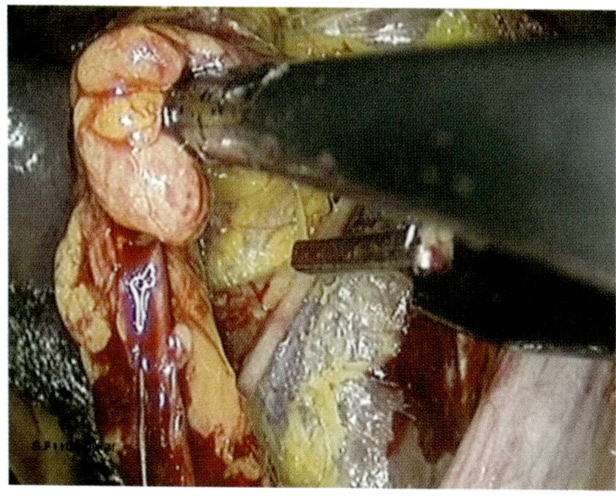

artery, vein and the obturator fossa should be devoid of any fibrofatty tissue. The psoas muscle along with the ilioinguinal nerve is the lateral limit of dissection. The same dissection is done on the other side. The entire nodal tissue is removed through the vagina.

Hemostasis is achieved and the wound is irrigated with normal saline. The vaginal closure is done abdominally with a 30 mm 2-0 vicryl introduced through the 10 mm working port and continuous interlocking sutures were taken. A nasogastric tube No. 16 is introduced through one of the 5 mm ports and is kept as a drain. The posterior peritoneum is not closed. The ports were removed under vision and the 10 mm port sites were sutured.

(Photographs courtesy: Galaxy Endoscopy Centre)

15 Laparoscopic Myomectomy

Preoperative Evaluation of the Patient

- History, examination
- Ultrasound for location, number of fibroids, any associated organic pathology like endometriosis, adnexal mass etc. (Transvaginal ultrasound is preferable). An abdominal ultrasound can be performed, especially in fundal fibroids
- Color Doppler to rule out uterine malignancy or a sarcomatous fibroid
- Limited MRI for uterus
- Routine investigations
- A hysteroscopy is always done before starting laparoscopy to exclude a submucous myoma. Submucous myomas more than 50% projecting into the cavity should preferably be removed hysteroscopically.

Preoperative Preparations

Usually no preparation. In cases of large fibroids or multiple fibroids, bowel preparation can be done.

Instruments and Equipments

The following are the additional laparoscopic instruments required for different types of myomectomy.

- 10 mm claw/tenaculum forceps
- 5 mm or 10 mm Myoma screw
- Unipolar diathermy needle
- Two 5 mm toothed graspers
- Two Needle holders
- Motorized morcellator
- CCL vaginal extractor - optional

Bowel Preparation

- Diet- One day prior to surgery soft diet till afternoon followed by liquid diet and then, nil by mouth for 8 hrs prior to surgery.
- Peglec powder- dissolve the pack in 2 liters of water to be given within 2-3 hrs on previous evening.

OR

- Exelyte solution 90 ml to be added in 300 ml of limca/fruit juice to be given on previous evening.

Prerequisites

1. Skilled laparoscopic surgeon; especially skilled in Laparoscopic suturing and morcellation.
2. Anesthetist, skilled and trained assistant, nursing staff.
3. A complete set of Operative Laparoscopy instruments, 5/10 mm myoma screw, and electromechanical morcellator.
4. Both monopolar and bipolar cautery, Harmonic if available.
5. Proper suturing set with needle holders, knot pushers for extra corporeal knots and scissors.
6. Injection vasopressin - 20 Units in 100 ml normal saline.

Position of the patient- same as laparoscopic hysterectomy

Procedure

- Placement of primary and secondary trocars depends upon the size and site of fibroid.
- Relation of fibroid with the uterus and fallopian tube should be carefully assessed after inserting primary trocar and then site of secondary trocars to be decided.
- Vasopressin 1 in 100 dilution is injected into fibroid at 3 to 4 sites to minimize bleeding (action will remain only for 20-30 min).
- Careful planning of incision is done.
- Incision is usually taken with a monopolar hook/spatula over the most bulging part of the myoma.
- Most preferred incision is transverse incision, as it will cut fewer vessels.
- Incision should be of sufficient depth, so that capsule of fibroid is visualized.
- With 2 Allis' forceps, cut edges are pulled apart so as to expose capsule of fibroid wall and make space for myoma screw insertion.

- Once the myoma screw is inserted, myoma is pulled outward and upward keeping counter traction on uterus downward with 2 Allis' forceps applied on the anterior lip the cervix.
- If one is in the right plane, myoma is usually extracted easily and there is minimal bleeding.
- Position of myoma screw is changed from time-to-time so that traction is applied next to cleavage line.
- Usually the base of myoma will have large feeding vessels, which should be cauterized and cut.
- Only active bleeders of the bed are cauterized which can be easily identified by underwater inspection.
- Undue cautery should be avoided, as it will give defective healing.
- Myoma after removal is parked at right paracolic gutter.

Closure of Uterine Flap

- Reconstruction of myoma bed is performed with Vicryl no. 1 suture
- Whether single or multiple layer closure is individual's decision-but the ultimate aim is to obliterate the dead space completely so as to avoid hematoma formation, which is another cause of weakening of scar.
- Start from one angle, first stitch is placed beyond angle either with intra-corporeal or extra-corporeal suture and then rest of defect is closed by taking deep continuous locking sutures and the end suture should be again beyond the angle of opposite side.
- If it is a single layer closure, ensure that stitches are deep enough to obliterate the dead space.
- We don't advocate multiple layer closure neither closure of endometrial layer.

Extraction of Myoma

- Myomas are extracted by electronic morcellation. Smaller myomas can be extracted by colpotomy.
- A meticulous lavage is given and hemostasis is checked.
- End result should be a clean pelvis.
- To keep a drain in the postoperative period is again an individual's choice.

MYOMECTOMY IN DIFFICULT SITUATIONS

Pedunculated Fibroid with a Broad Base

- Instead of transverse incision, circular incision should be taken at the base of fibroid in a circumferential manner.
- With myoma screw, myoma is pulled up and enucleated after cauterizing base of the pedicle.

Broad Ligament Myomas

- Majority of broad ligament myomas are removed by a posterior incision unlike at laparotomy where division of round ligament and removal by anterior route is preferred.
- The oblique incision is made in the broad ligament parallel to the vessels.
- A myoma screw is now inserted and traction is applied slowly while a grasper is used for retracting the broad ligament.
- Any bleeding vessels are coagulated then and there.
- After complete enucleation, broad ligament is inspected for complete hemostasis.
- A drain is kept in the pelvis and observed.
- There is no need to suture the broad ligament back.

TIPS

- In case of multiple fibroids where the shape of the uterus is distorted, round ligaments help in identification
- As far as possible, incision should be taken anteriorly than on posterior wall. Self pre-operation USG always helps to enhance surgical performance on table especially in cases of multiple myomas. One can decide the number of myomas that can be taken out through a single incision. There is no tactile sensation in laparoscopy so small myomas hidden under large myomas, if known beforehand, can be removed successfully.
- We don't advocate use of pre-op GnRH analogues to reduce the size of myoma but is practiced by few endoscopic surgeons.
- Traction on uterus downwards with Allis´ forceps applied to anterior lip of cervix and upward counter traction on myoma with myoma screw, next to cleavage line will facilitate dissection.
- Myomas up to 5-6 cm can be delivered with colpotomy.

- Proper serosal approximation, hemostasis, clean pelvis at the end, early mobilization will help in prevention of postoperative adhesions..
- Instillation of vasopressin, speedy surgery, skillful and rapid suturing, good knot tying techniques will help to minimize bleeding.
- Occassionally one can encounter excessive bleeding from vasopressin injection so one should keep in instilling vasopressin even while withdrawing the needle as shown in below.

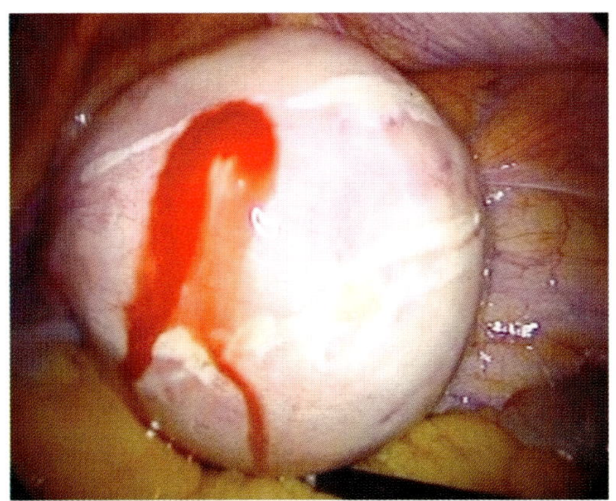

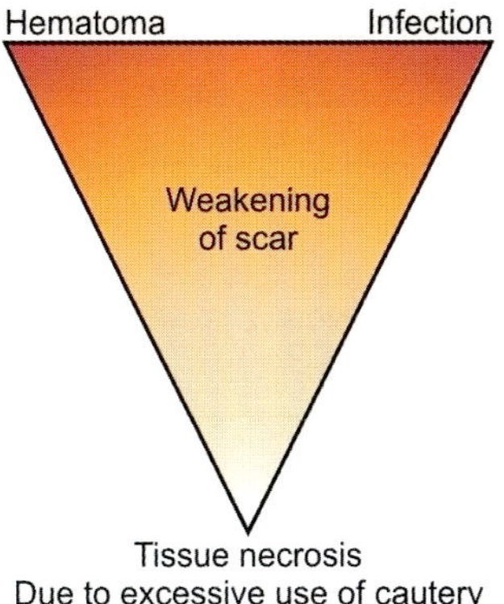

> *The technique of laparoscopic myomectomy has to be modified according to the type, location, number and degenerative changes undergone by the myoma. It also has to be modified according to the experience of the surgeon and instruments available.*

LAPAROSCOPIC MYOMECTOMY

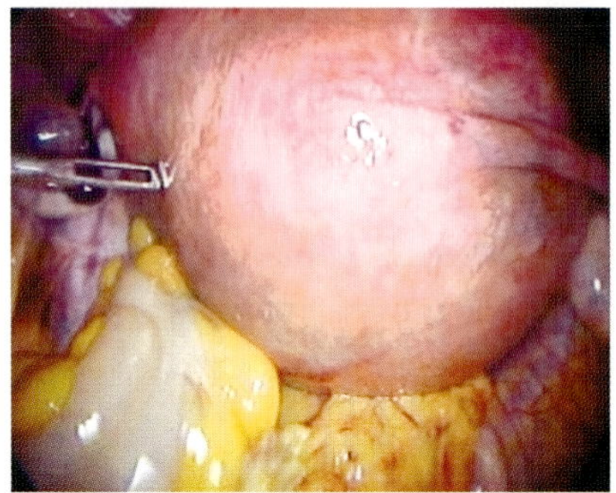

Intramural myoma

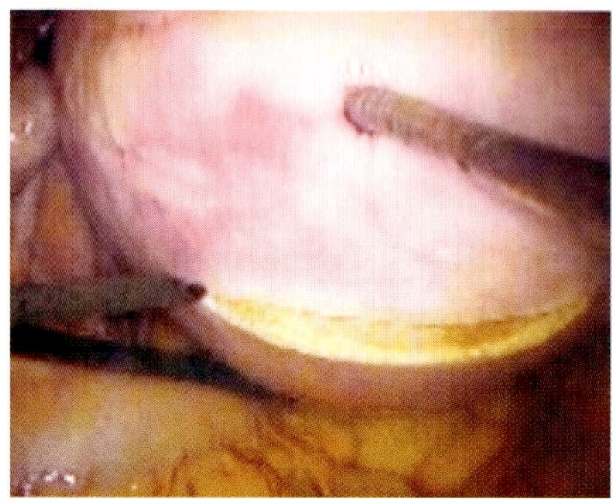

Incision with monopolar hook after vasopressin instillation

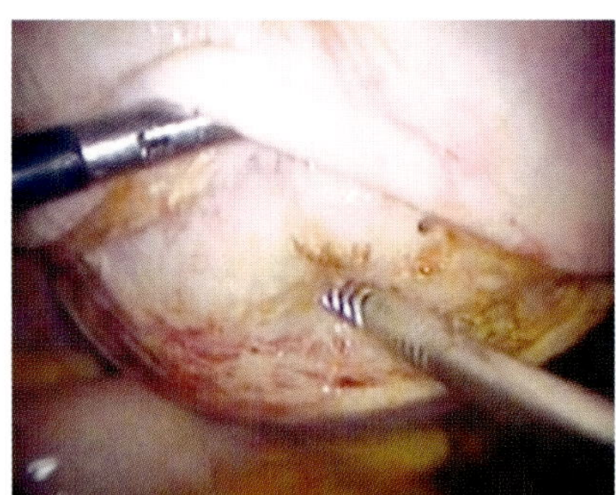

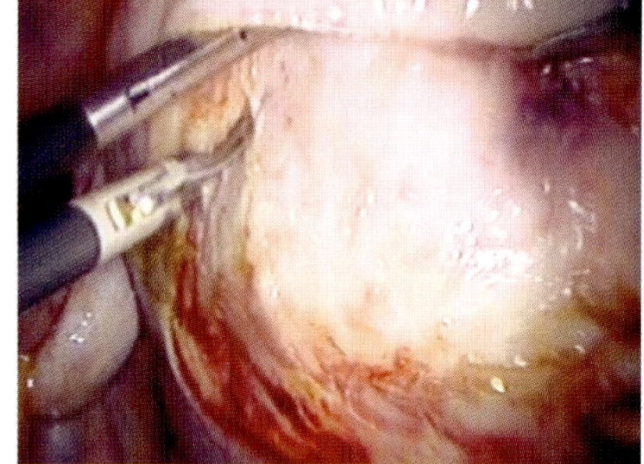

Enucleation in process

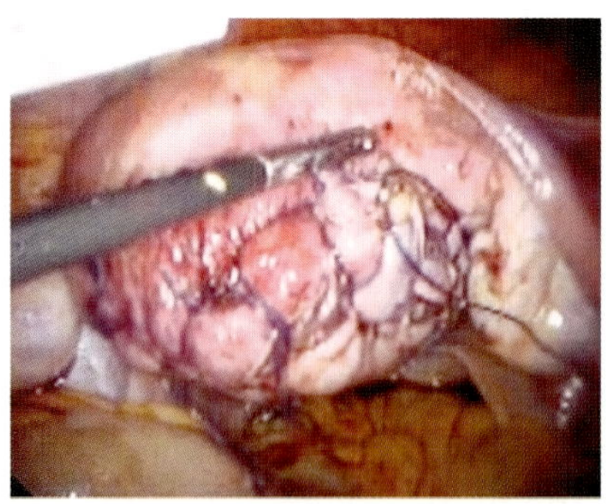

End result

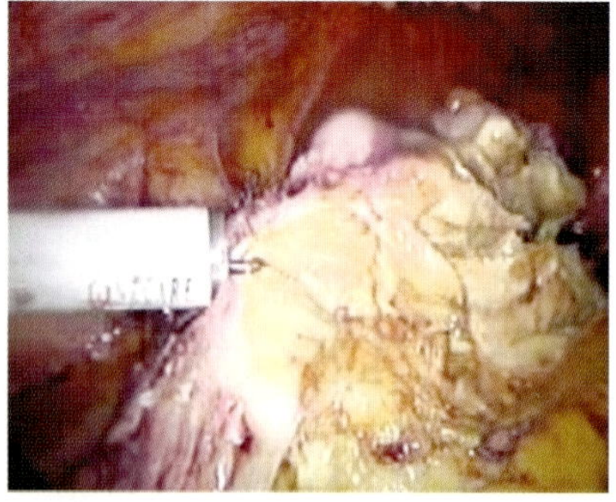

Morcellation

(Photographs courtesy: Ruby Hall IVF and Endoscopy Centre)

REMOVAL OF LARGE POSTEROCERVICAL FIBROID

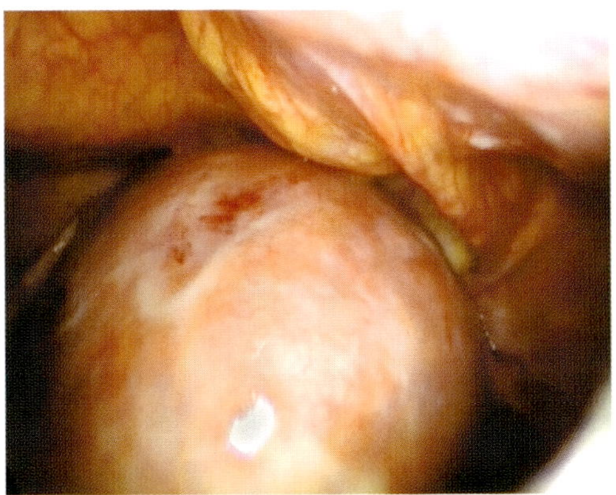

Panaromic view

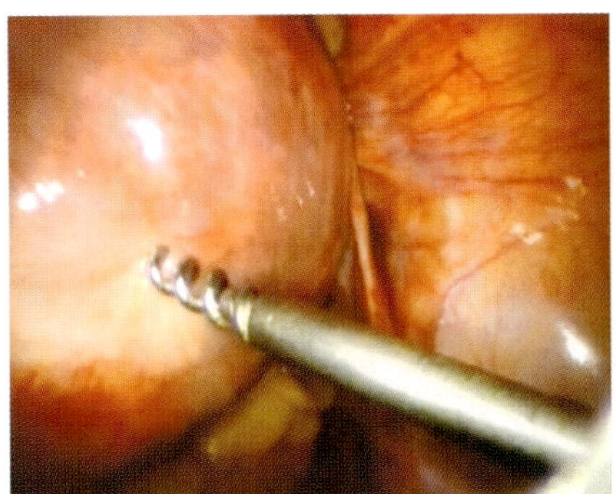

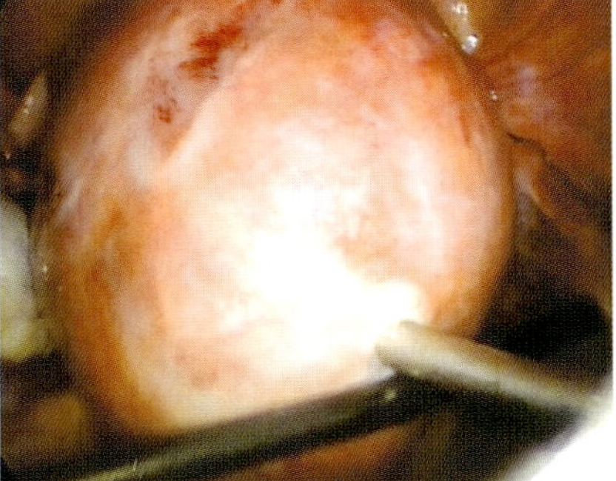

Myomectomy made easier by deimpacting myoma with myoma screw. This step makes myoma accessible and easier for further extraction in routine way

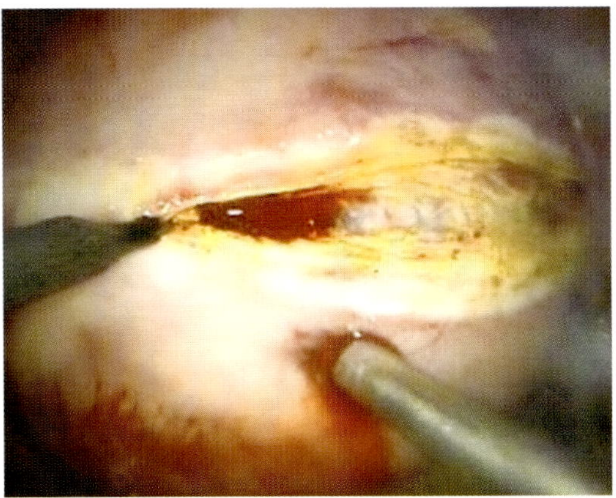

Incision with monopolar hook

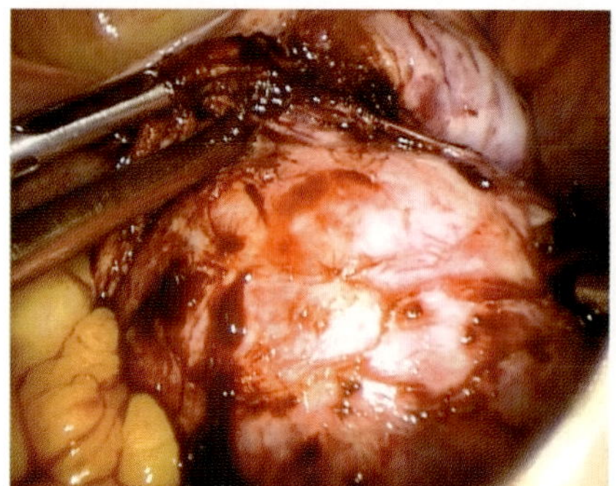

Enucleation in process

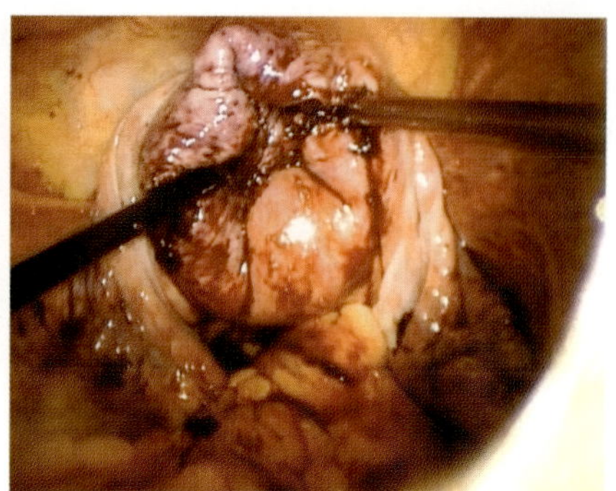

Myoma bed compressed to allow stoppage of capillary oozing

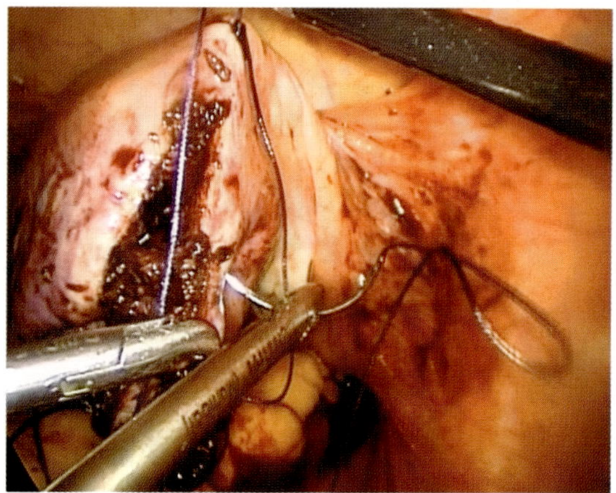

Right angular stitch

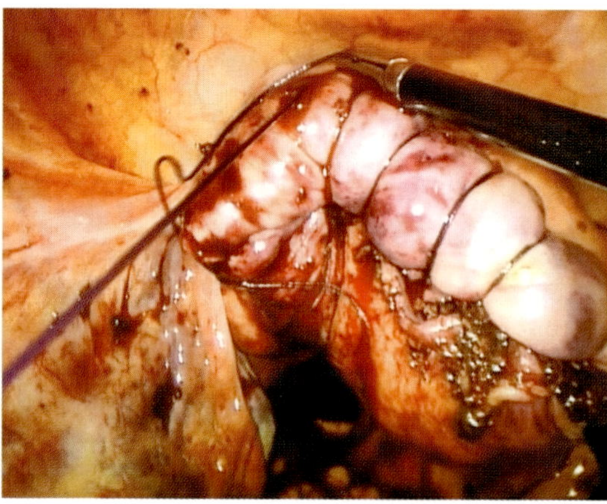

Continuous locking sutures

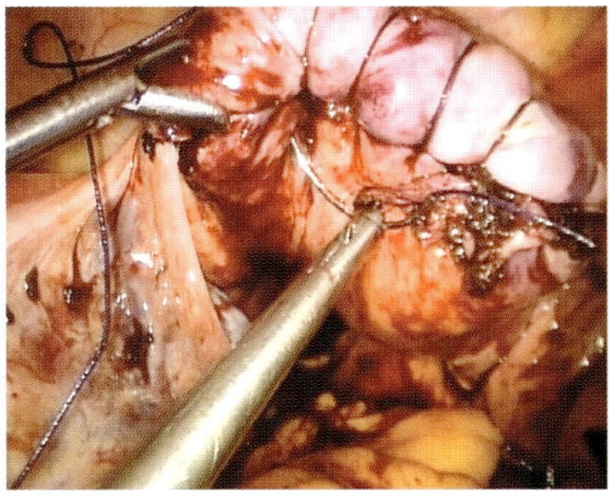

Left angular stitch

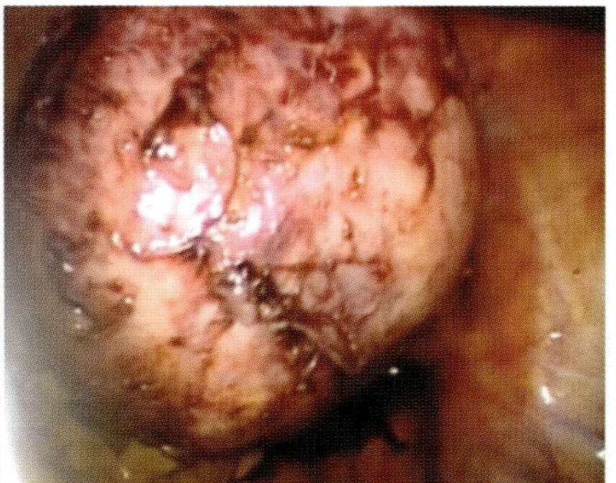

Enucleated large myoma

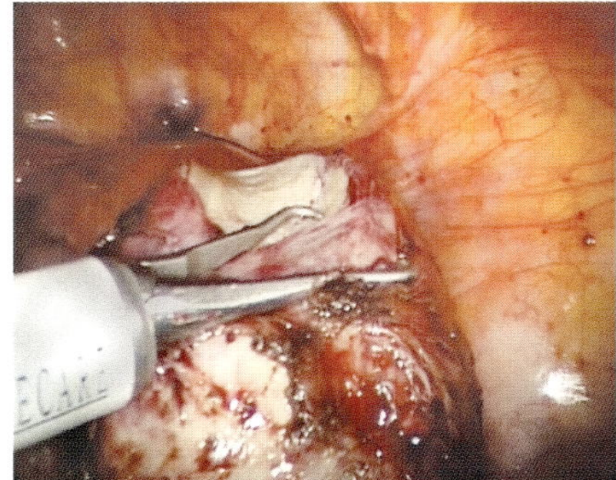

Morcellation in progress

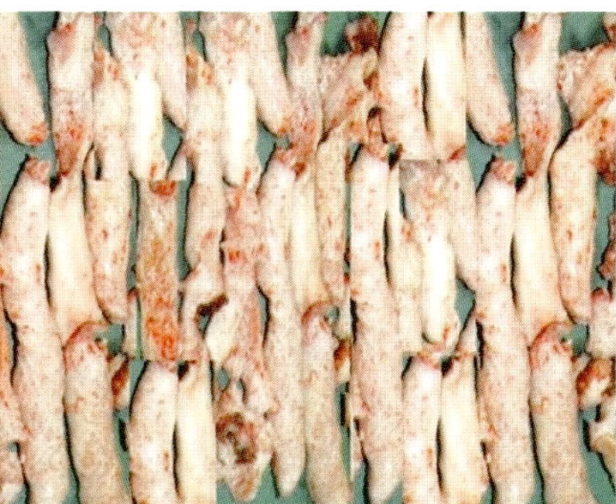

Morcellated pieces

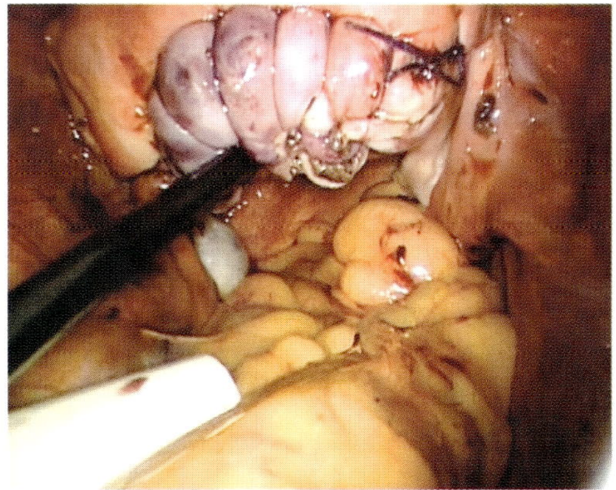

End result has to be clean pelvis with good hemostasis

(Photographs courtesy: Ruby Hall IVF and Endoscopy Centre)

REMOVAL OF SMALL POSTEROCERVICAL FIBROID

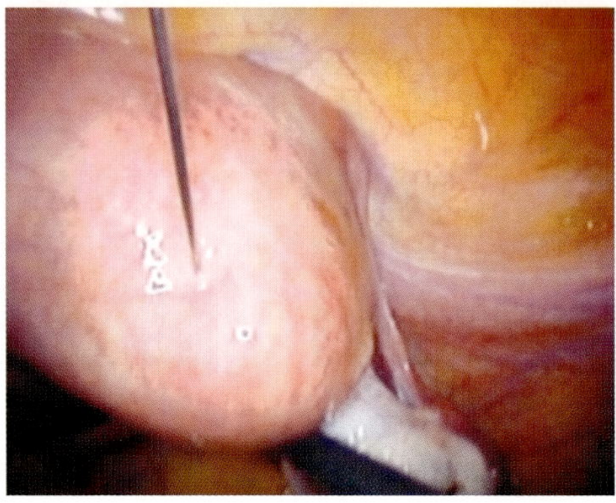

In case of smaller posterior cervical fibroid accessibility can be achieved by just lifting and supporting myoma with grasper for vasopressin injection

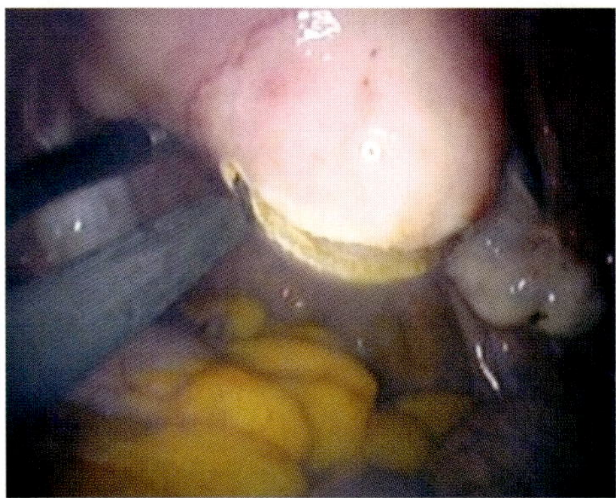

Incision with monopolar hook

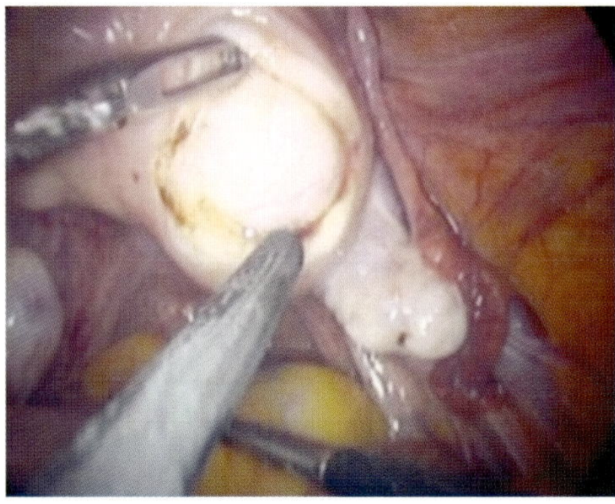

Separation of capsule of fibroid

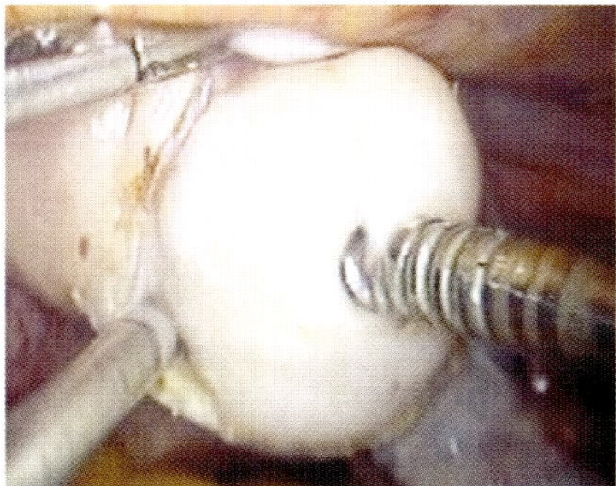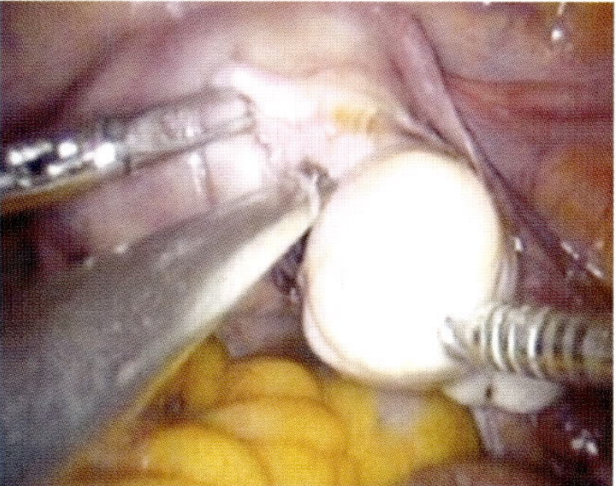

Enucleation in process

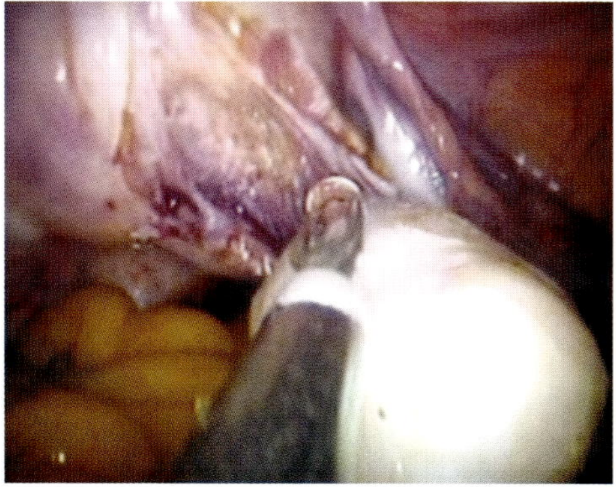

Enucleation completed

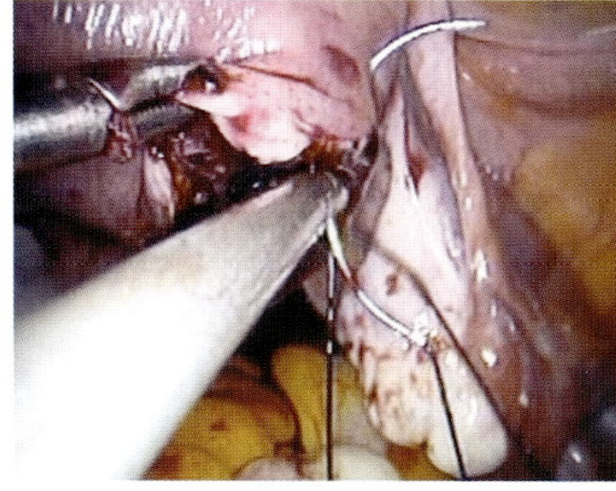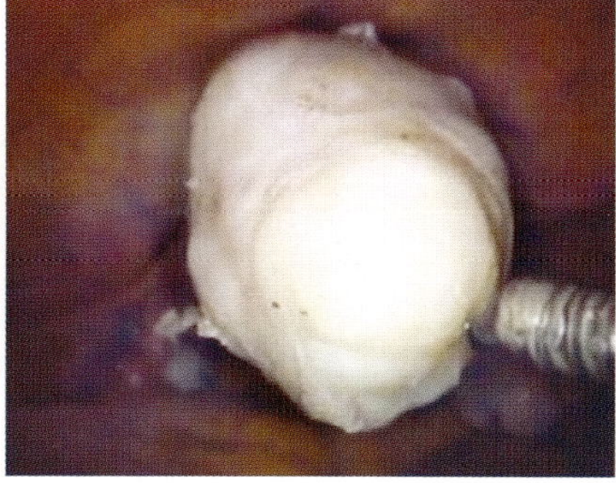

Suturing

Enucleated myoma of this size can be
removed through colpotomy

(Photographs courtesy: Ruby Hall IVF and Endoscopy Centre)

MYOMECTOMY WITH VERTICAL INCISION

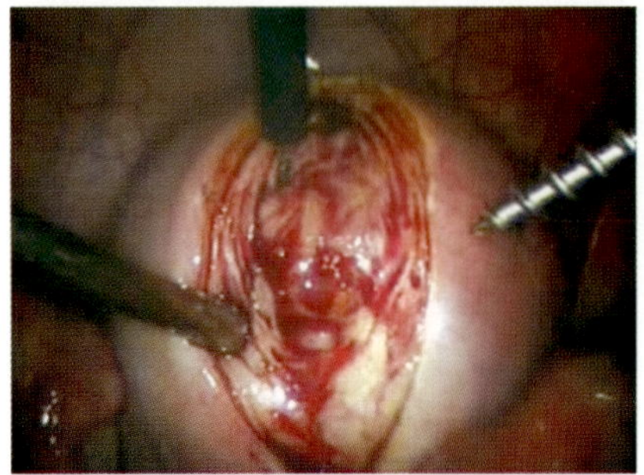

Incising the myometrium

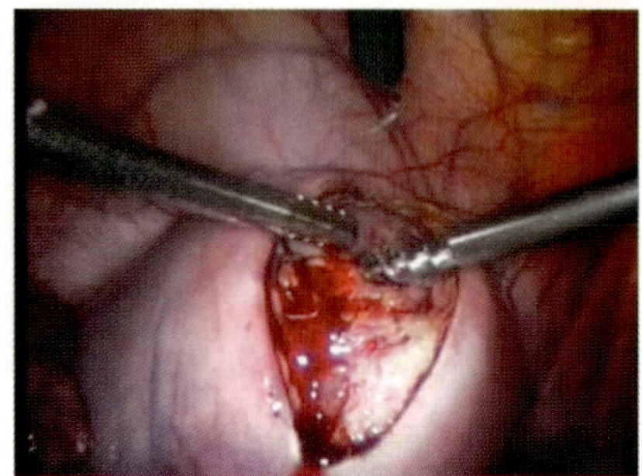

Enucleating the myoma

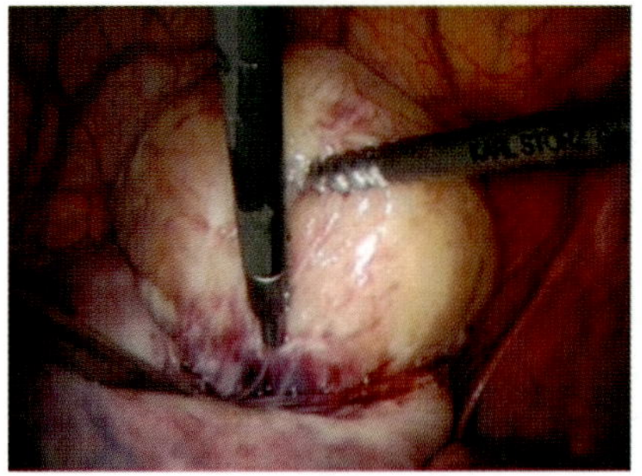

Coagulation of vessels of myoma bed

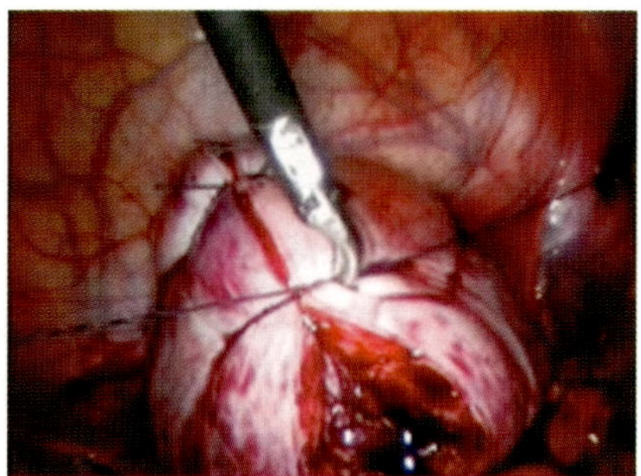

Re-approximating the myometrium
using intra-corporeal sutures

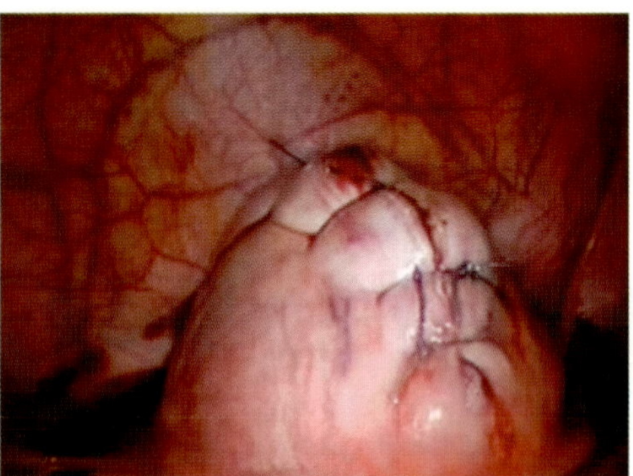

End result

(Photographs courtesy: Dr PG Paul)

VARIOUS MYOMAS

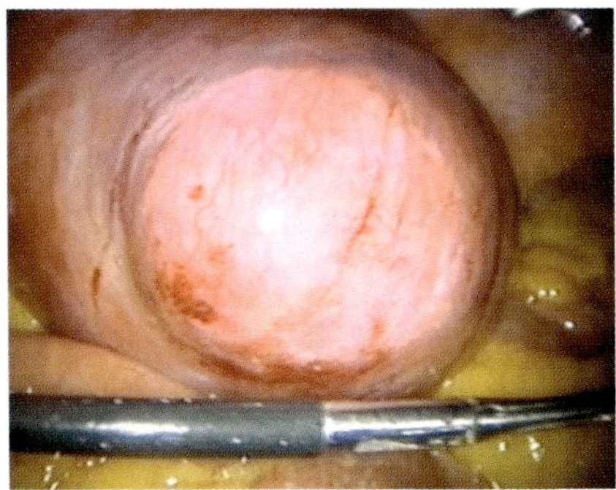

Myoma above myoma

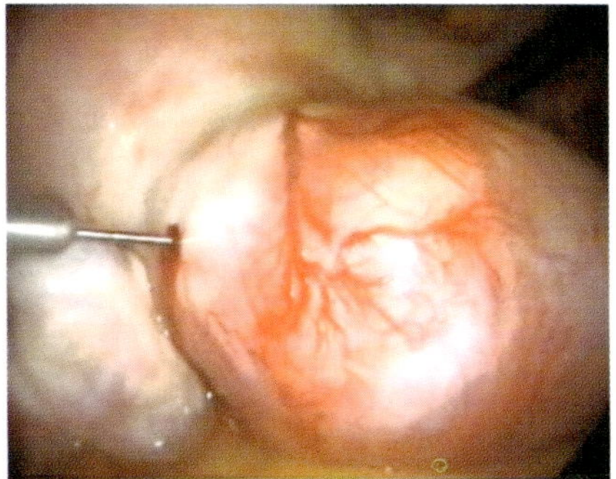

Vascular myoma
(Photograph courtesy: Dr Prakash Trivedi)

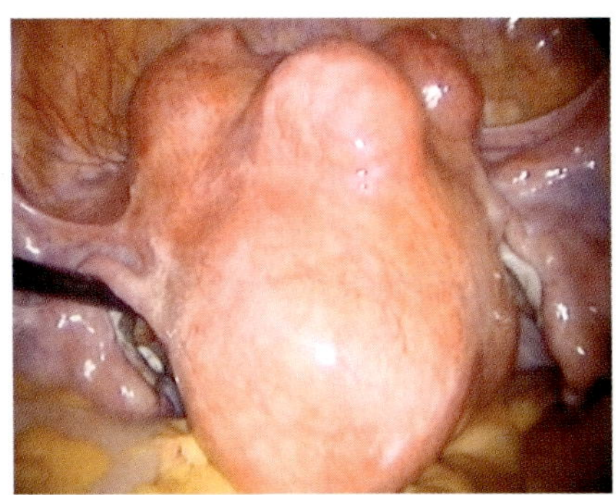

Multiple myomas

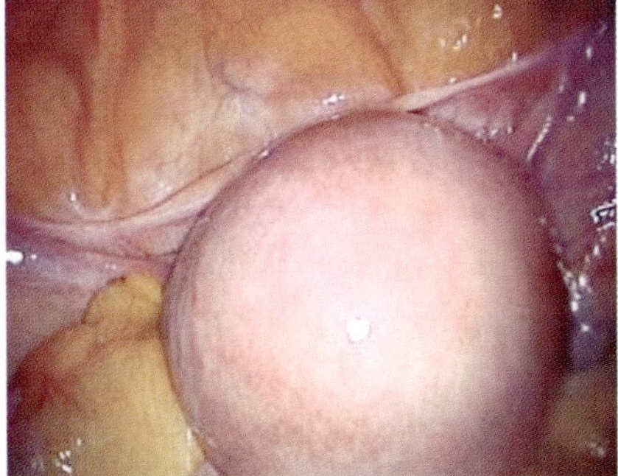

Fundal intramural globular myoma

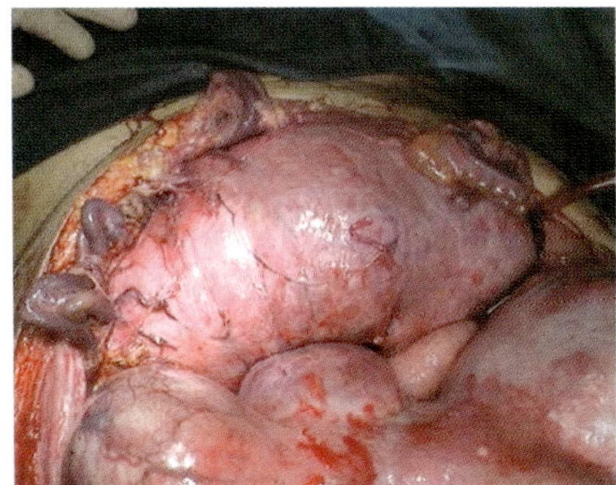

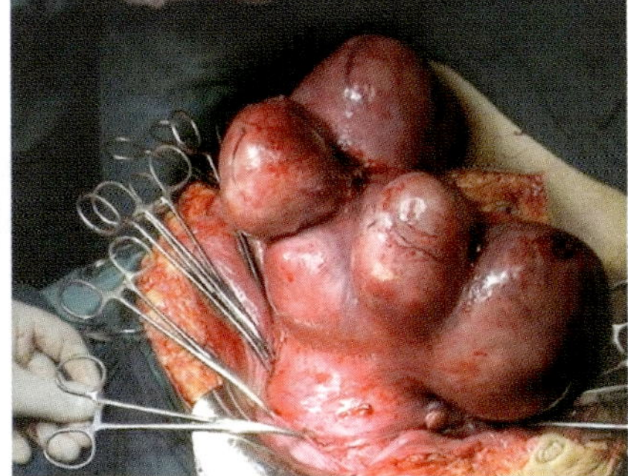

Few myomas can not be tackled by laparoscopy

(Photographs courtesy: Ruby Hall IVF and Endoscopy Centre)

16 Laparoscopic Management of Benign Ovarian Mass

Preoperative Evaluation

- Diagnosis with a thorough history and clinical examination (per vaginal, per rectal)
- Routine blood investigation
- Tumor markers - Ca125/ CEA/ alpha fetoprotein/ Beta HCG
- Transvaginal sonography
- Color Doppler to rule out malignancy

After confirming that the ovarian cyst is benign, laparoscopic ovarian cystectomy can be done.

Preoperative Preparation

No specific preparation is required.

Laparoscopic Ovarian Cystectomy

A standard 10 mm laparoscope is introduced with 3 side ports, 2 on the left side and one on the right side.

Intraoperatively, cell washings from the pelvis and upper abdomen should be collected and sent for evaluation to rule out malignancy.

Characteristics of the mass, age of the patient should be seen and decision taken, whether to do oophorectomy or cystectomy.

In ovarian cystectomy, it is necessary to remove the cyst intact with minimal trauma to the residual ovarian tissue.

- If a cyst is larger than 10 cm in size, then first with 18-guage needle fluid in pouch of Douglas is aspirated and sent for cytologic examination.
- Cyst wall is identified and separated from ovarian tissue by applying two claw forceps on the cyst wall and ovarian wall each, and pulled apart.

- Claw forceps are advanced from time-to-time next to the cleavage line for proper dissection and to avoid tearing of healthy ovarian tissue
- Cyst is punctured and opening is increased so as to accommodate suction irrigation cannula. Fluid is sucked out and inner cyst wall is examined. Bipolar forceps is used to control the bleeding at the base of the capsule.
- A densely adherent cyst may require sharp dissection to completely free the cyst wall.
- After removing or excising the cyst, the cyst can be removed intact by following methods:
  1. Removal in Endobag/Lapsac
  2. Removal in a probe cover or non lubricated sterile condom
  3. Colpotomy

Polycystic Ovarian Drilling

- Ovary is stabilized by holding its ligament with nontraumatic grasper.
- Insulated PCOD needle is passed through left upper port and placed perpendicular to ovarian surface with power set at 20-40 watts in cutting mode.
- Ovary at prominent follicle is then punctured with 4-6 punctures for 2 seconds, 1 cm away from each other in each ovary at the depth of 2-3 mm to prevent deep penetration.
- Then ovaries are lavaged with ringer lactate solution. Any bleeding points at punctured site are seen under water flow and tackled. Thorough lavage at the end, will avoid postoperative adhesion.

TIPS

- During drilling, area close to the ovarian pedicle should be avoided to prevent jeopardizing ovarian blood supply.
- 4-6 holes are sufficient for achieving Hypoandrogenism.
- Hysteroscopy should be done in all the cases since fair number of PCO's have concomitant uterine septum.

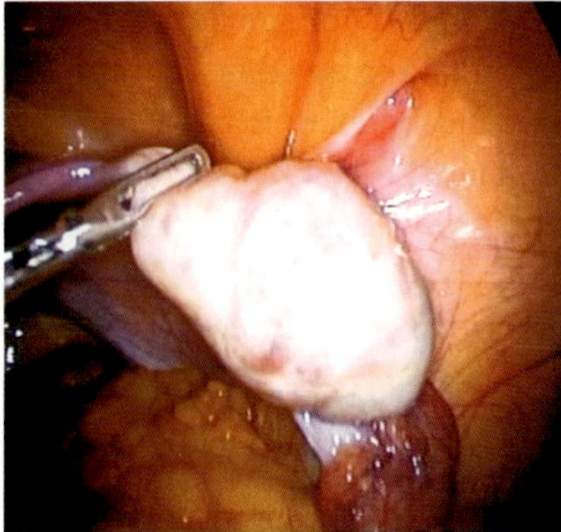

Right polycystic ovary

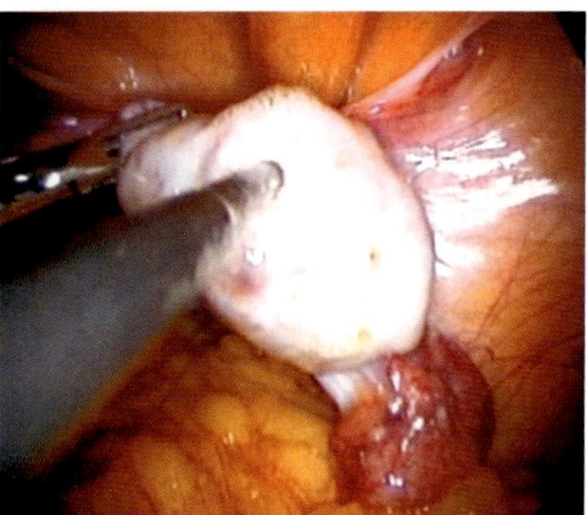

Cysts punctured with insulated PCO drilling needle

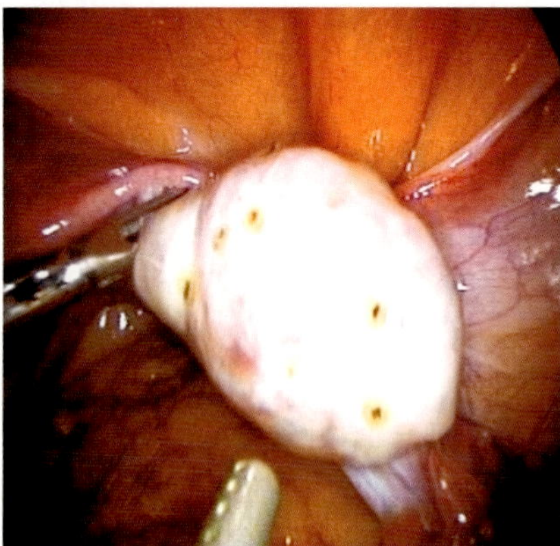

End result

(Photographs courtsey: Ruby Hall IVF and Endoscopy Centre)

SIMPLE OVARIAN CYSTECTOMY AND REMOVAL WITH COLPOTOMY

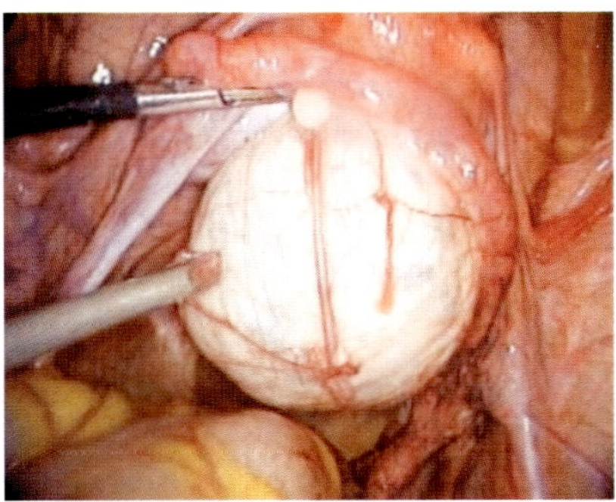

30 years old female with left ovarian cyst ~ 7 cm. not responding to oral contraceptive pills. Tumor markers and Doppler normal

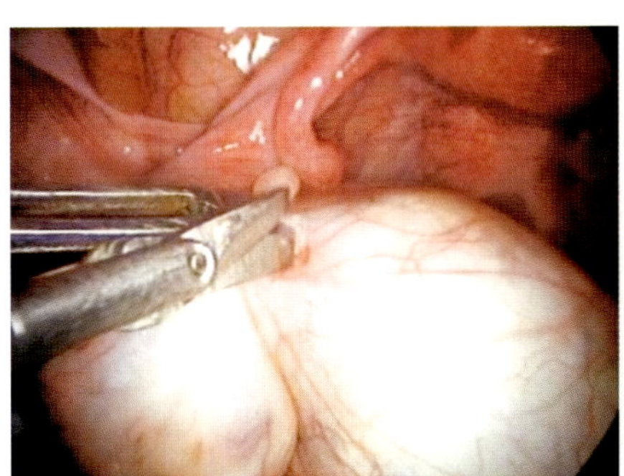

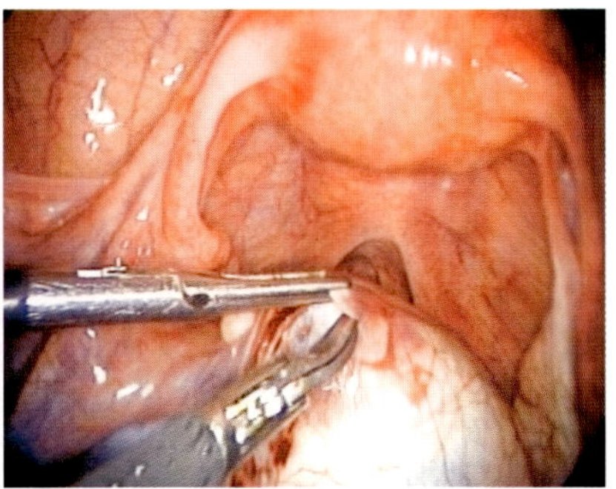

Cyst wall incised with scissors and dissected

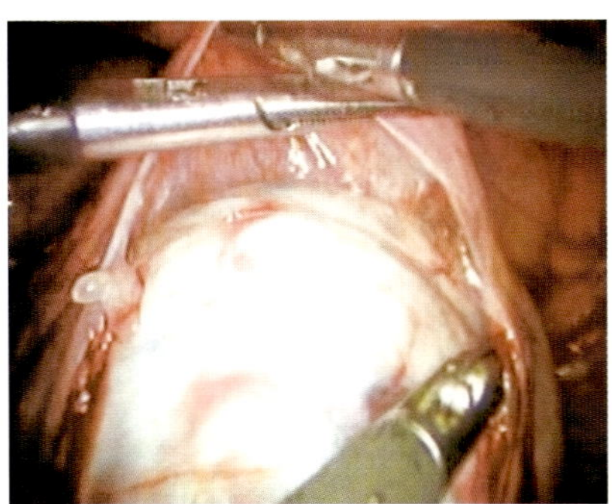

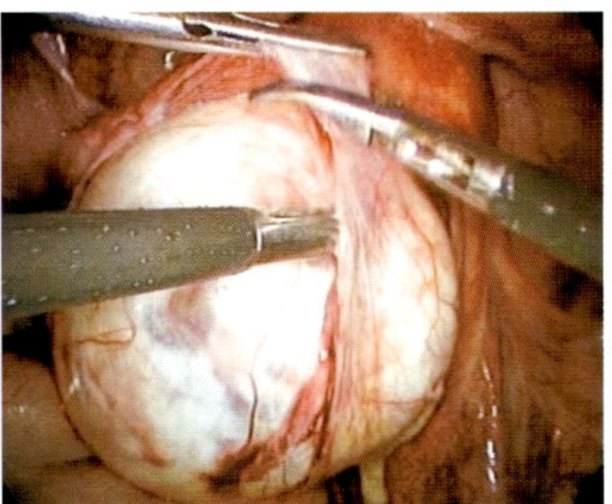

Enucleation of cyst in toto

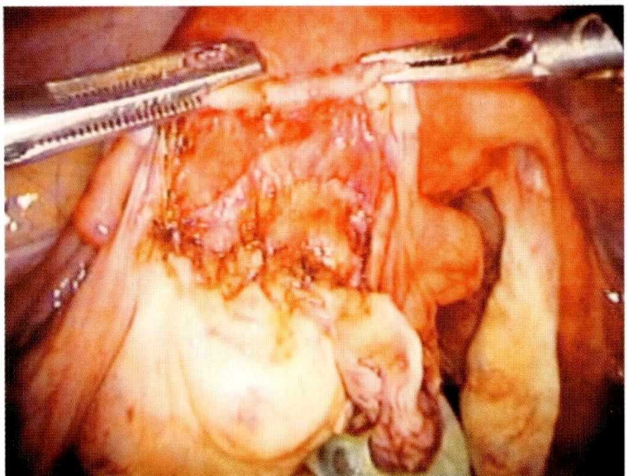

Base of the cyst cauterized

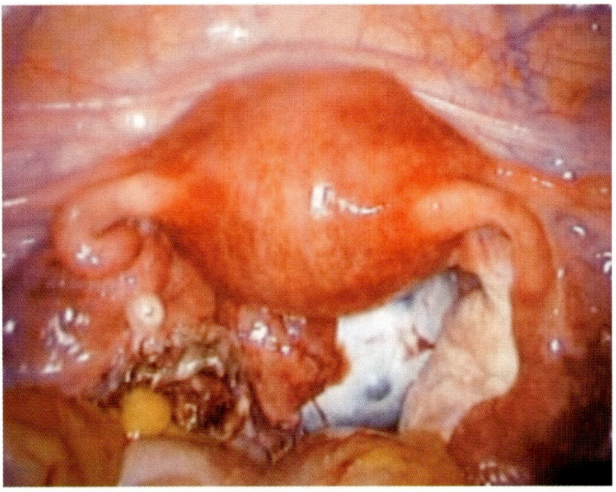

End result – cyst in POD

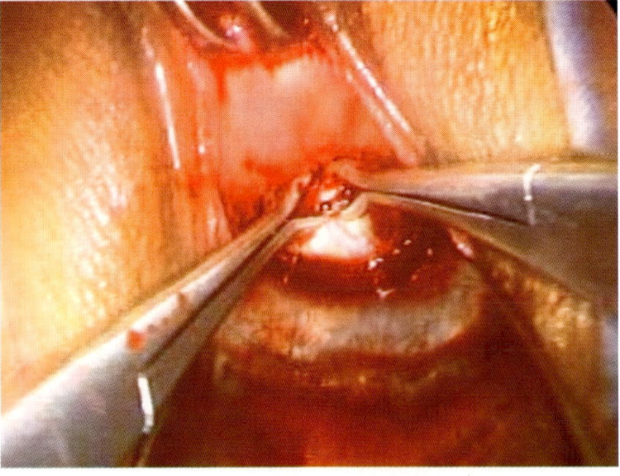

Cyst extracted through colpotomy

(Photographs courtesy: Ruby Hall IVF and Endoscopy Centre)

EXCISION OF BENIGN ADNEXAL MASS AND EXTRACTION IN ENDOBAG

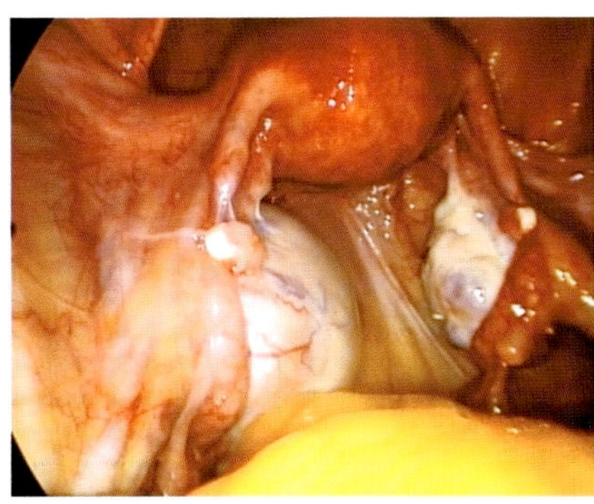
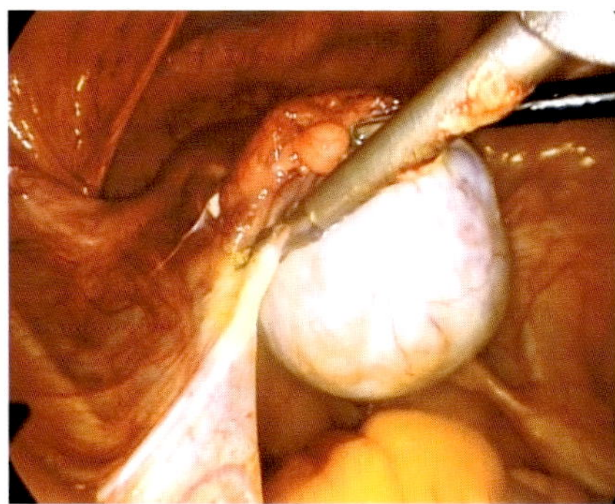

No adhesions with lateral pelvic wall and pouch of doughs

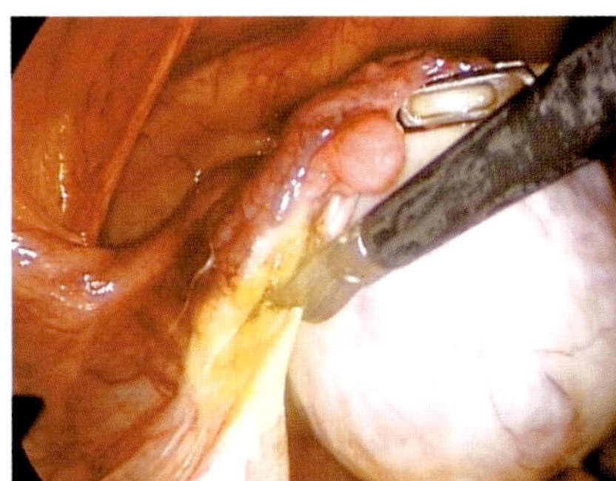
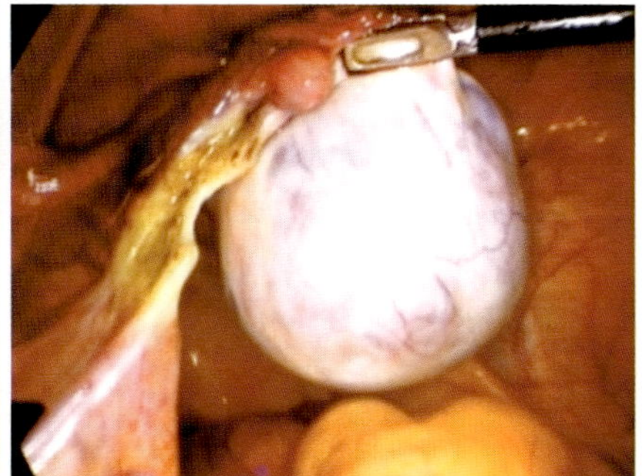

Infundibulopelvic ligament cauterized and cut

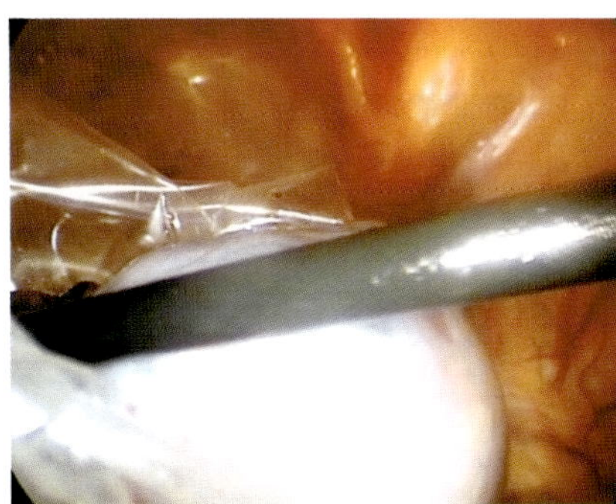
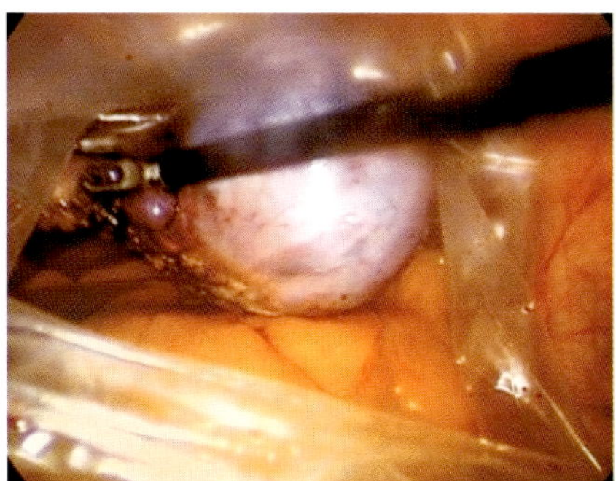

Adnexa removed in endobag

(Photographs courtesy: Ruby Hall IVF and Endoscopy Centre)

42-yr-old female with huge multicystic right ovarian cyst. Tumor markers & color Doppler studies – Benign Cystadenoma.

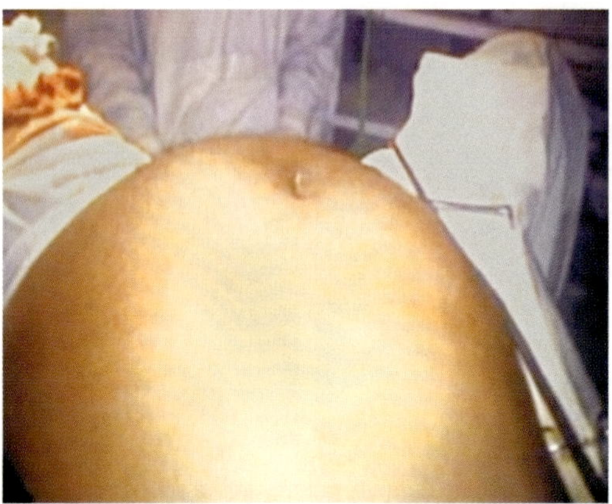

Patient on table – obvious distension of lower abdomen with huge ovarian cyst

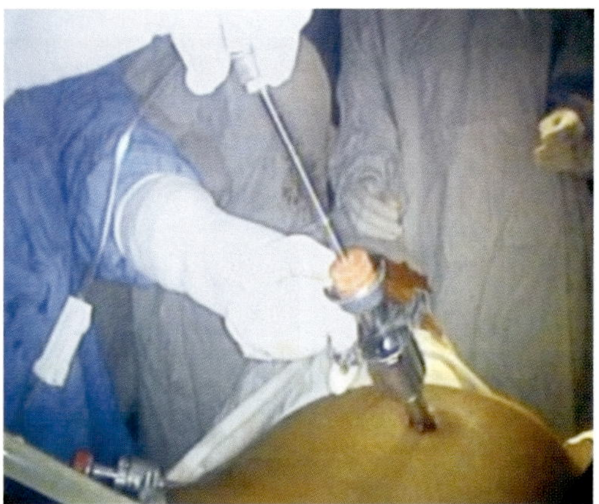

Direct trocar entry into the ovarian cyst under vision
through video telescope at palmer's point

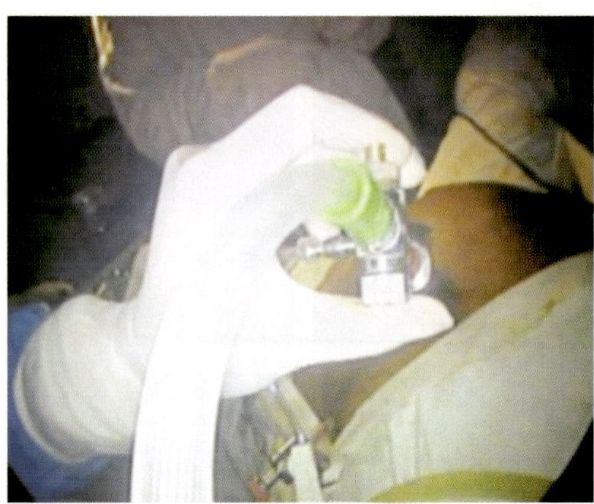

Suction of the cyst fluid

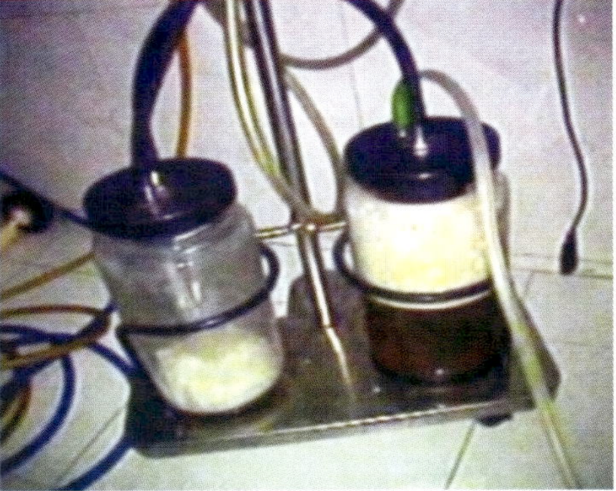

Suction bottles showing collection of the cystic fluid in process

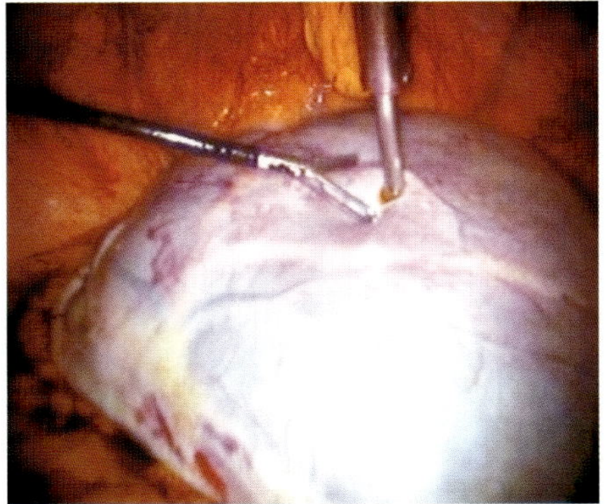

Endoscopic view of cyst fluid being aspirated

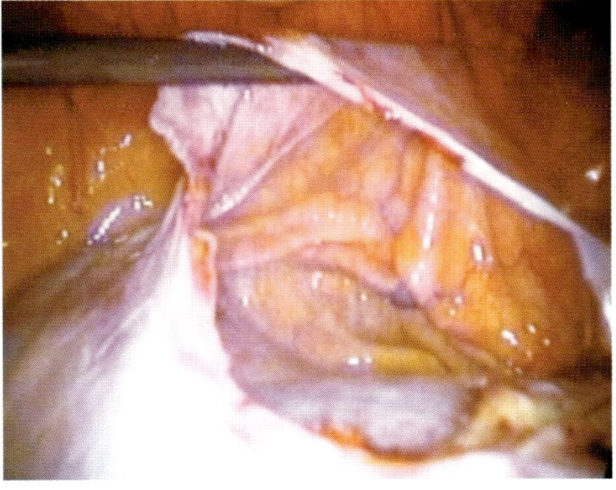

Cystoscopy showing benign inner cyst wall

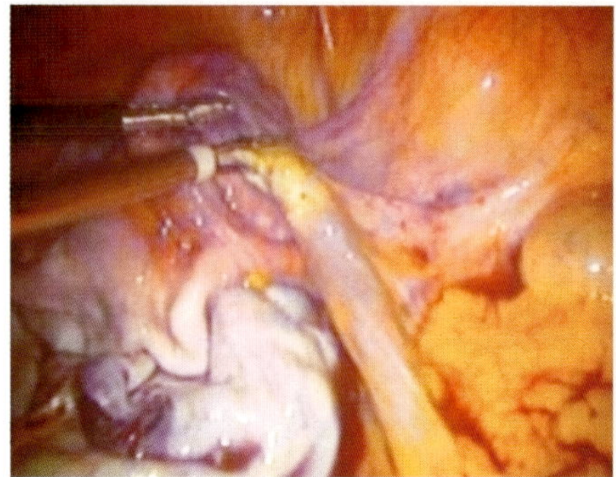

Right adnexectomy being performed

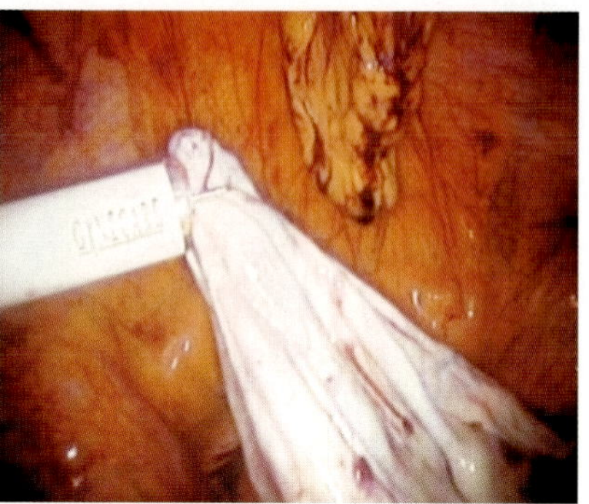

Morcellation of adnexa
with huge cyst wall

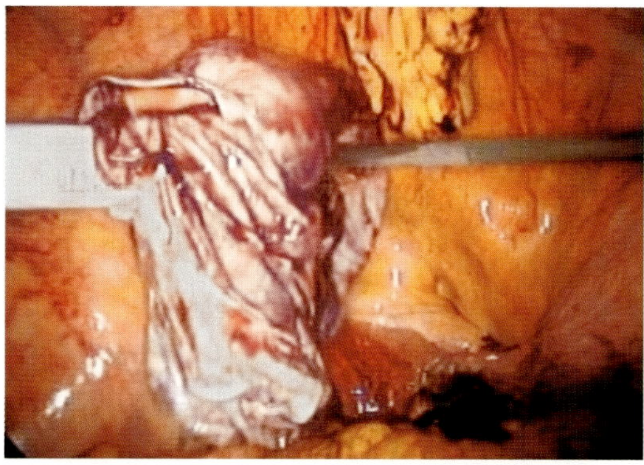

Cyst morcellation in process

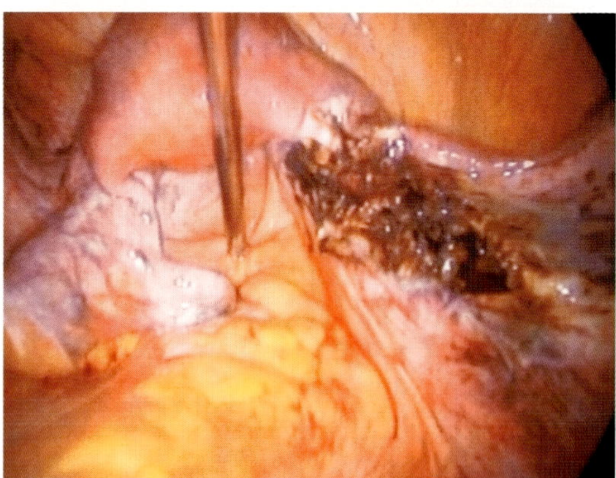

Thorough lavage given
End result — clean pelvis

(Photographs courtesy: Ruby Hall IVF and Endoscopy Centre)

45-year-old female presented with acute pain in the lower abdomen. USG revealed a twisted huge left ovarian cyst. Tumor markers and sonography confirmed Benign nature of the cyst.

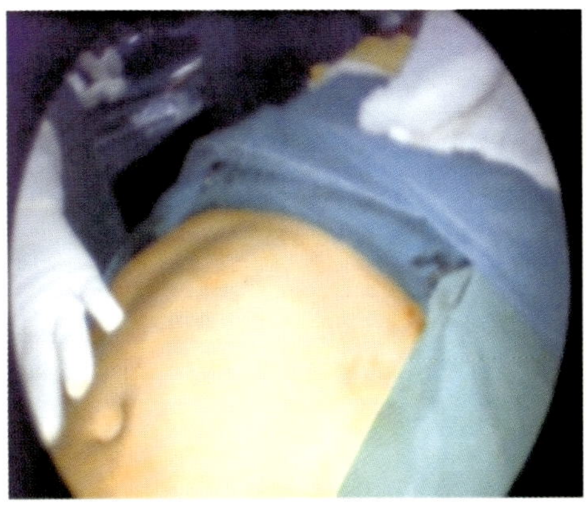

Huge ovarian cyst — note the obvious abdominal distention

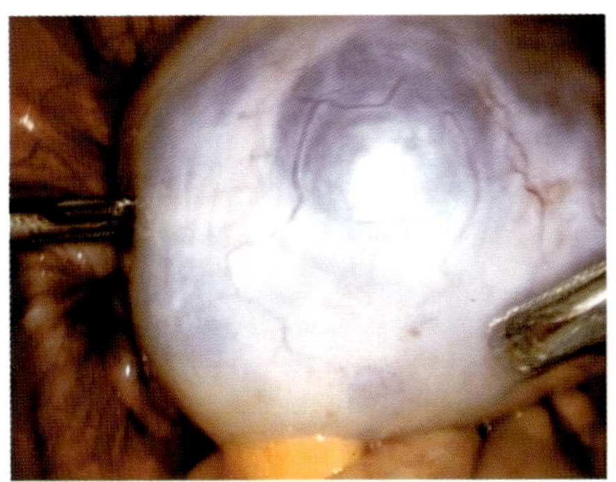

Endo view of cyst

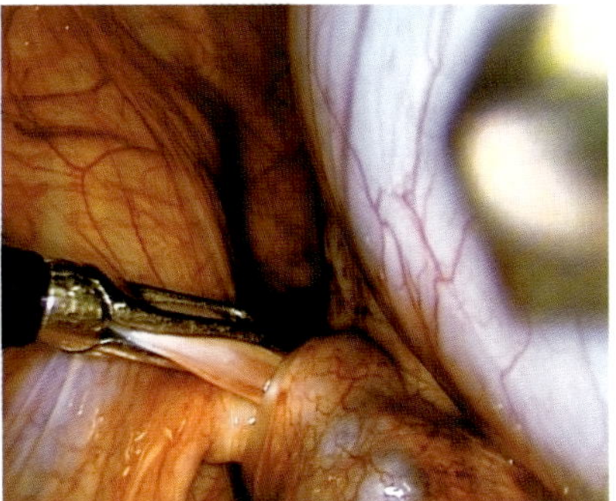

Twist noted

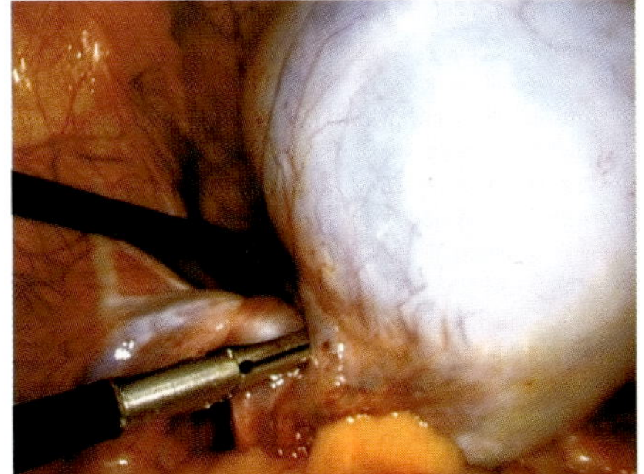

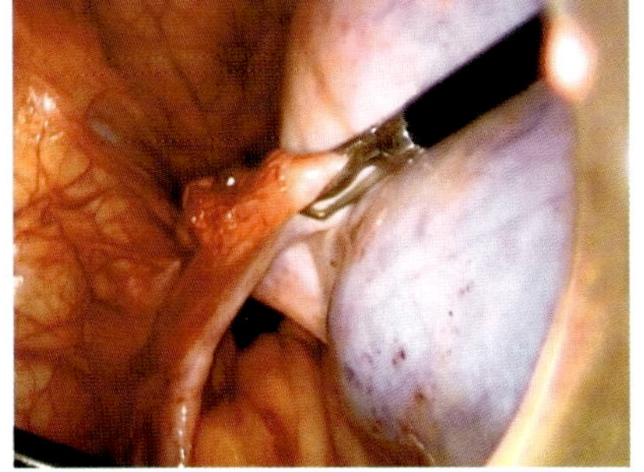

Detorsion completed and adnexectomy performed

(Photographs courtesy: Ruby Hall IVF and Endoscopy Centre)

REMOVAL OF HUGE OVARIAN CYST

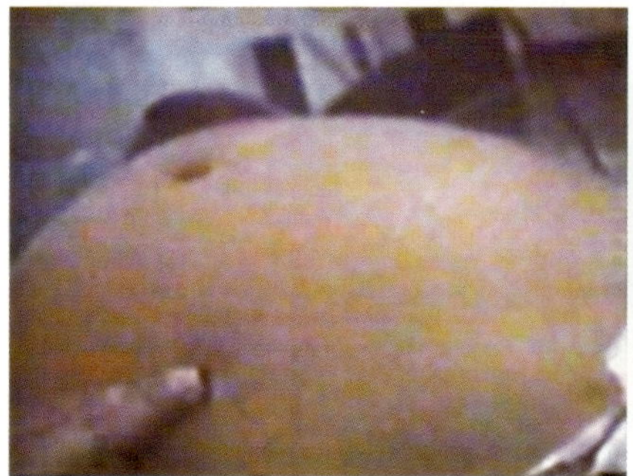

Large benign ovarian cyst

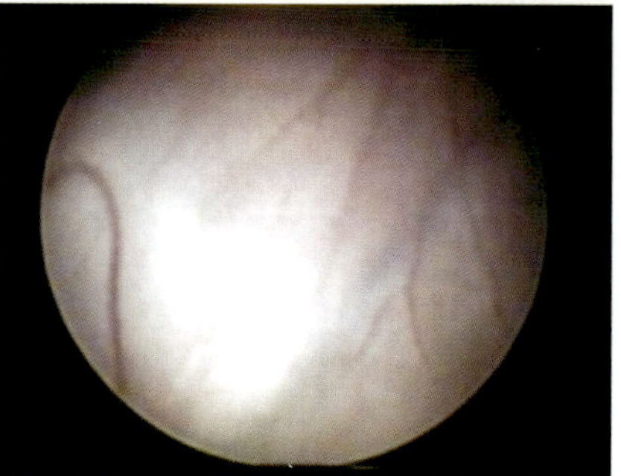

Cyst from inside

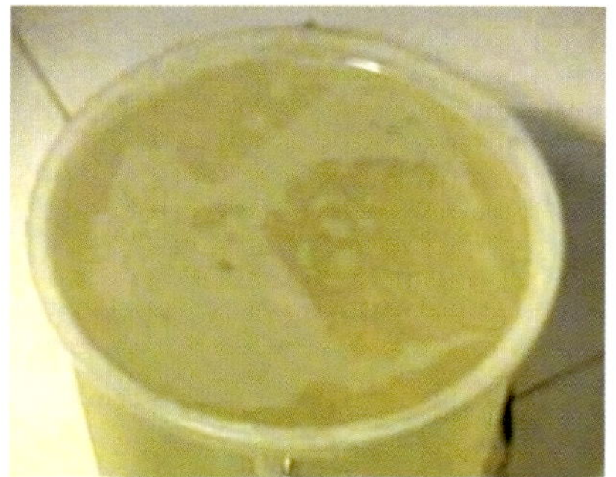

Aspirated cyst fluid

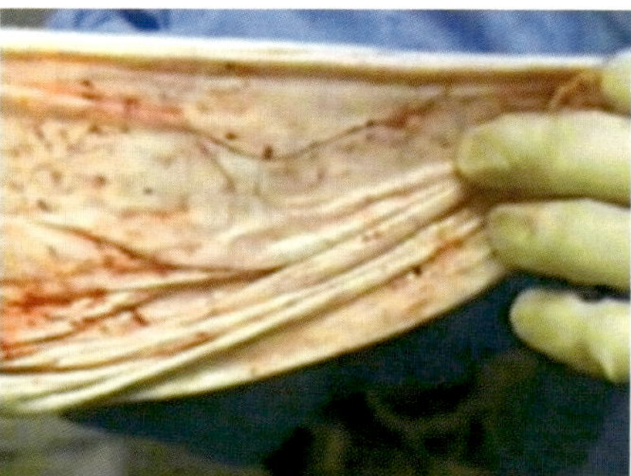

Peeling of the cyst wall

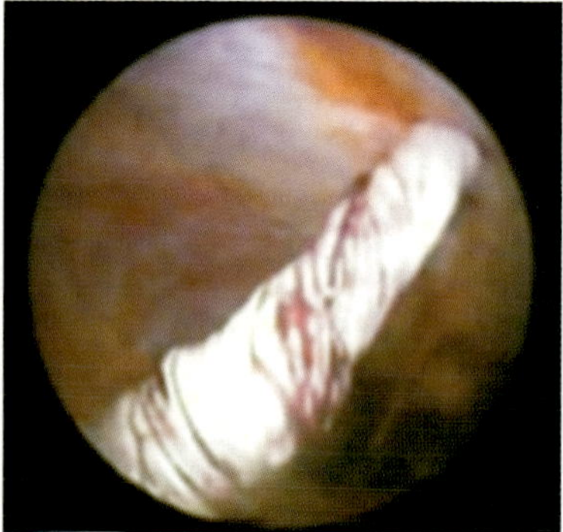

Cyst wall removed from the side port

(Photographs courtesy: Dr Prakash Trivedi)

BENIGN CYSTIC TERATOMAS

- Teratomas often can be excised intact.
- But if the cyst ruptures, the resulting contamination would be greater than if the cyst was opened and aspirated.
  Development of the plane is very important, sharp cut is taken on cortex and then plane is created either with hydro-dissection or scissors, further enucleation of cyst is performed.
- After the cyst is excised, the base is coagulated with the help of bipolar forceps if bleeding is present.
- The edges of the ovary are left open to heal.
- Suturing is avoided since this causes unnecessary bleeding, collection of the blood in the ovarian cortex and postoperative adhesion.
- After laparoscopic removal, the tumor is retrieved through posterior colpotomy incision, if cyst is less than 6 cms and larger cyst is retrieved in a lapsac.
- In case, the cyst ruptures, the abdominal cavity should be cleaned off sebaceous material and hair, which may be cumbersome.

TIPS

- In case of large defects, sutures can be taken inside the ovary with no. 2-0 delayed absorbable material.
- Incomplete removal of the material may cause peritonitis.

23-year-old unmarried girl, known case of dermoid had left sided oophorectomy by laparotomy at the age of 18, came to us with right sided 3 ovarian dermoid. It was very important to perserve ovarian tissue as much as possible.

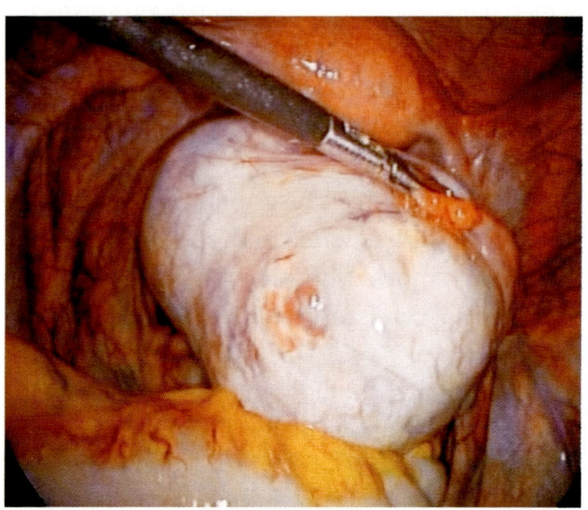

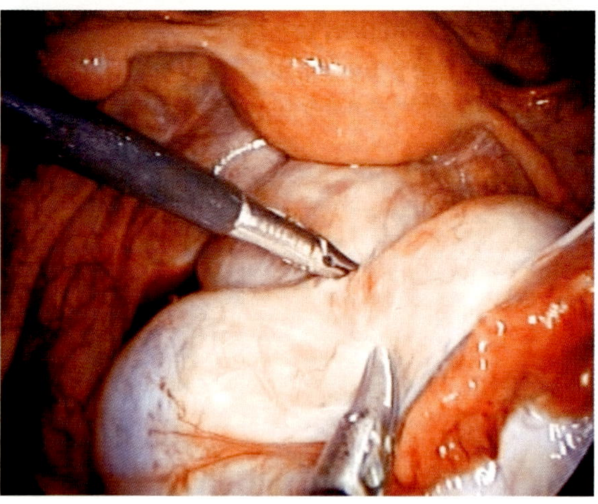

Right ovarian dermoids. Note – absence of left ovary

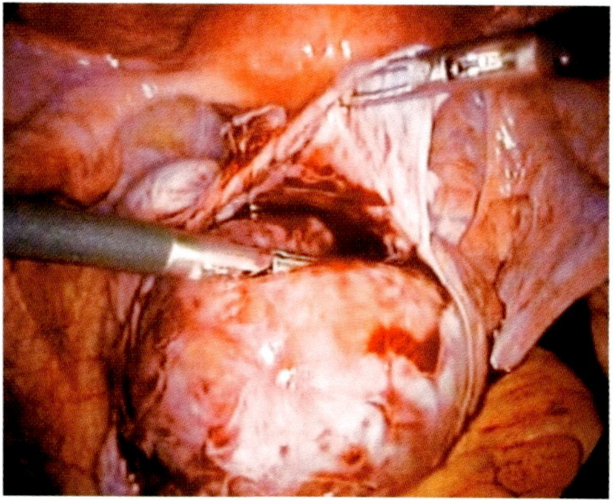

Dermoid cysts excision in process

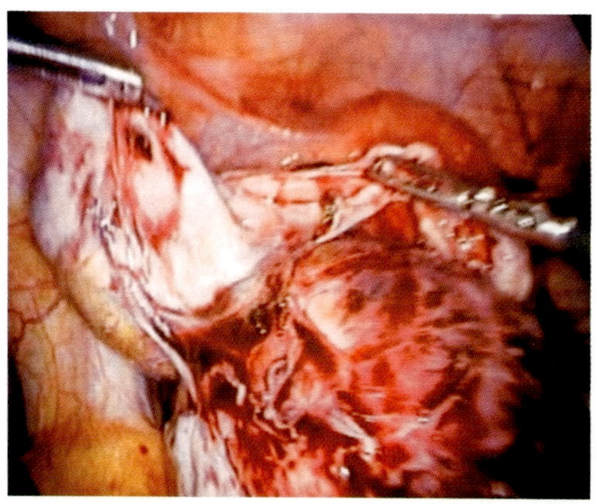

Second dermoid cysts excision in process

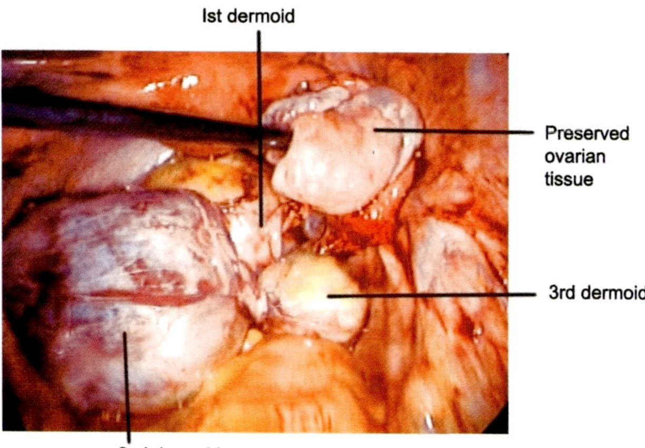

All 3 dermoids removed and placed in the POD.
Adequate amount of ovarian tissue preserved

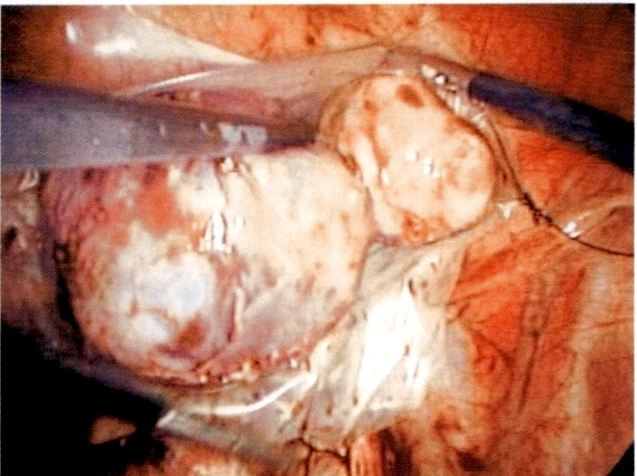

Dermoid cysts placed in endobag

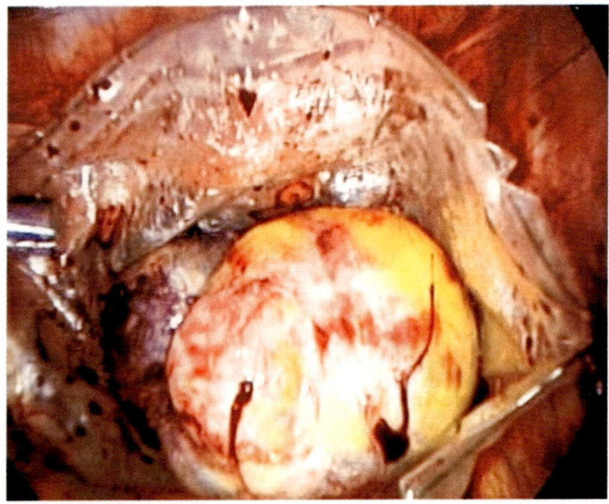

Dermoid cysts placed in endobag

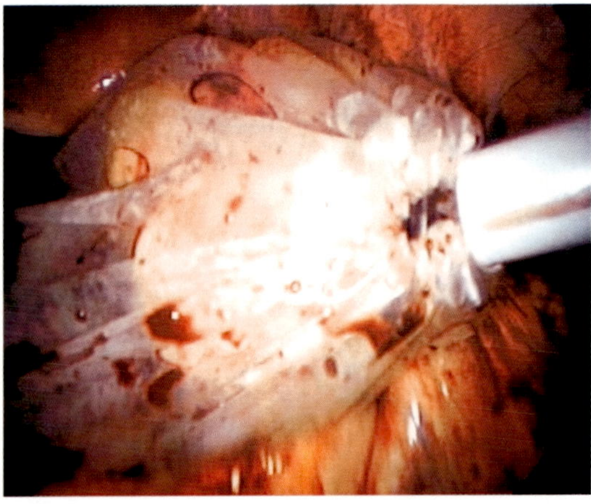

Endobag being extracted through the secondary 10 mm port

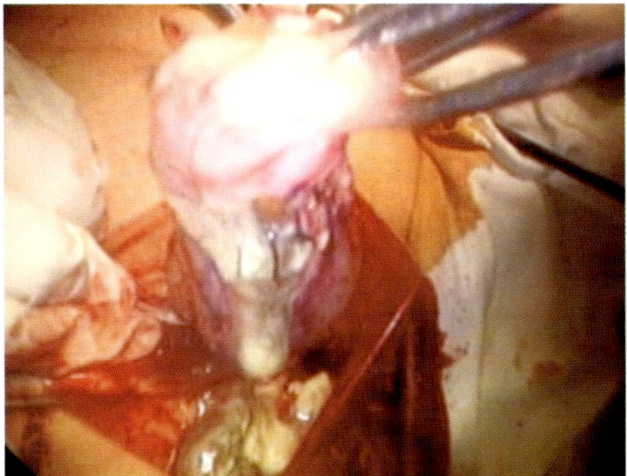

External view of dermoid cyst getting removed. Precaution
has to be taken to keep endobag intact to avoid spillage

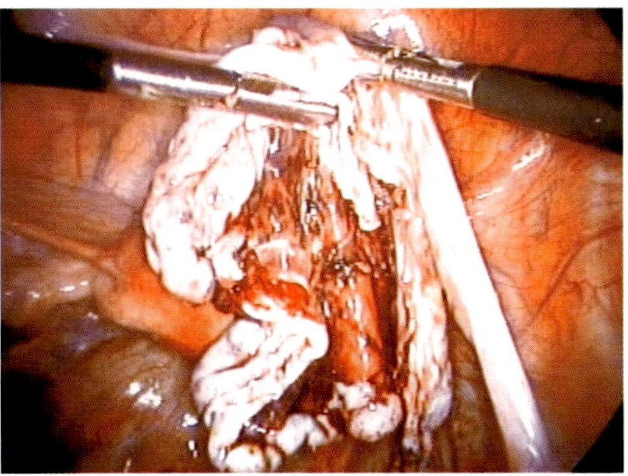

Good amount of healthy ovarian tissue is preserved and the edges
of the ovary are left open to heal

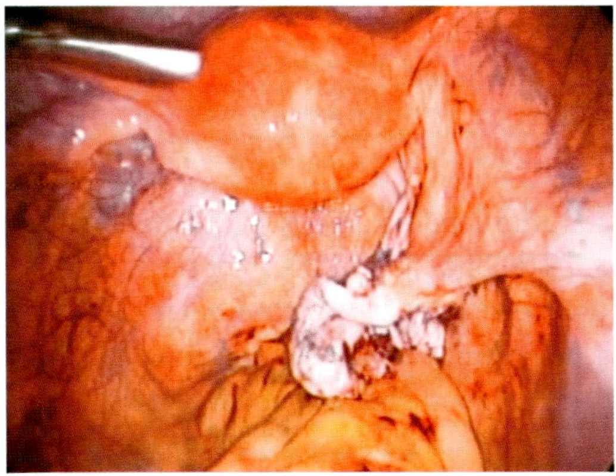

End result

(Photographs courtesy: Ruby Hall IVF and Endoscopy Centre)

17 Laparoscopic Management of Tubal Ectopic

UNRUPTURED ECTOPIC

Preoperative Evaluation

- Diagnosis by thorough history and USG.
- No other preoperative preparation needed for unruptured ectopic.
- Ruptured ectopic can be tackled laparoscopically if the patient is hemodynamically stable.

Preoperative Preparation

Blood needs to be organized as per patient's condition.

Important Instruments

- One 10 mm and two/three 5 mm trocars
- Two non-traumatic graspers
- Bipolar forceps
- Monopolar microneedle
- Suction irrigation cannula

SALPINGOSTOMY

- A standard 10 mm laparoscope is introduced with three side ports, two on the left side and one on the right side.
- 5-10 cc of vasopressin in 1:100 dilution can be instilled in mesosalpinx with laparoscopic needle at the site of ectopic pregnancy (though this is not practiced by many endosurgeons).
- With a non traumatic grasper, the tube is stabilized proximal to the ectopic mass.

- A linear cut is given with a monopolar microneedle on the antemesenteric border of the ectopic mass by using a cutting cautery current.
- Usually the ectopic mass will extrude out, otherwise it is squeezed out by holding fallopian tube with two nontraumatic graspers proximal and distal to the ectopic mass. It is then gently removed.
- Copious lavage is also given through the salpingostomy incision so that blood clots can be washed through the fimbrial end.
- If there is any bleeder at the incision site, it is seen under water flow and cauterized precisely with bipolar.
- The ectopic mass can be removed through the 5 mm port.
  * Milking of ectopic pregnancy in the ampullary region is not advised. But if the ectopic is at the fimbrial end, it can sometimes be milked out of the fimbrial end.
  * Linear salpingostomy is not successful in case of the isthmic ectopic pregnancy.

TIPS

- The suture at the linear salpingotomy does not offer any advantage over the non suture technique.
- If the ectopic has occurred due to the narrowing of the proximal part of fallopian tube, which is not corrected, there are chances of repeat ectopic in the same tube.

UNRUPTURED ECTOPIC

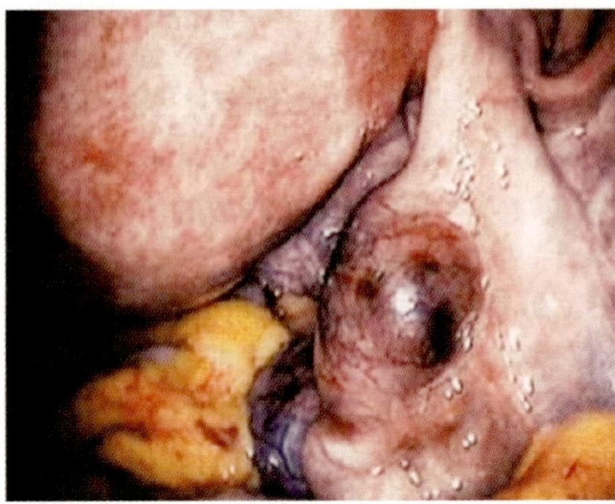

Right tubal unruptured ectopic pregnancy

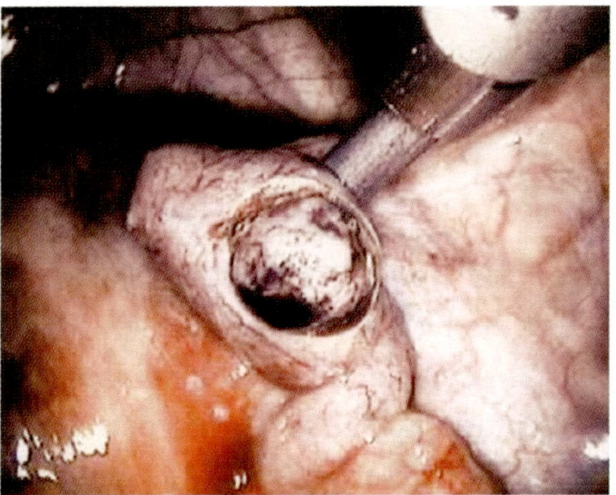

Ectopic tissue seen protruding after linear incision with
needle using monopolar cutting current

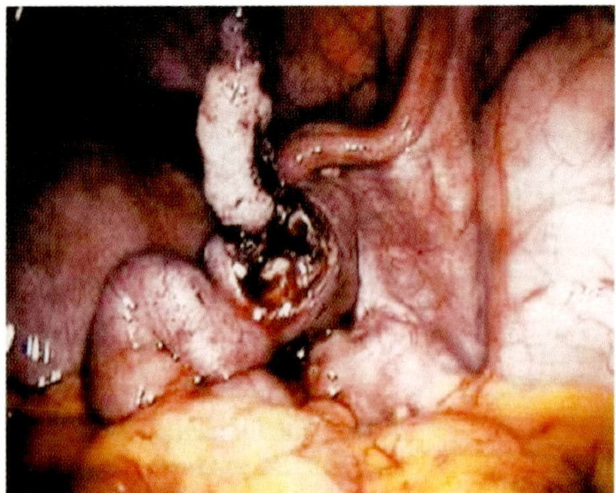

Ectopic tissue removed with non-traumatic grasper

(Photographs courtesy: Ruby Hall IVF and Endoscopy Centre)

SALPINGECTOMY

Indications

- Isthmic pregnancy
- Ruptured ectopic
- Recurrent ectopic
- Associated hydrosalpinx
- Damaged tube.

Procedure

- Fallopian tube to be excised is held at the distal end and is lifted up to visualize mesosalpinx of the fimbrial end, which can be cauterized precisely without damaging the blood supply to the ovary.
- Serial cauterization and cutting is done so as to remove the whole length of the tube.
- Removal of specimen- 5 mm telescope is passed through secondary port and 10 mm grasper is passed through the primary port and the specimen is removed always under vision.
- Usually blood is squeezed on the bowel loops from the specimen while removing the specimen out through the primary port, which should be sucked.

RUPTURED ECTOPIC

Instruments

- Two 10 mm and two/three 5 mm trocars
- Two nontraumatic graspers
- Bipolar forceps
- Monopolar needle
- 10 mm suction irrigation cannula

Procedure

- If patient is hemodynamically stable, one can proceed with laparoscopic salpinectomy.
- If one is familiar with direct trocar insertion, it is preferred, as it will save time.
- If a bleeding spurter is seen, it should be held with nontraumatic forceps and cauterized first.

RUPTURED ECTOPIC

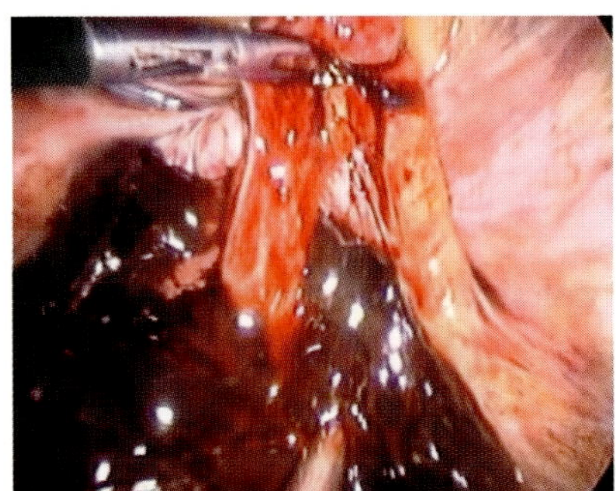

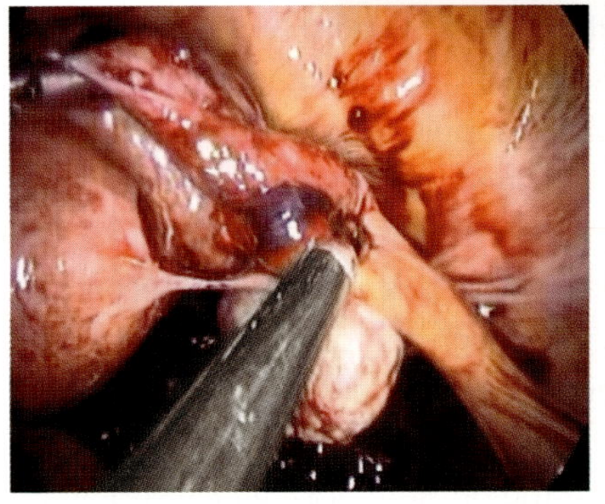

Salpingectomy in progress

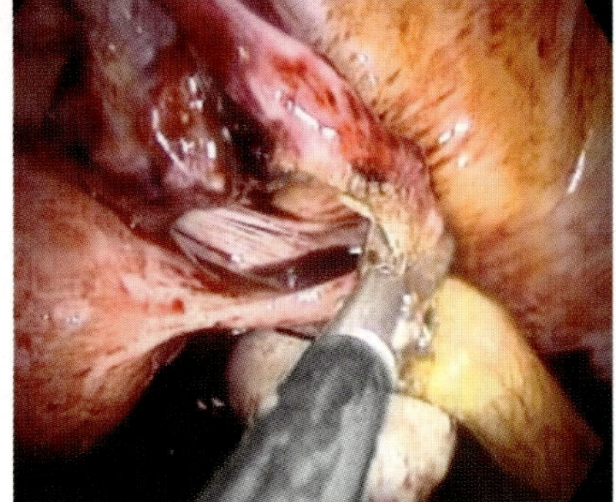

Salpingectomy complete

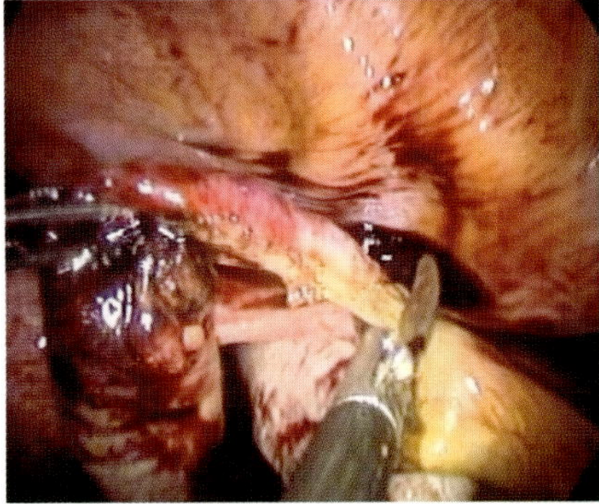

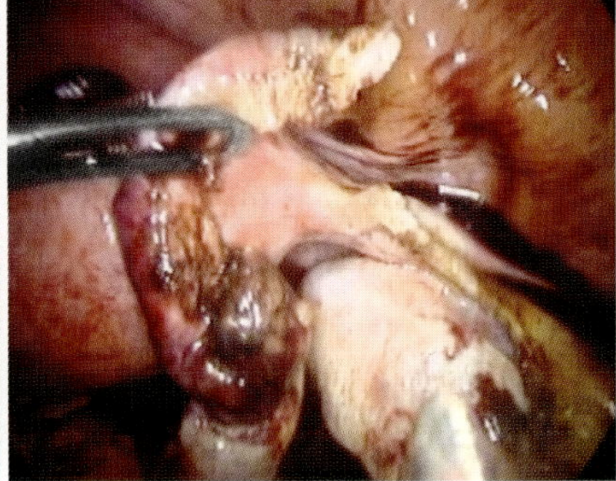

- Rest of the procedure-salpingectomy is performed as usual.
- To hasten the speed of removal of blood clots from peritoneal cavity, 10 mm suction cannula is used.
- Thorough lavage should be given to remove all blood and blood clots from the peritoneal cavity,which at times may be tedious. But this is an important step otherwise adhesions may be formed.
- Drain can be kept from the side port for 12 hours.

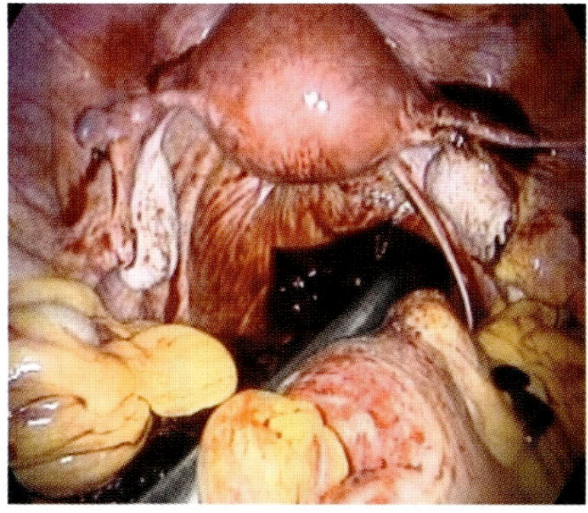

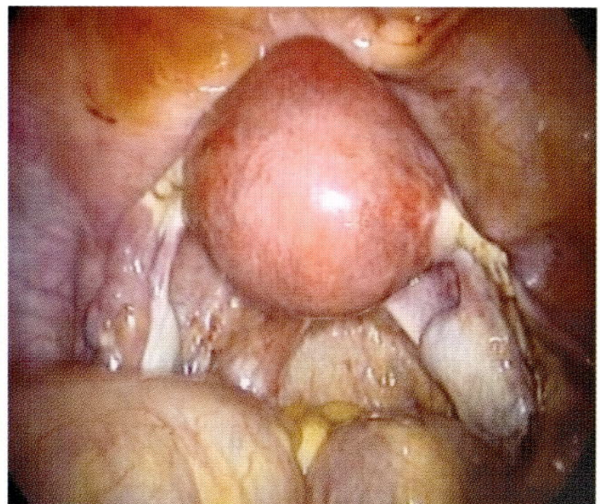

Left side associated hematosalpinx so
left cornu blocked as patient was for IVF

End result

ECTOPIC PREGNANCIES AT VARIOUS SITES

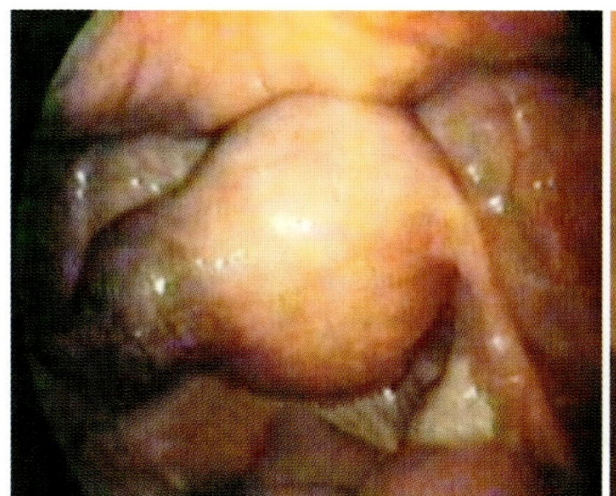

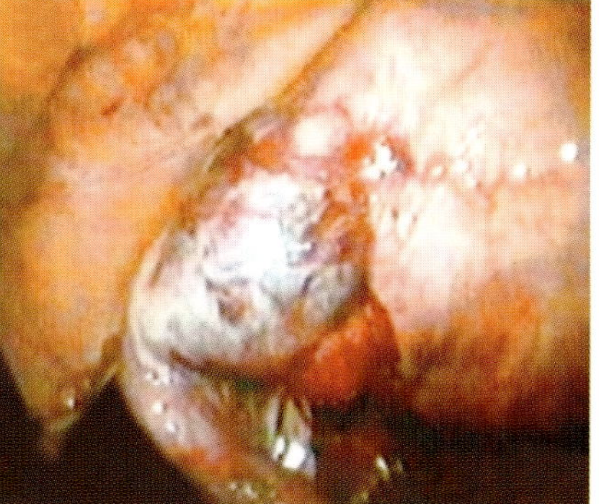

Interstitial ectopic

Isthmic ectopic

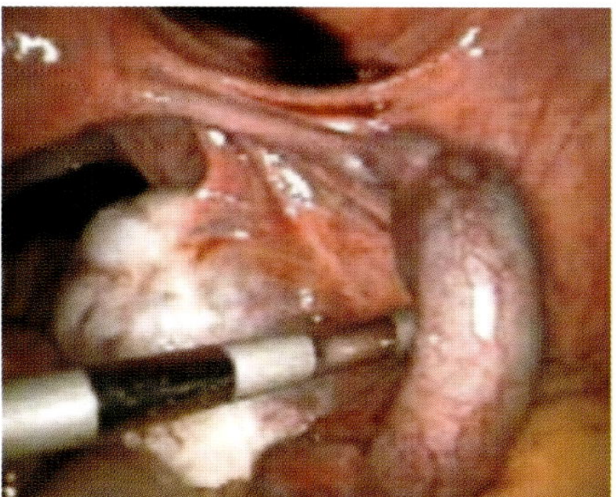

Ampullary ectopic

OVARIAN ECTOPIC

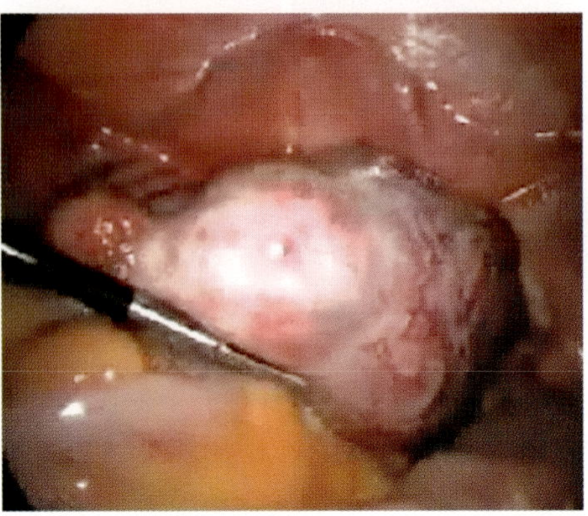

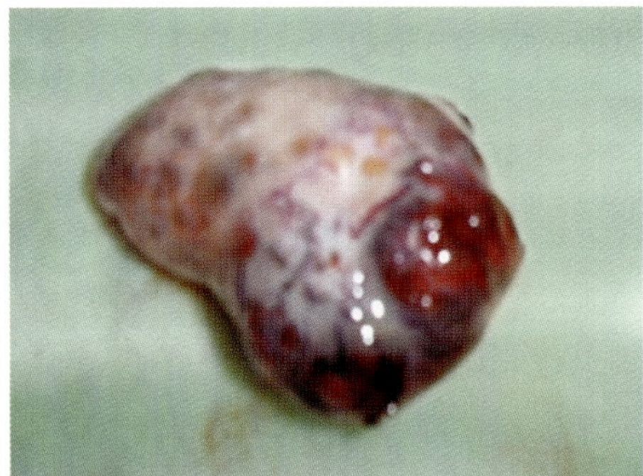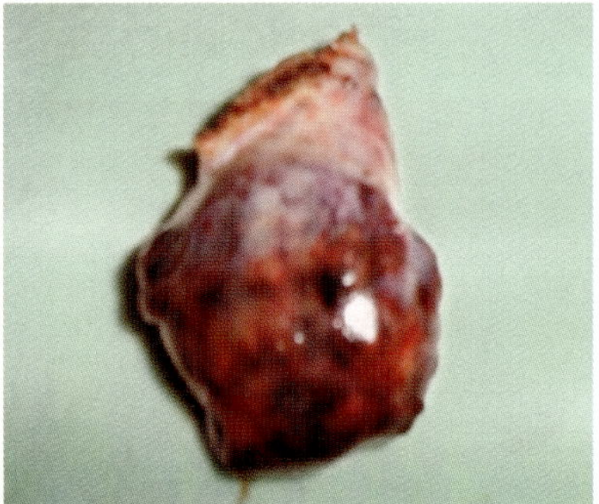

Since ectopic was highly vascular had to remove the mass in toto

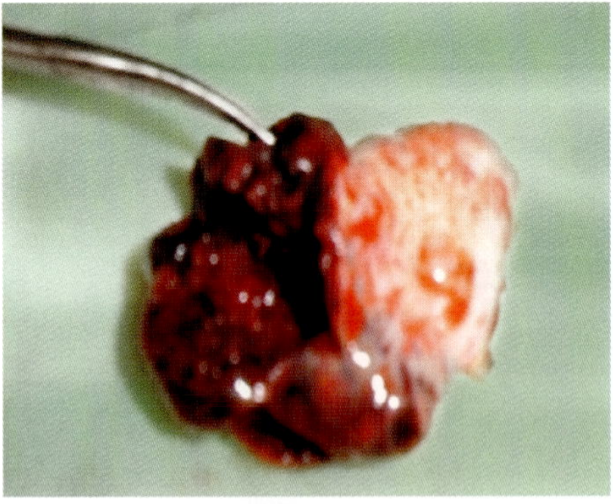

Cut section

(Photographs courtesy: Ruby Hall IVF and Endoscopy Centre)

Laparoscopic Salpingectomy

Preoperative Evaluation

History and examination of patient.

Preoperative Preparation

No specific preparation as such is needed.

Criteria for Salpingectomy in an Infertile Patient

- Written consent.
- Hydrosalpinx more than thumb size or easily seen on sonography.
- Hematosalpinx or pyosalpinx.

Instruments

- 5 mm zero degree laparoscope
- 10 mm zero degree laparoscope
- Single chip/three chip camera
- Bipolar forceps
- 10 mm tooth grasper
- Two nontraumatic graspers
- Suction irrigation system

Procedure

- 3 port laparoscopic entry
- The pathological tube is held with the nontraumatic grasper and the mesosalpinx is coagulated very near to the tube (so that ovarian blood supply is not compromised) with bipolar and cut with scissors. (If one has Harmonic energy source, surgery becomes simplified as

cauterization and cutting will happen simultaneously and also lateral thermal spread is minimal.)

- Removal of specimen - 5 mm videoscope is passed through upper secondary port and 10 mm grasper with 10 mm reducer is passed through 10 mm primary port and the specimen is removed through it.
- Thorough lavage is given at the end and hemostasis is confirmed.

TIPS

- Utmost care should be taken to avoid damage to the ovarian blood supply by staying close to the fallopian tubes.

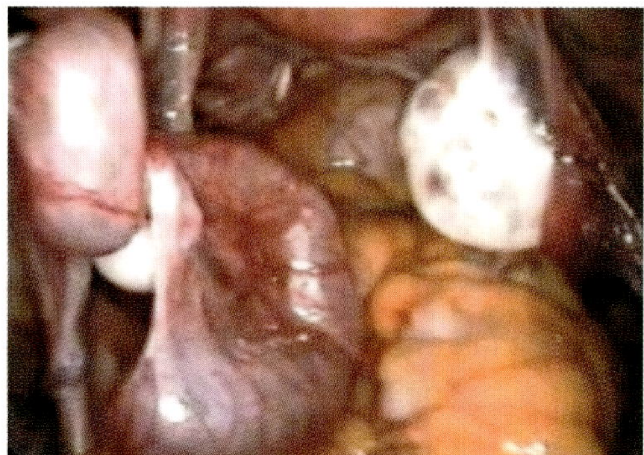

Left hydrosalpinx

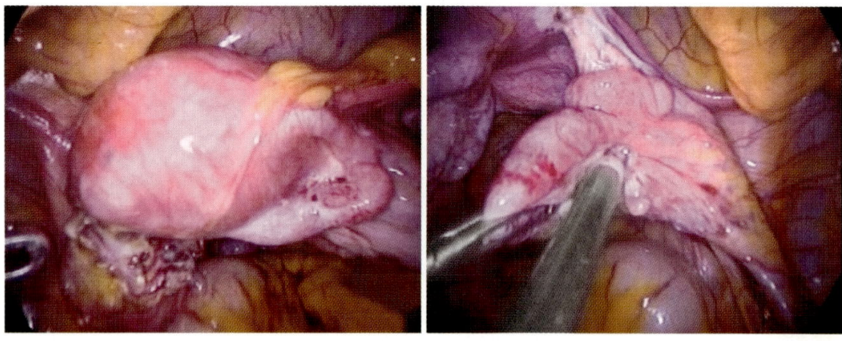

Right tuberculous salpingitis

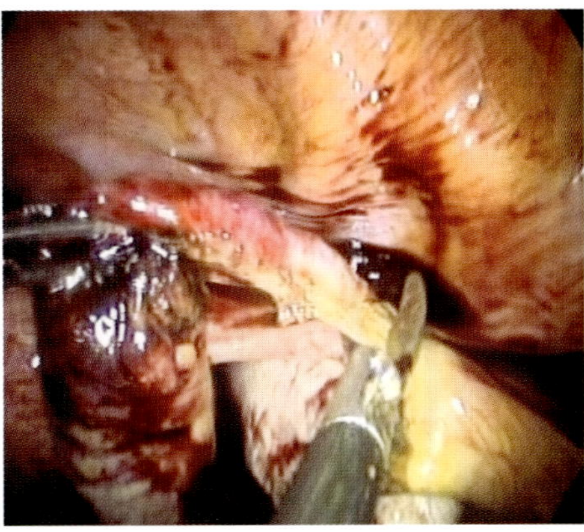

Right salpingectomy for ectopic pregnancy
with incision line next to mesosalpinx

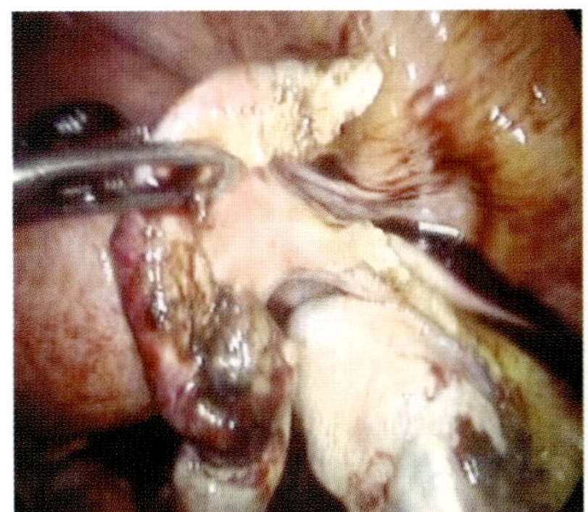

Right salpingectomy completed

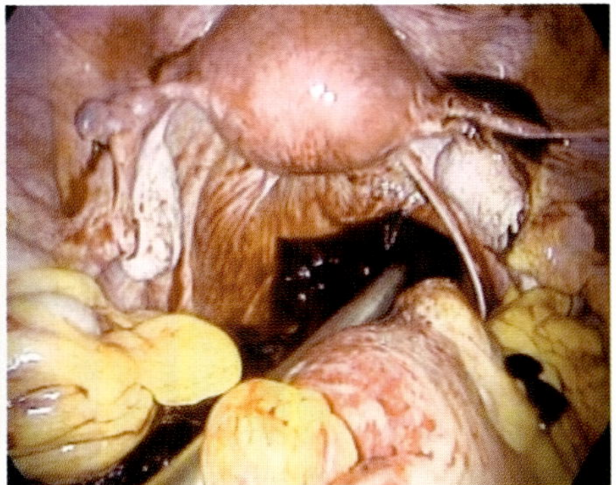

Thorough suction and irrigation,
left hematosalpinx also seen

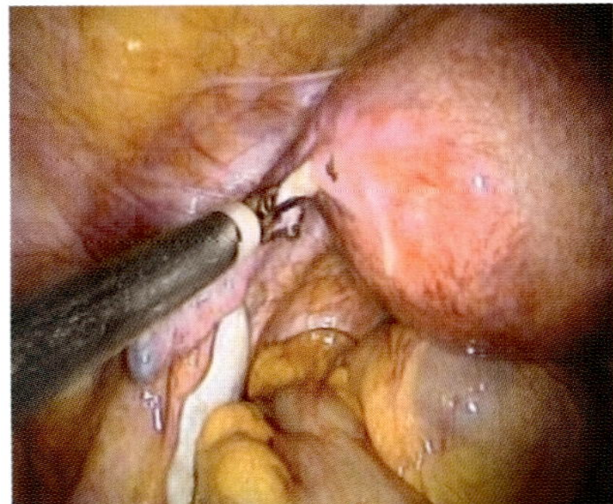

Patient for IVF, left cornual end cauterized, as found to have hematosalpinx

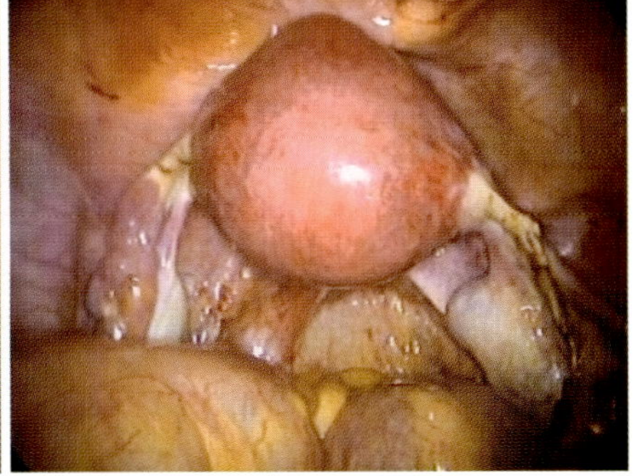

End result – clean pelvis

(Photographs courtesy: Ruby Hall IVF and Endoscopy Centre)

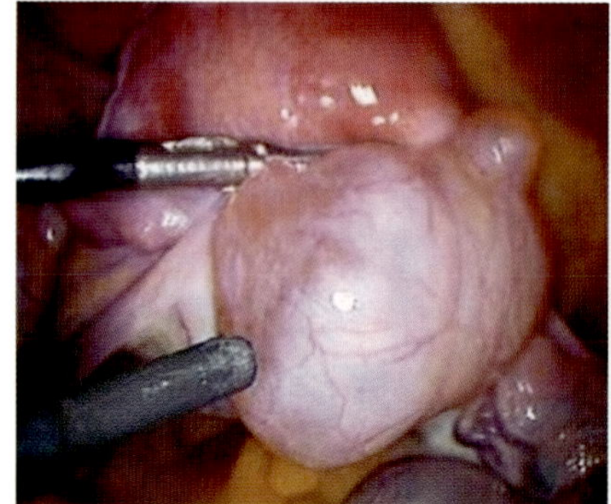

Left hydrosalpinx

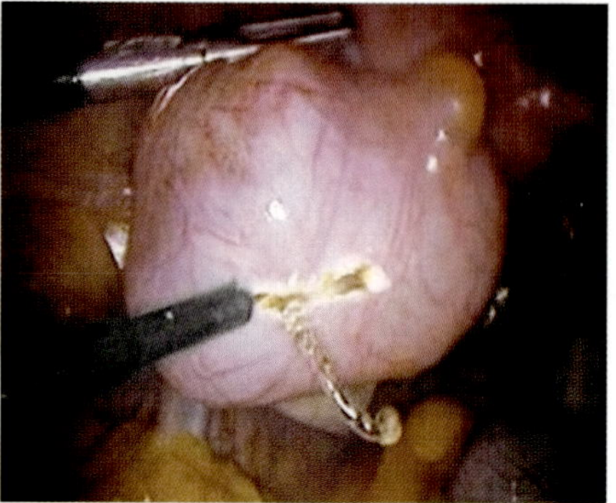

Left hydrosalpinx drained

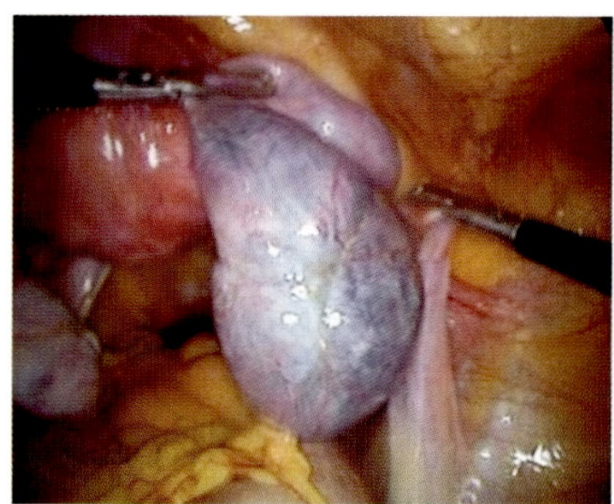

Right hematosalpinx

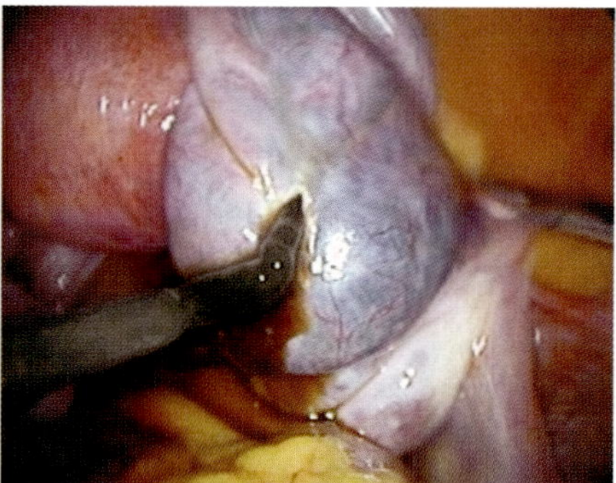

Hematosalpinx drained

LAPAROSCOPIC STERILIZATION

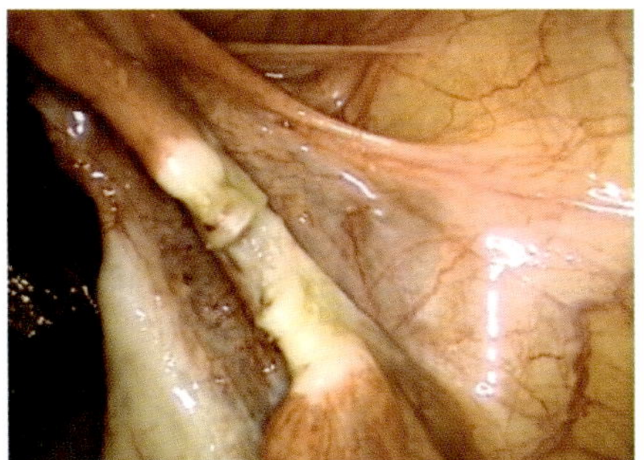

Right fallopian tube cauterized

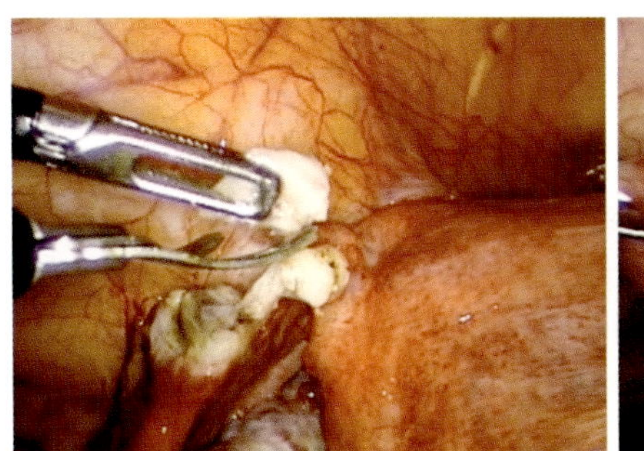

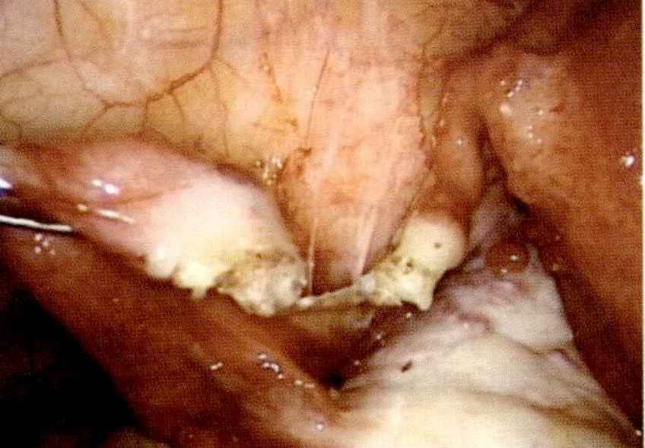

Right fallopian tube cauterized and cut

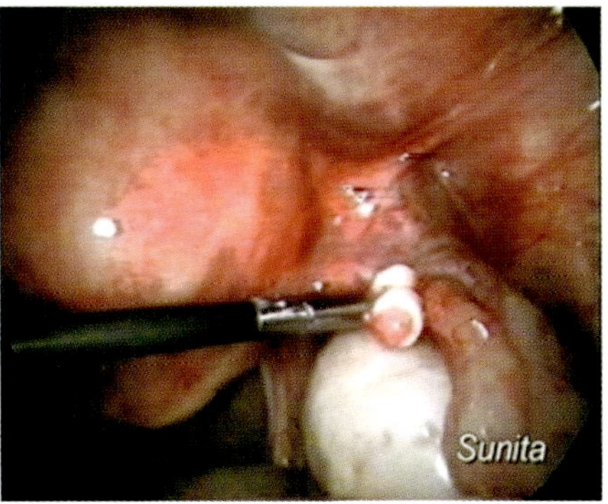

Sterilization with sialistic bands

(Photographs courtesy: Ruby Hall IVF and Endoscopy Centre)

19 Laparoscopic Management of Hydrosalpinx

Preoperative Evaluation

- Diagnosis by thorough history and ultrasonography.
- Ultrasonography should reveal a normal uterine cavity with good ovarian volume.
- Normal male factor.
- Normal female hormonal assays and documentation of ovulation.
- Salpingoscopy - It should be performed at the time of laparoscopy. Major and minor mucosal folds are to be seen along with any intraluminal adhesions or strictures.

Preoperative Preparation

- No other preoperative preparation needed for fimbrioplasty.

Important Equipments

- 10 mm zero degree laparoscope
- Single chip/three chip camera
- Monopolar needle
- Bipolar forceps
- Nontraumatic graspers
- Suction irrigation system

Surgical Steps

- Distended fimbrial end is stabilised with two nontraumatic graspers (Maryland's forceps are better) passed through the lower left and right contralateral ports.
- A monopolar needle is passed through the left upper port.

- Distended fimbrial end is punctured with monopolar needle with cutting current between 20-40 Watts, fluid is drained and cruciate incision is taken from the puncture site in all four directions (Figs 19.1 to 19.3)
- The fimbrial ends are then everted and the ends are coagulated with the lowest possible power setting so as to coagulate only the serosa. This is done to avoid re-agglutination. (some Endoscopic surgeons do evert the fimbria by endosuturing) (Figs 19.4 and 19.5).
- Methylene blue dye is injected and spillage is confirmed.
- Thorough lavage is given and hemostasis achieved.
- Under surface of diaphragm is checked for any adhesions.

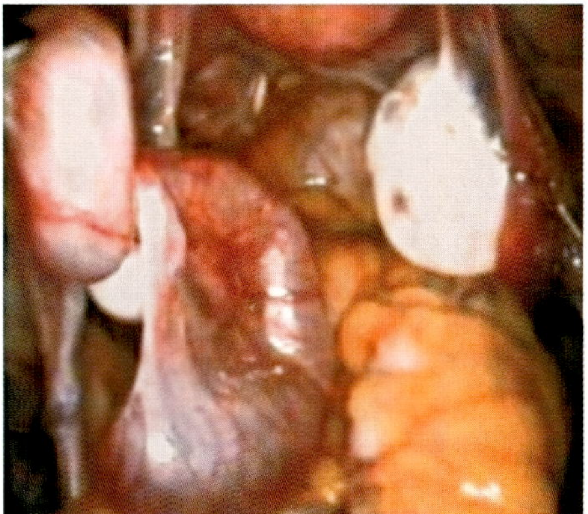

Fig. 19.1: Left hydrosalpinx

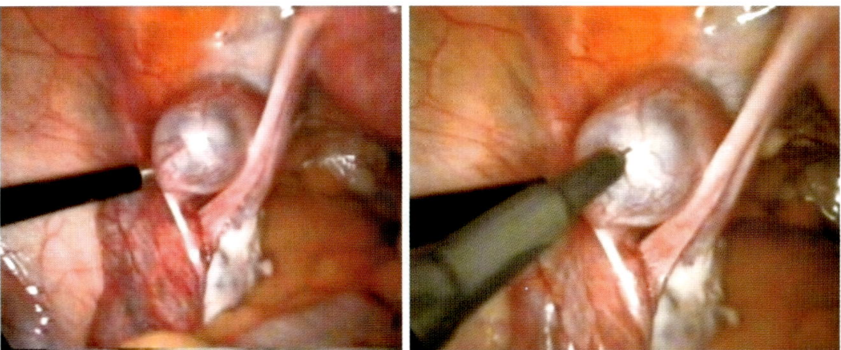

Fig. 19.2: Puncture with monopolar needle

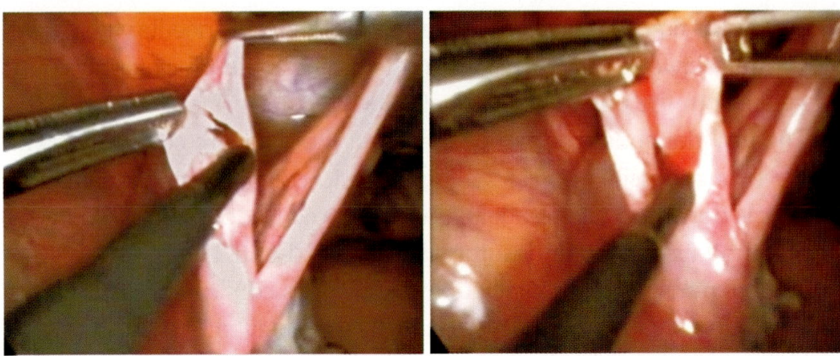

Fig. 19.3: Cruciate incision in progress

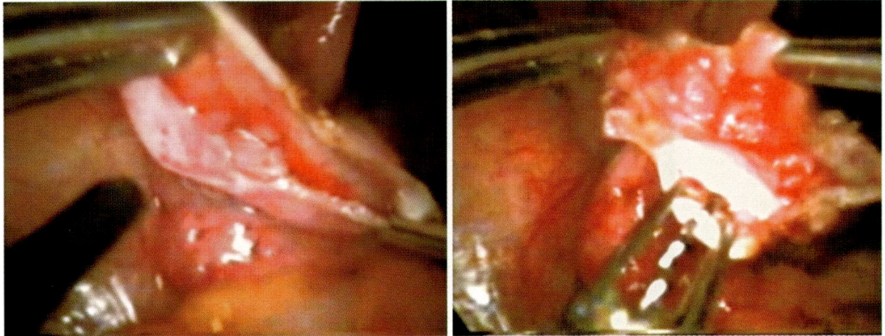

Fig. 19.4: Flattened fimbria seen inside the lumen

Fig. 19.5: Cauliflower fimbrial end, end result

TIPS

- When the fimbria are encapsulated and hidden, the antimesentric border is incised to remove the fibrotic bands and expose the fimbria.
- After fimbrioplasty, a close watch should be kept on ectopic pregnancy.
- We recommend Hysterosalpinoscintigraphy after 6 weeks to know functional patency of the fallopian tubes. (i.e. ciliary movements).

(Photographs courtesy: Ruby Hall IVF and Endoscopy Centre)

20 Laparoscopic Tubo-Tubal Anastomosis

Laparoscopic microsurgery is a new discipline that synergizes the potential of classical microsurgery and laparoscopy. It can overcome the deficiencies in each of the techniques. Advent of microsurgical technique began by Swolin in 1967. First microsurgical reversal of the sterilization was done by Gomel and Winston in 1977.

Preoperative Evaluation

- Semen analysis: to rule out male factor.
- Day 3 Serum FSH level to know the ovarian reserve.
- HSG to know the length and condition of the proximal tube.
- Saline infusion sonography and hysterosalpingography may be helpful.
- Details about the previous tubectomy.

Indications

- Reversal of tubal sterilization procedure
- Mid-tubal block secondary to various pathology
- Tubal occlusion secondary to ectopic pregnancy treatment
- Failed tubal cannulation for proximal tubal block
- Failed previous macrosurgical sterilization reversal

Contraindications

Absolute Contraindications

- Aged 40 years or older
- Decreased ovarian reserve or ovarian failure
- Tubal infertility not amenable to tubal reconstruction
- Extensive tubal damage

- Hydrosalpinx with a diameter of more than 3 cm
- Inadequate proximal or distal tubal segment for reanastomosis
- Projected tubal length of less than 3 cm after the reconstruction procedure
- Extensive pelvic/peritubal adhesions
- Abnormal uterine cavity
- Any contraindication to pregnancy or surgery
- Severe male factor infertility or male sterility which otherwise needs ART treatment.

Equipments and Instruments

Magnification, Resolution and Digital Enhancement

- 25-40X magnification is essential to identify healthy mucosa of the fallopian tube. 10-15X magnification is adequate for microsuturing.
- Use of endoscope, digital three chip camera with monitor has a 'Multiplier Effect' and the magnification can be achieved up to 20-25X.

Microinstrumentation

- It is collectively known as 'Koh ultramicro series' (Fig. 20.1).
- Terminal serration of the jaw is specially treated so that microsuture material does not get crushed.
- Handle design should be such that least friction and maximum transmission of hand movement occur to the instrument tip. 130° angle between handle and shaft of the instruments provides better movements.

Sutures, Needles and Energy

- More rigid needles are better for micro-endosuturing.
- The suture material should be 6-0 to 8-0 polypropylene, depending upon the surgeon's experience of material handling and preference.
- Electrosurgery: 15-20 W for cutting and 15 W for fulguration, use minimum cautery to preserve sub-tubal vasculature (Fig. 20.12).
- *Handlin's Uterine Manipulator* is a fine disposable instrument (Fig. 20.2), which allows administration of the dye and manipulation of the uterus without causing any significant trauma.

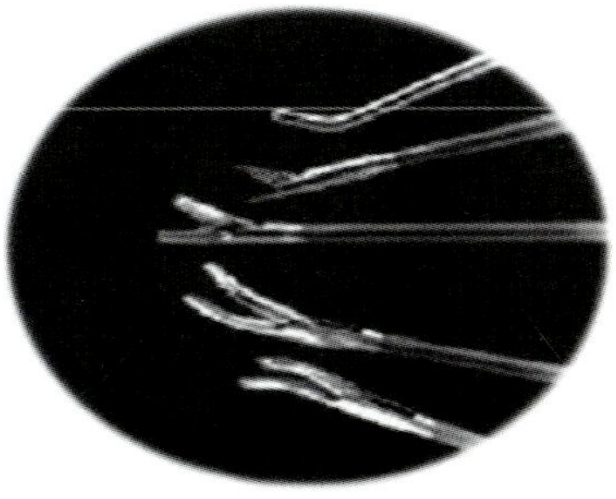

Fig. 20.1: Koh ultramicro series

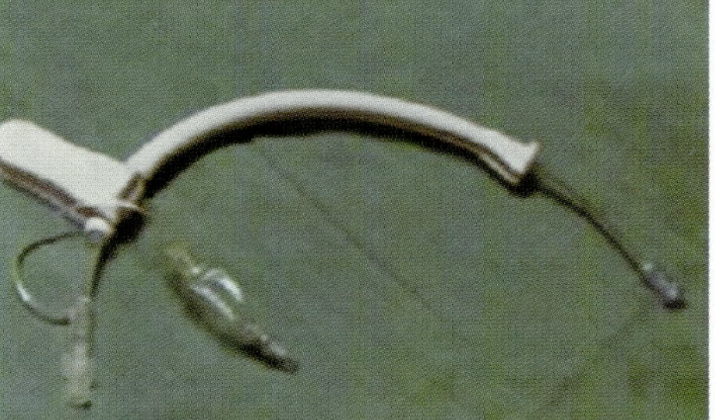

Fig. 20.2: Handlin's uterine manipulator

Selection of Cases

Length of Tubal Damage in Various Methods of Ligation

Type of TL	Length of Damage	Case Type
Monopolar diathermy	50 mm	Unfavorable
Filshie's clip (Fig. 20.3)	4 mm	Most favorable
Bipolar diathermy (Fig. 20.4)	30 mm	Intermediate
Falope Ring TL (Fig. 20.5)	40 mm	Unfavorable
Pomeroy's method	30 mm	Intermediate
Hulka clip	7 mm	Favorable

Other non suitable cases are pathological tubes with PID, Salpingitis Isthmica Nodosa and Failed tubal cannulation.

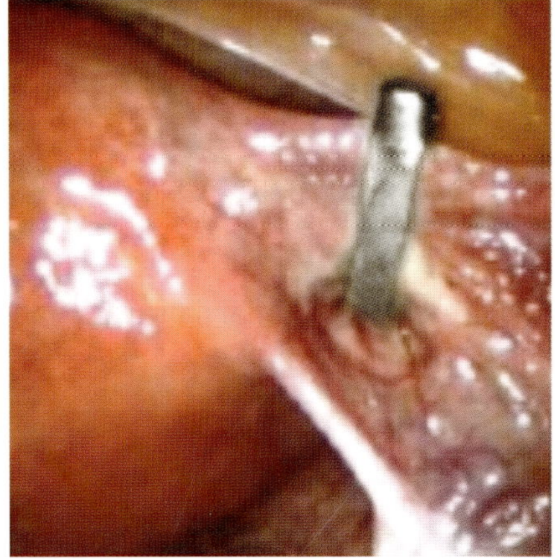

Fig. 20.3

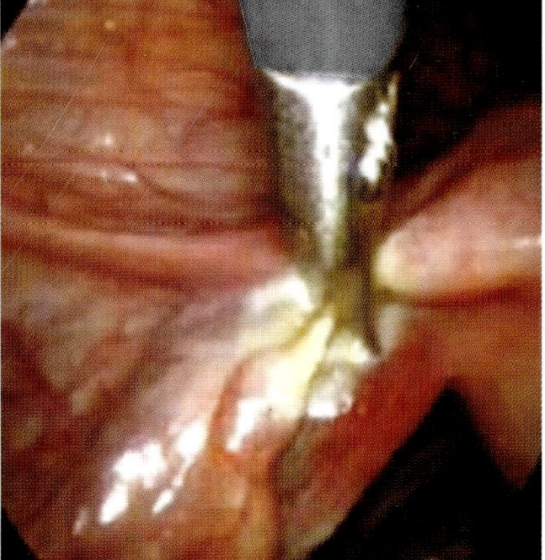

Fig. 20.4

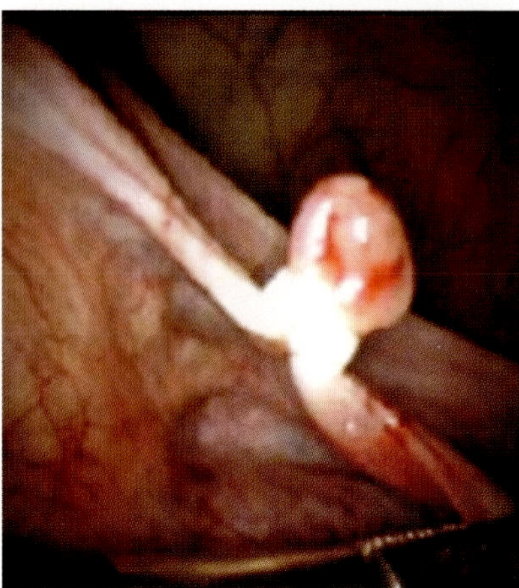

Fig. 20.5

Intra-operative Evaluation

Before proceeding for the tubal reconstruction one must evaluate the inside of the tube, so as to be confirmed that the anastomosis is going to be fruitful or not at all worthwhile. This involves Salpingoscopy and Falloposcopy.

- Salpingoscopy allows direct inspection of tubal mucosa in the ampullary part.
- The degree of tubal mucosal damage is probably the major factor in establishing the prognosis for tubal surgery.
- Brosen's classification is useful for evaluation according to degree of mucosal atrophy and mucosal adhesions.

Salpingoscopy Grade 1: (Fig. 20.6) Normal intra-luminal findings with healthy Major (Primary) and Minor (Secondary) folds.

Salpingoscopy Grade 2: (Fig. 20.7) Mucosal nuclear staining with Methylene blue dye.

Salpingoscopy Grade 3: (Fig. 20.8) Tubercles Minimal flattening and minimal adhesion (↓) of endosalpinx.

Salpingoscopy Grade 4: (Fig. 20.9) Moderate flattening of endosalpinx with intraluminal adhesion.

Salpingoscopy Grade 5: (Fig. 20.10) Severe flattening of mucosa with severe inter-luminal adhesions.

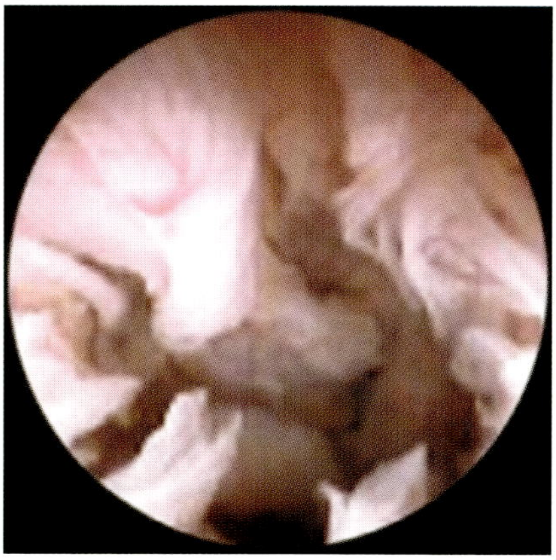

Fig. 20.6

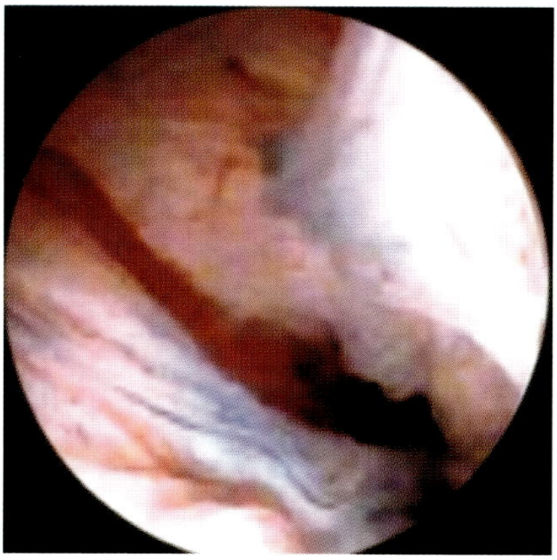

Fig. 20.7

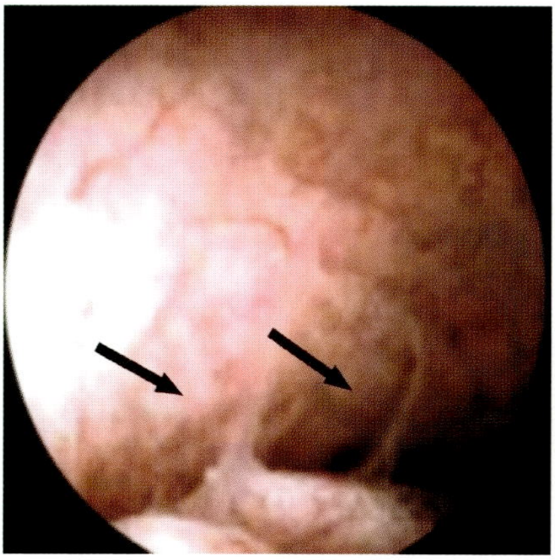

Fig. 20.8

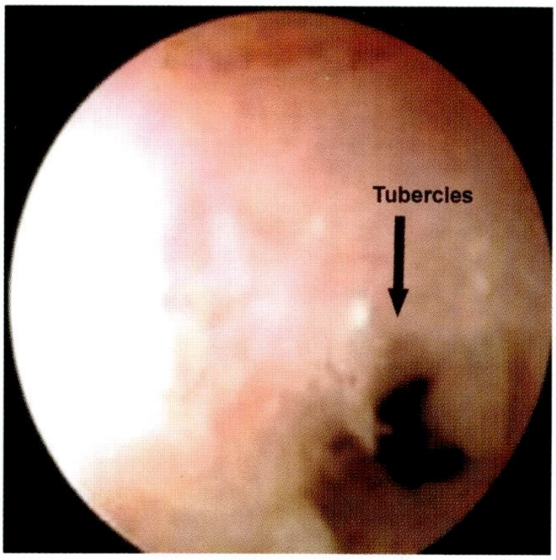

Fig. 20.9

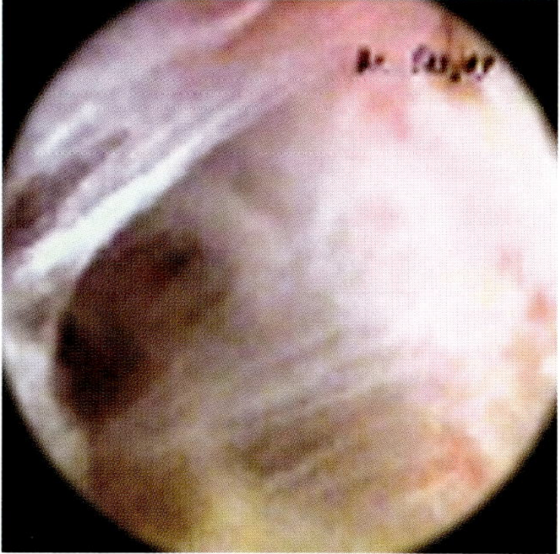

Fig. 20.10

Surgical Technique (Fig. 20.11)

Total 5 ports are used

- 10 mm laparoscope through the primary umbilical port.
- Four ancillary ports, two 5 mm and two 3 mm.
- The lower pelvic port of 5 mm is placed 4 cm medial and above the anterior superior iliac spine i.e. Ipsilateral Port.
- Contralateral port of 3 mm size placed exactly opposite to ipsilateral port.
- Another ipsilateral port of 3 mm is para-umbilical and laterally in the anterior axillary line.
- One 5 mm central port, 2-3 cm above the pubic symphysis.

'The position of the ports is critical in enabling fluent two handed operating as well as suturing. The so-called 'fulcrum effect' is virtually eliminated by adopting specific port positions.'

Port Positioning Sub-tubal Vessels

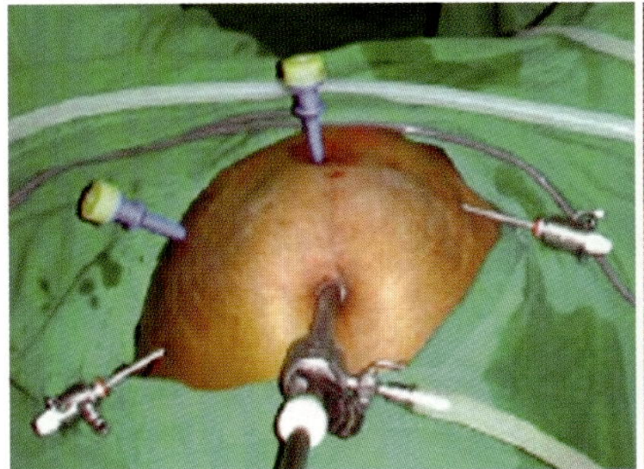

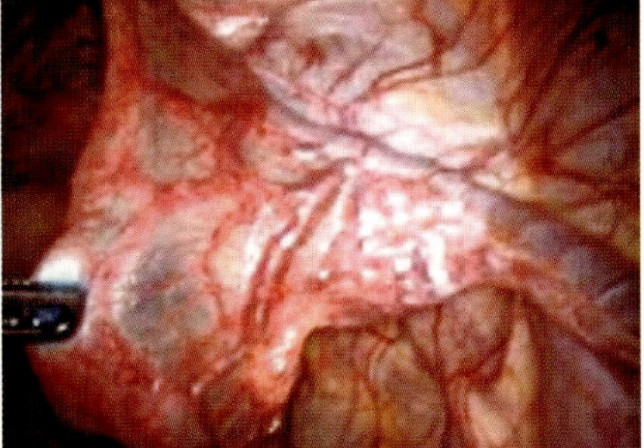

Fig. 20.11   Fig. 20.12

Important Surgical Steps

The surgical procedure involves transection of the tubal stumps and removal of scar tissue, approximation of the mesosalpinx, anastomosis of the muscle and mucosa, and approximation of the serosal layer.

Procedure

- Dilute vasopressin is infiltrated into the mesosalpinx for hemostasis and hydrodissection.
- It is very important to prepare the tube in two layers for a good anastomosis. Inclusion of any scarred portion in anastomosis can lead to poor healing.

- The site of tubal obstruction is identified and held with a fine grasper. A circular incision is made on the serosa of the proximal stump about half a centimeter from the probable site of transection with a fine monopolar needle. Sharp scissors are used to excise the obstructed portion of fallopian tube leaving a smooth edge to the patent lumen.
- It is important that the dissection is halted at the level of the mesosalpinx to avoid injuring the blood vessels and compromising the vascularity of the tube.
- Chromopertubation is performed through the cervix to check the patency of the proximal stump.
- The distal segment is also prepared in 2 layers in a similar manner. The patency of the segment is also checked by retrograde Chromopertubation.
- The mesosalpinx is approximated with a 6-0 polypropylene suture. Tube is then approximated which is most difficult and important step.

First Layer, the mucosal-muscularis layer.

- Most important is 6 O'clock position stitch.
- To keep the knot outside the lumen, stitches are taken from outer to inner side on proximal end and vice versa on distal end.
- Rests of the stitches are taken at 12, 3, and 9 O' clock position in the similar manner.
- After approximation of the inner layer, chromopertubation should demonstrate tubal patency.
- The serosa is then approximated with two or three interrupted 7-0 sutures.

Second layer, the sero-muscularis layer;

- Sutured with 6-0 polypropylene.
- Thorough peritoneal irrigation with Ringer's lactate solution throughout the operation.
- Postoperative care is the same as for any other laparoscopic surgery. The patient is usually discharged on the evening of surgery or the first postoperative day.

TYPES OF ANASTOMOSIS

Isthmo-Isthmic Anastomosis

- Lumen size is 500 μm-1 mm
- Equal lumen size and thick muscularis allows technically easier and better anastomosis.

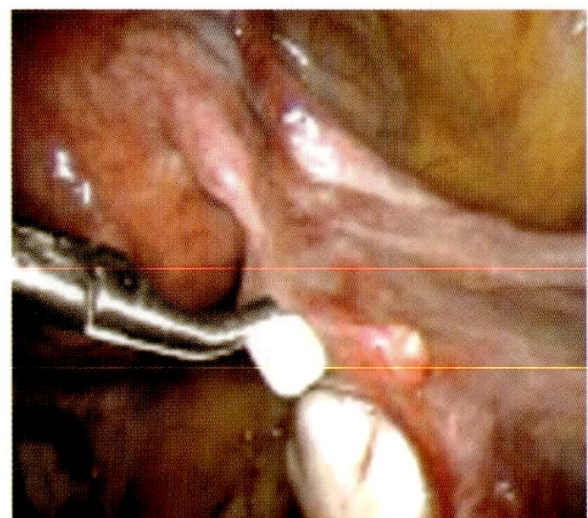

Falope ring excision

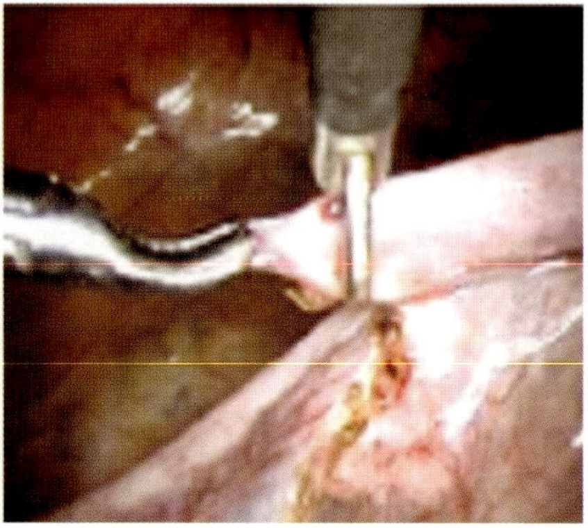

Refreshening of edges

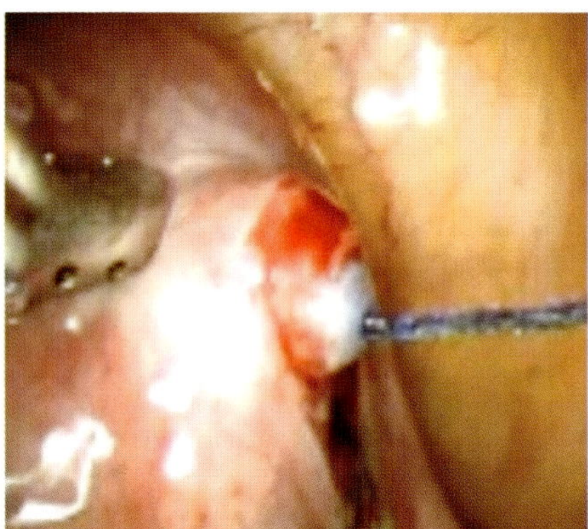

Free dye flow

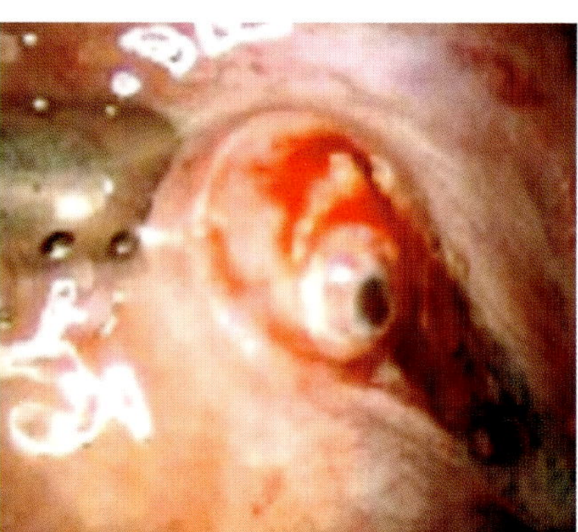

Magnified view

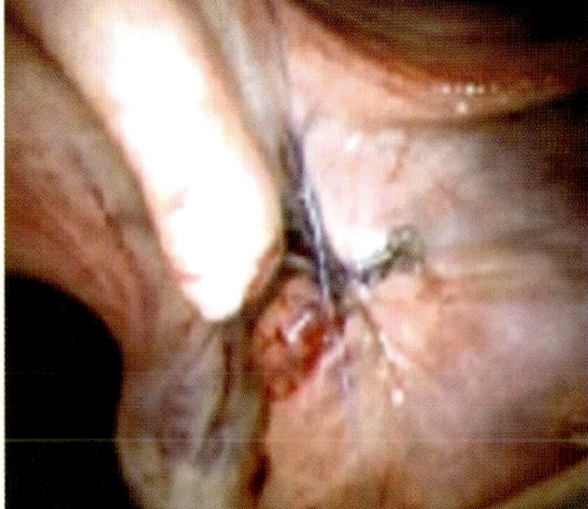

Mesosalpinx stitch

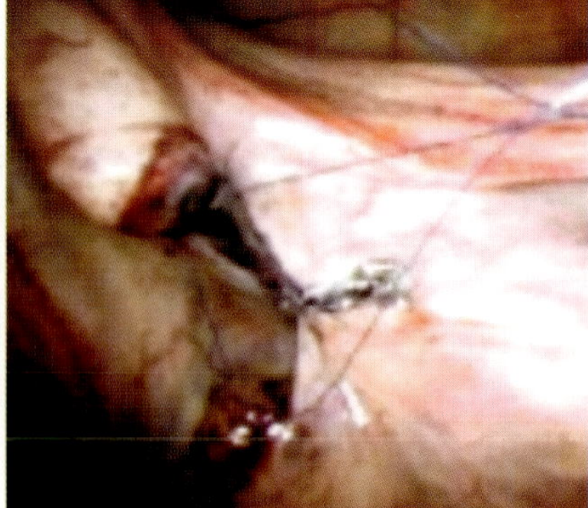

6 O'clock stitch

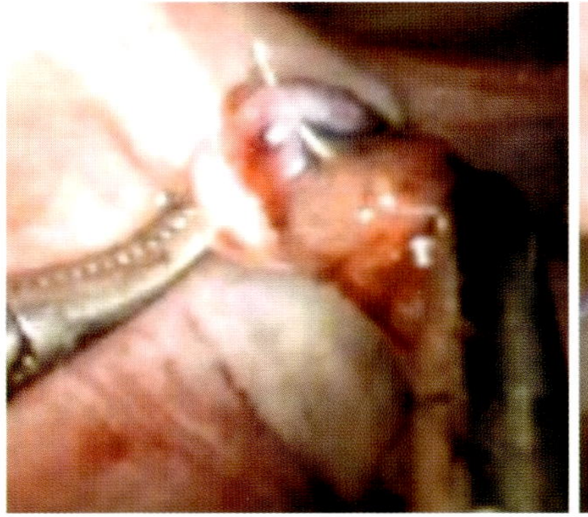

12 O'clock stitch

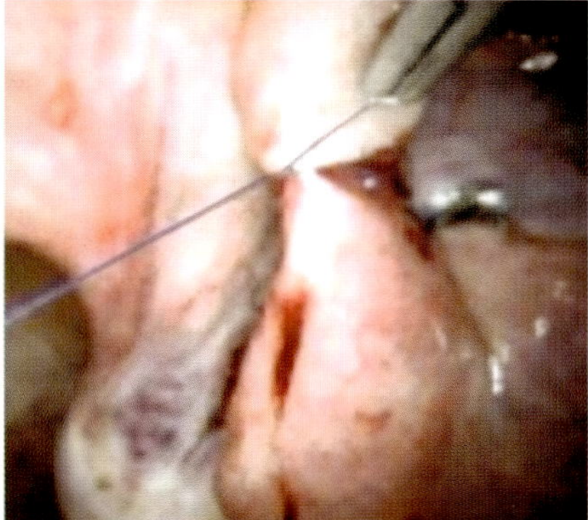

Second layer

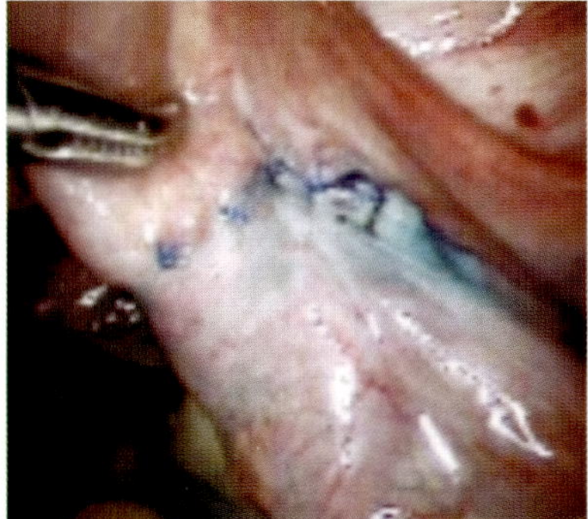

No leak at the site of anastomosis

Isthmo-Ampullary Anastomosis

- Luminal disparity is the potential problem which can be adjusted by cutting the isthmic end.

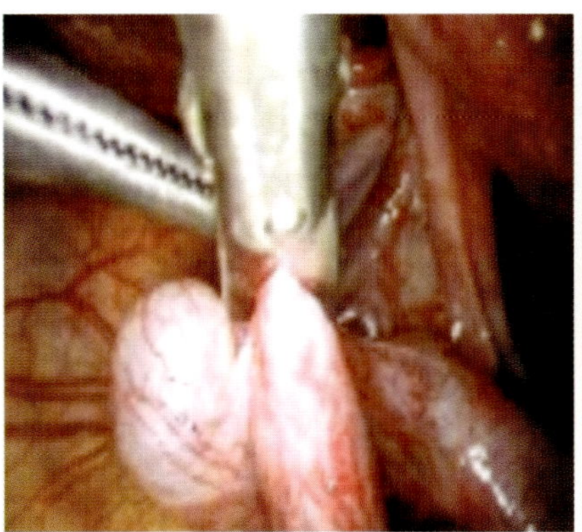

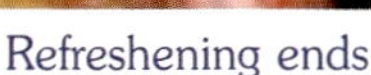

Refreshening ends

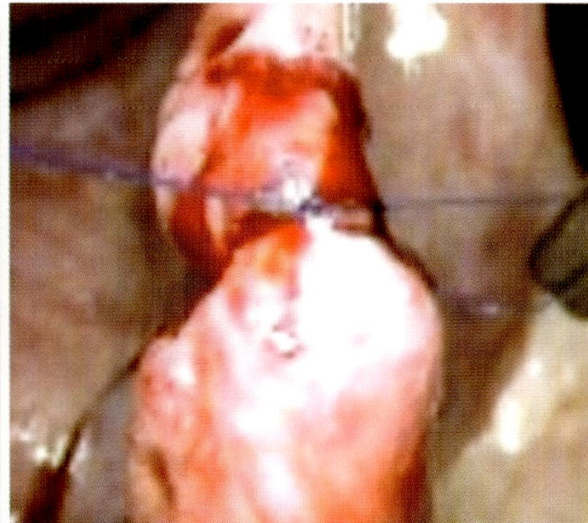

First layer

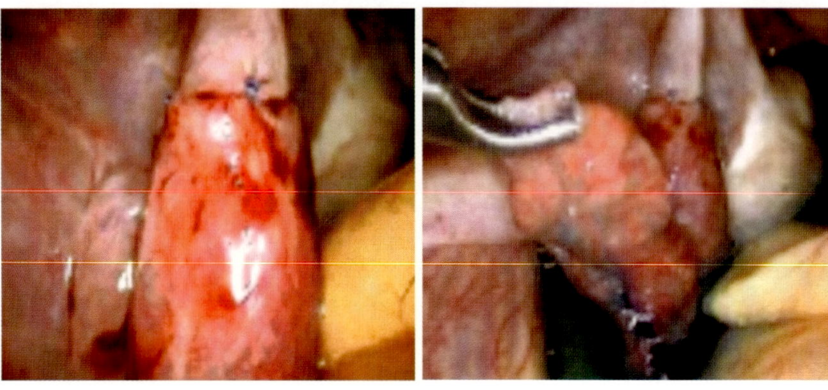

Second layer　　　　　　　　　　　Free spill

Ampullo-Ampullary Anastomosis

Technically difficult anastomosis due to thin muscularis and tendency for mucosal folds prolapse.

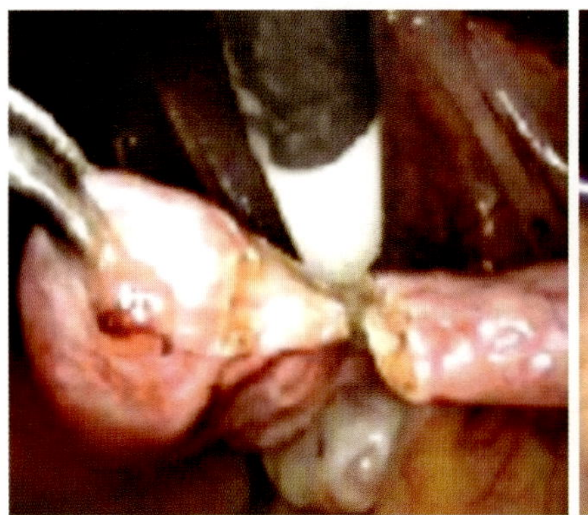
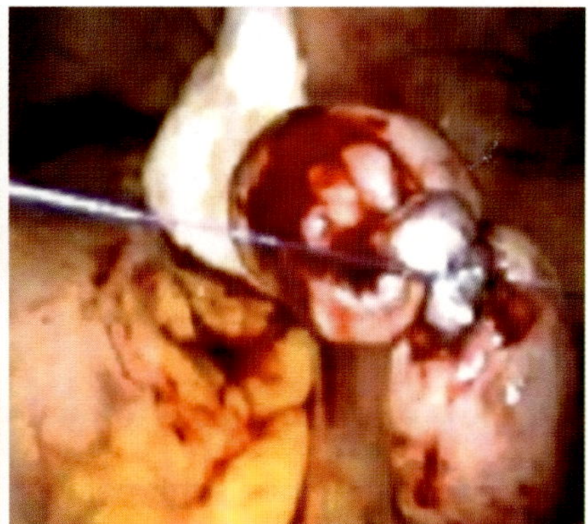

Refreshening ends　　　　　　　　　First layer

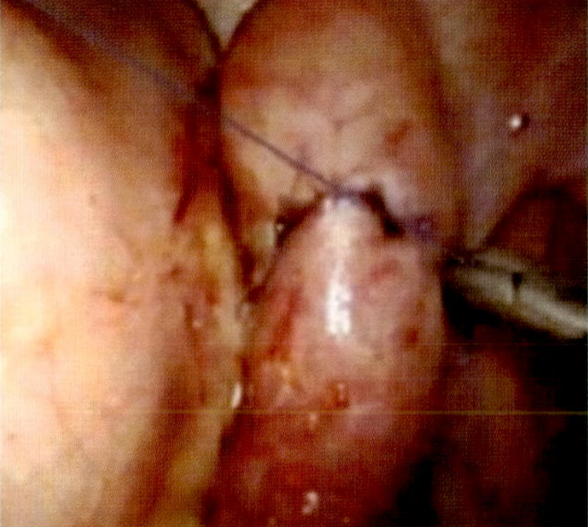

Second layer

Tubo-Cornual Anastomosis

Wedge excision in the cornual end mobilises good length of interstitial tube.

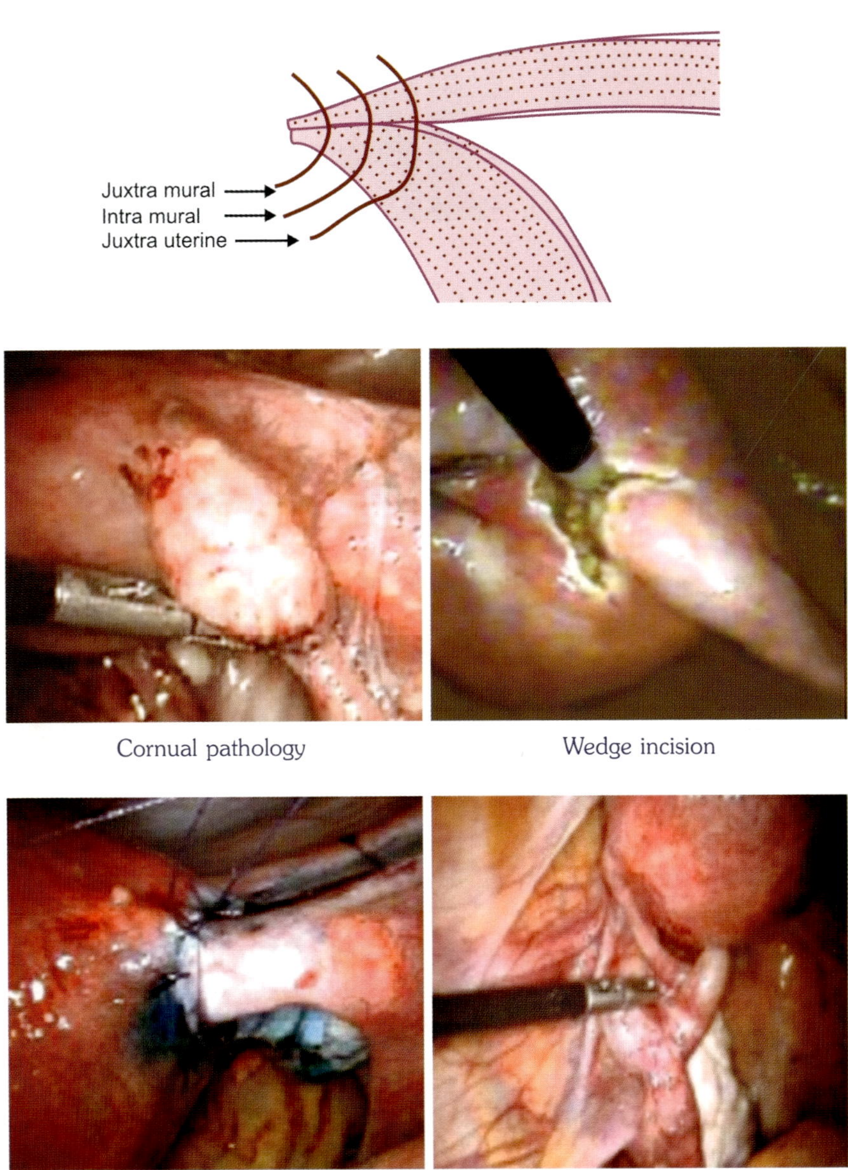

Cornual pathology

Wedge incision

Interstitial anastomosis

Mild hydrosalpinx

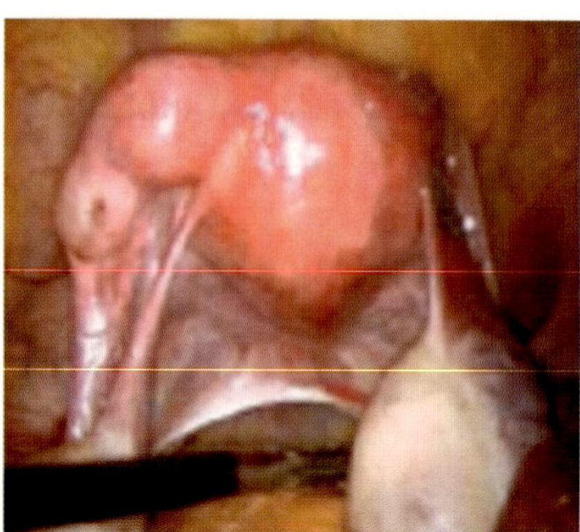

Cornual pathology

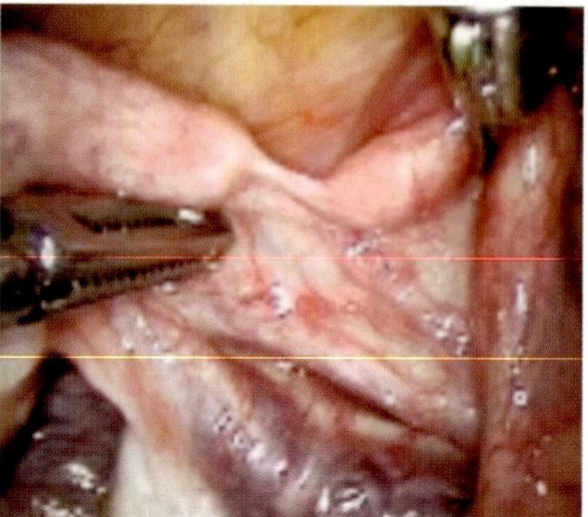

Proximal tubal block

Pathological Tubes

Salpingoscopy plays a key role in decision making for reconstructive surgery of such tubes.

TIPS

- Pregnancy rates are comparable with open tubal re-canalization.
- Salpingoscopy is very helpful in presence of pathological block.
- In cases of ectopic pregnancies segmental excision is best option as compared to salpingostomy or total salpingectomy, if the ectopic sac is < 2 cm of size.
- More cost-effective than IVF in the long run.
- Single step treatment as compare with IVF which may require multiple steps in each cycle.
- Make sure that the incision does not extend beyond the mesosalpinx.
- Ensure the right angled cut of the tubal ends for better alignment and approximation.

(Photographs courtesy: Dr Sanjay Patel)

21 Laparoscopic Management of Endometrioma

PREOPERATIVE EVALUATION

Thorough history with investigations like USG, Ca 125

PREOPERATIVE PREPARATION

Bowel Preparation

- Diet- One day prior to surgery soft diet till afternoon followed by liquid diet and then, nil by mouth for 8 hrs prior to surgery.
- Peglec powder- dissolve the pack in 2 liters of water to be given within 2-3 hrs on previous evening.

OR

- Exelyte solution 90 ml to be added in 300 ml of limca/fruit juice to be given on previous evening.

IMPORTANT EQUIPMENTS

- 10 mm 0° laparoscope
- 5 mm laparoscope
- 5 mm atraumatic grasping forceps, toothed grasping forceps, microdissecting forceps and other standard operative endoscopy instruments
- Good suction irrigation cannula (5 mm)
- Monopolar needle
- Bipolar forceps
- Scissors
- 10 mm grasper (for extraction of specimen)
- Rectal and vaginal probe
- Lapsac bag
- Rumi/Hulka's uterine manipulator

Position of the Patient

Patient is placed in a low modified lithotomy position on the Allen's stirrups with adjustable and padded leg rest.

Port Placement

Standard port placement (refer to chapter on port placement).

A 10 mm 0° laparoscope or occasionally 30° laparoscope is introduced through primary port. CO_2 is used for pneumoperitoneum at a rate of 3-9 litres/min with a pressure cut off at 15 mm Hg.

Trendelenberg's position is always given after primary port placement. Whether endometrial cyst wall ablation or cystectomy depends upon:

- Size of the endometrioma
- Feasibility of excision
- History of previous surgeries for endometrioma
- Symptomatology- whether pelvic pain or infertility

Usually,

- Endometrium < 3 cm- Ablation of cyst wall
- Endometrium > 3 cm- Cystectomy

ABLATION OF CYST WALL

- After seeing the site of endometrioma, its relation with adjacent organs- ureters, bowel and lateral pelvic wall, and the point at which the endometrioma should be punctured is decided (Fig. 21.1).
- Usually ovary is adherent and does not need stabilization, little lifting may be needed before puncturing
- Endometrioma is punctured with a needle with monopolar cautery current (Fig. 21.2).
- Chocolate material is completely drained. The incision is extended so as to visualize the inner cyst wall. Thorough inspection of inner cyst wall is an important step (Figs 21.3 and 21.4).
- A small cyst wall piece is taken and sent for histopathological examination
- Rest of the cyst wall is ablated with bipolar cautery/laser.
- Thorough lavage should be given.
- Always aim at a clean pelvis as the end result
- Ovarian wound is left open to heal (and not sutured)

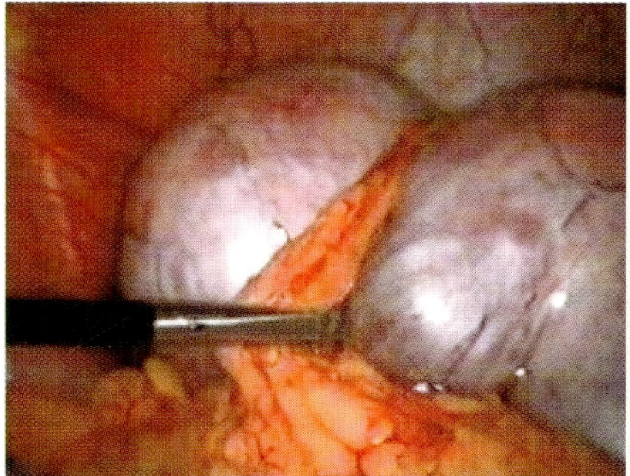

Fig. 21.1: Huge endometriomas

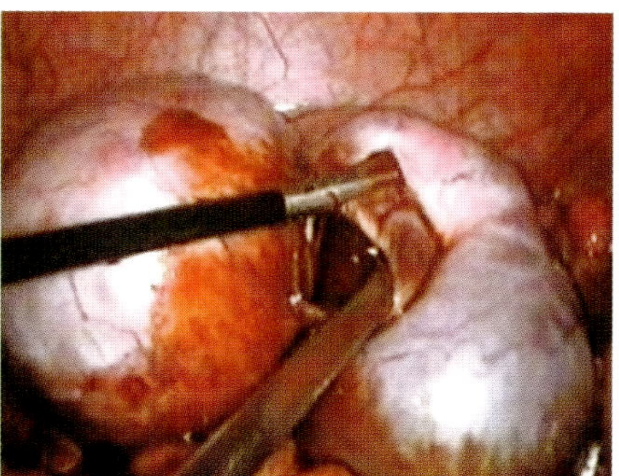

Fig. 21.2: Puncture and suction of chocolate fluid

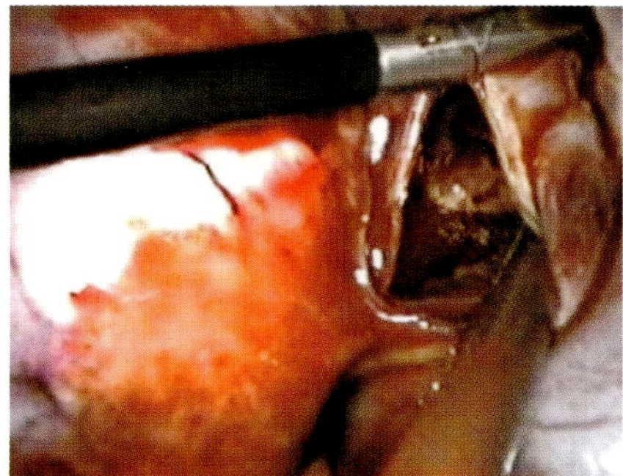

Fig. 21.3: Extending the incision

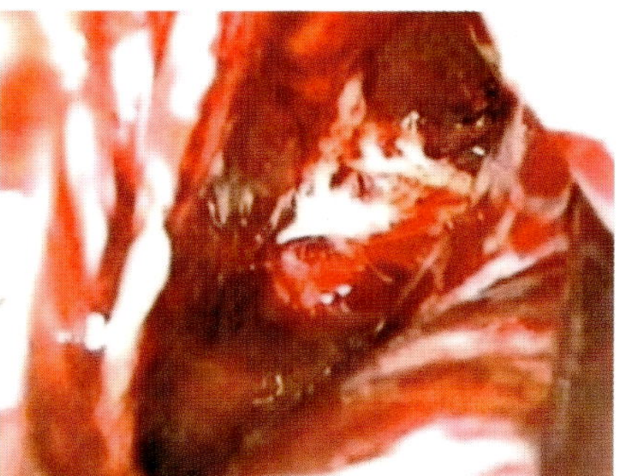

Fig. 21.4: Cystoscopy i.e. inspection of the cyst wall

CYSTECTOMY

- Again the point of puncture is decided and the endometrioma is punctured with the monopolar needle.
- The incision is extended with scissor or the same monopolar needle so as to accommodate suction irrigation cannula.
- Suction cannula is inserted into cyst and the chocolate material is completely drained out. This avoids excessive spillage of chocolate material in the lower abdomen especially in case of a large cyst.
- The incision is further extended.
- Inner cyst wall is inspected thoroughly (Fig. 21.4).
- Cyst wall is identified and separated from ovarian tissue by applying two claw forceps on the cyst wall and ovarian wall each, and pulled apart (Figs 21.5 and 21.6).

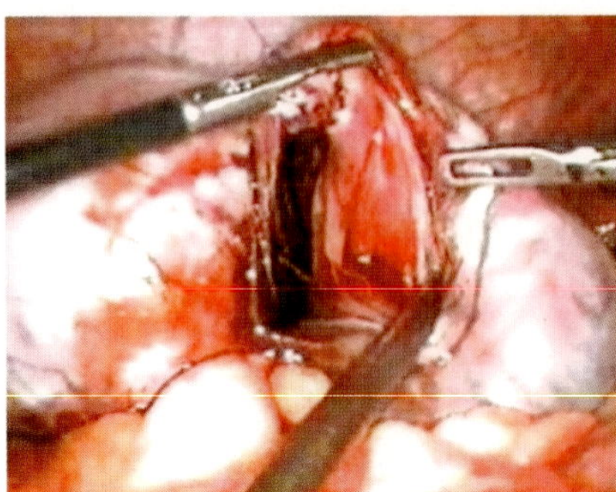

Fig. 21.5: Creating plane

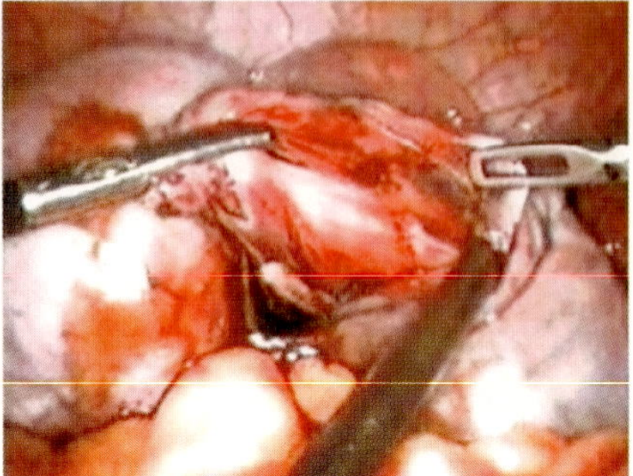

Fig. 21.6: Cystectomy in process

- Claw forceps are advanced from time to time next to the cleavage line for proper dissection and to avoid tearing of healthy ovarian tissue.
- Once the cyst wall is excised completely, the bed is observed for any active bleeder under water.
- With simple grasper the pressure is applied on the ovarian tissue to stop oozing.
- During this time, through the other port, suction cannula is inserted and the pelvis is thoroughly lavaged.
- Usually capillary oozing stops with pressure and only active bleeder seen under water flow can be cauterized with bipolar.
- Avoid excessive cauterization of the bed as it will further reduce ovarian reserve.
- Removal of cyst wall- 5 mm telescope is passed through secondary port and 10 mm grasper is passed through the primary port and the specimen is removed always under vision. If specimen is small, it can be removed by withdrawing it in 10 mm reducer passed through primary port, but if it is bulky, either cut in 2 pieces and remove as above or remove in Lapsac.
- Cauterization of any endometriosis spots if present in pelvis should be performed.
- Thorough lavage should be given and a clean pelvis as an end result should be achieved (Figs 21.7 and 21.8).
- Again, reconstruction of ovarian bed is not necessary but in cases of large endometrioma, simple 2 or 3 stitches to approximate the opposite walls can be taken to avoid adhesions.

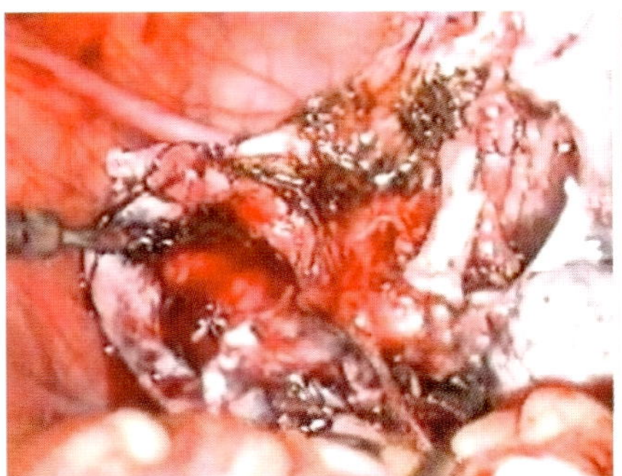

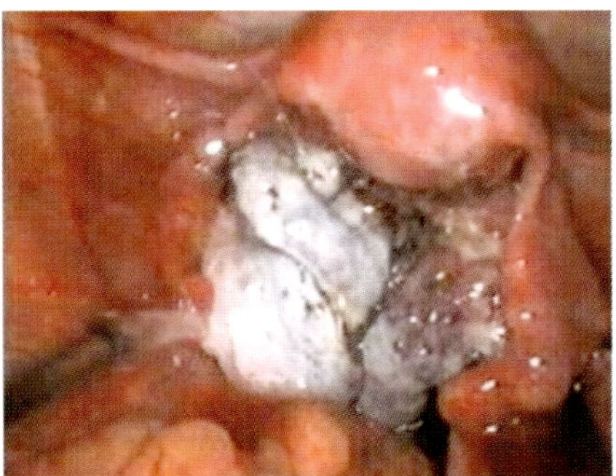

Fig. 21.7: Coagulation of bleeders to achieve hemostasis

Fig. 21.8: End result

Postoperative Care

- All patients should be discharged by evening, as early mobilization is equally important in reducing postoperative adhesions.
- Immediately, after laparoscopic drainage, 3 injections of GnRH analogues (once every 4 weeks) or 3 months depot injection can be given. 2nd look laparoscopic surgery may be advocated.

TIPS

- Good Trendlenberg position, adequate pneumoperitoneum and bowel preparation will keep bowel away from the field.
- Before proceeding for the surgery, if there are pelvic adhesions they should be removed either with sharp scissors or ultrasicion.
- During adhesiolysis in patients with extensive endometriosis, try to go from the lateral pelvic wall to the medial, and proceed from identifiable tissue organs to unidentified ones.
- Always aim at conserving ovarian tissue and minimizing postoperative adhesions.

(Photographs courtesy: Ruby Hall IVF and Endoscopy Centre)

Laparoscopic management of endometrioma with extensive adhesions.

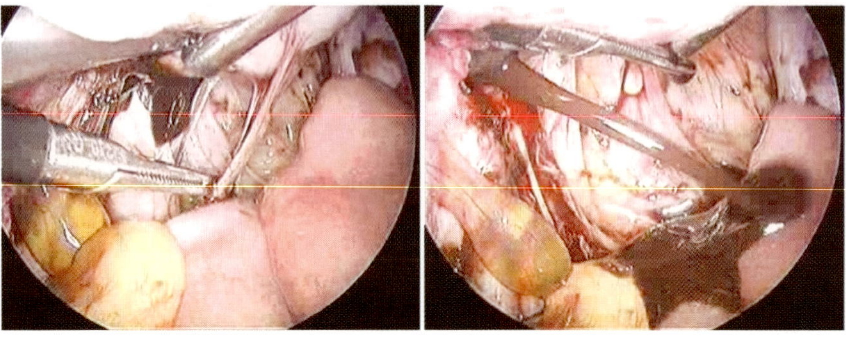

Endometrioma opened   Chocolate material is drained

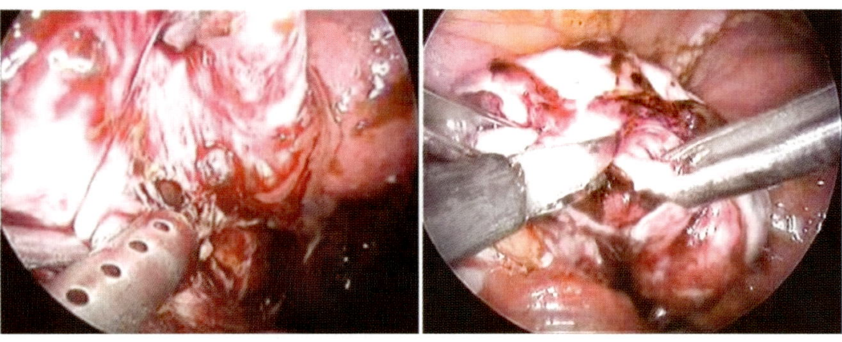

Opening of the endometrioma   Relaxing incision

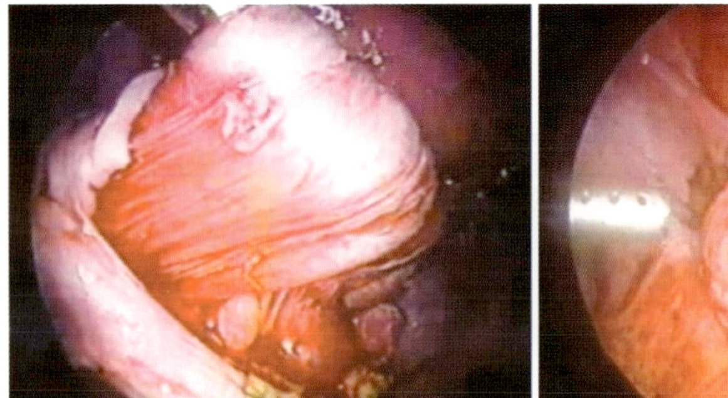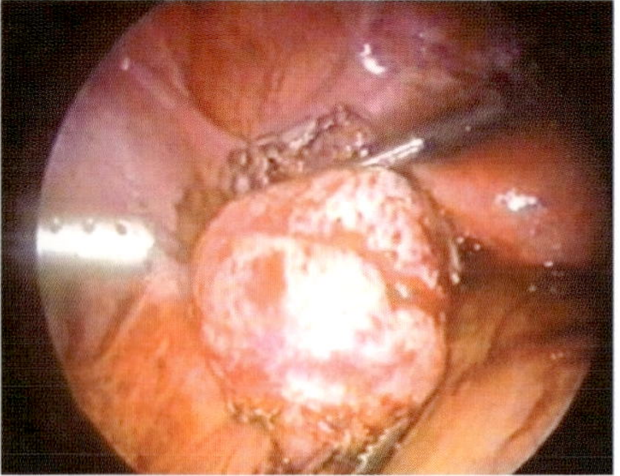

Peeling of cyst wall   Evertion to expose cortex

(Photographs courtesy: Dr Prakash Trivedi)

22   Salpingoscopy

It is the endoscopic examination of the mucosal folds of the distal segment (ampullary portion) of the fallopian tube which has an important role in the investigation of infertility.

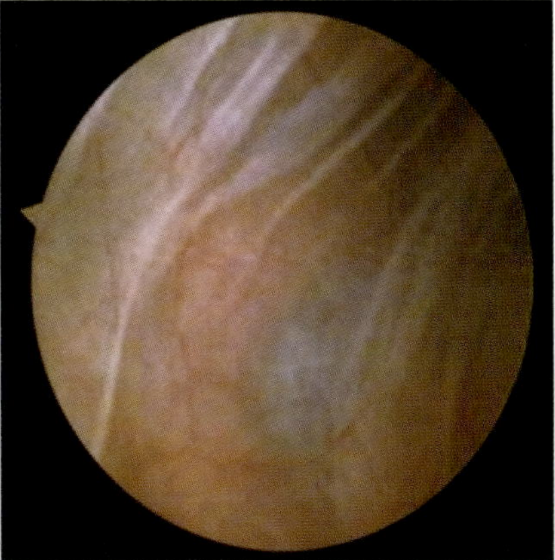

INSTRUMENTS AND PROCEDURE OF SALPINGOSCOPY

Salpingoscopy is performed under laparoscopic guidance. Two separate laparoscopic cameras (Karl Storz, Tuttlingen, Germany) each with separate monitors should be used.

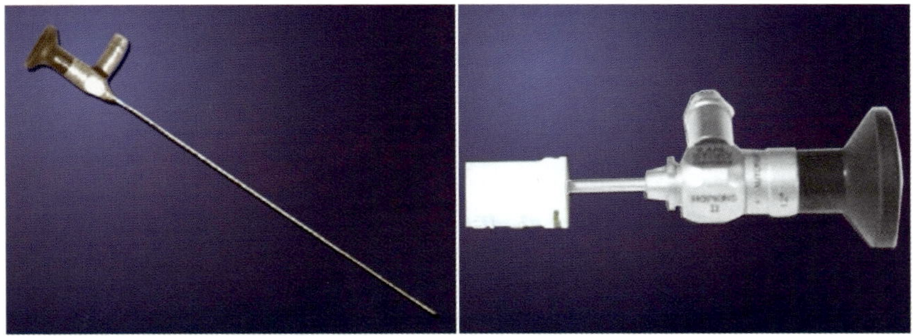

Figs 22.1 and 22.2: Telescope 2.9 mm

Salpingoscopy is performed using 2.9 mm diameter telescope with 12° angle (Figs 22.1 to 22.4). 2.9 mm telescope with diagnostic sheath is 4 mm in diameter.

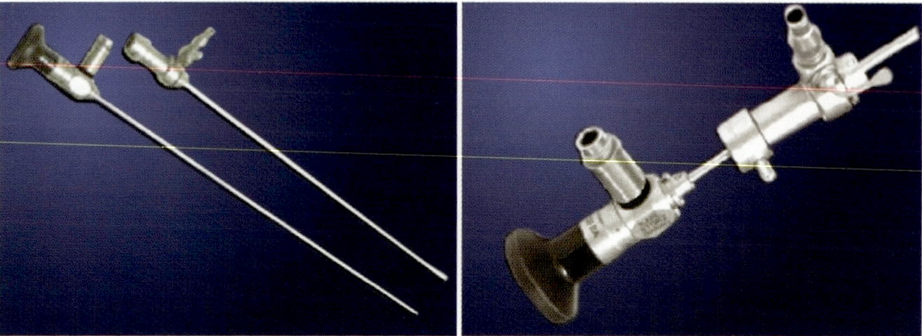

Figs 22.3 and 22.4: Telescope with diagnostic sheath (4 mm)

- Normal saline is used for distension of the fallopian tubes without any positive pressure.
- Occasionally dilatation of the fimbrial end is performed using a retrograde dye tester instrument (Figs 22.5 and 22.6) or a 5 mm Maryland grasper (Figs 22.7 and 22.8).
- Retrograde dye tester is a hollow, light and smooth conical tip instrument. It was actually designed to be used at laparoscopic tubal recanalisation for retrograde dye test.

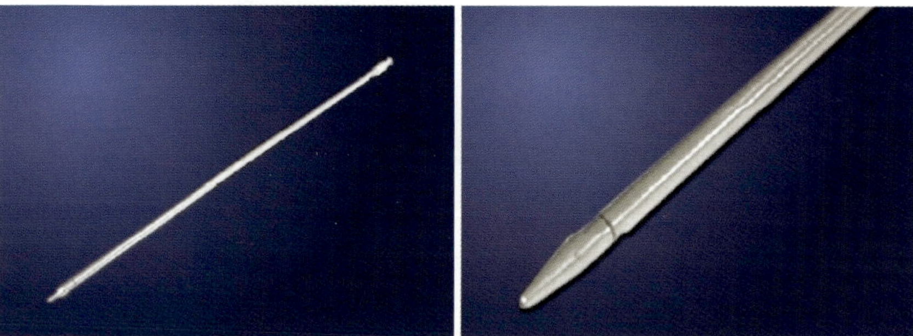

Figs 22.5 and 22.6: Retrograde dye tester

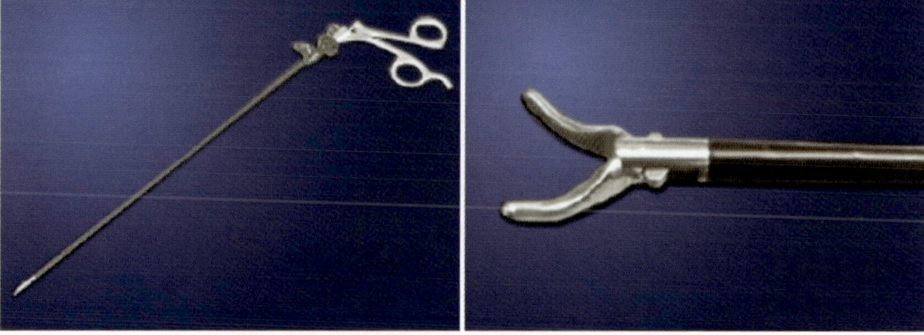

Figs 22.7 and 22.8: Maryland grasper

Extreme caution and gentleness is required in handling fimbriae as they play the most important role of ovum pick up and are indeed very delicate structures (Figs 22.9 and 22.10).

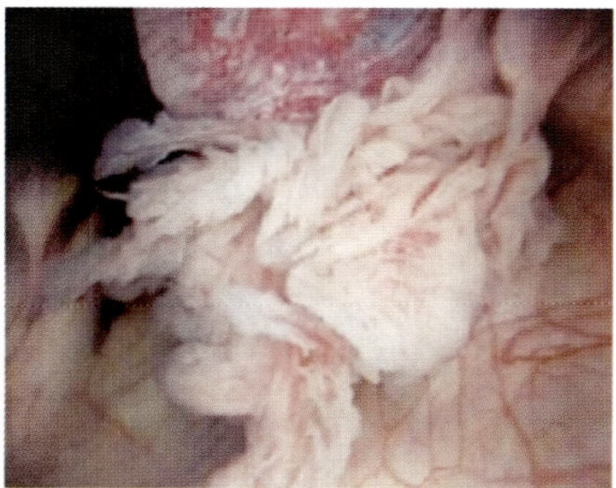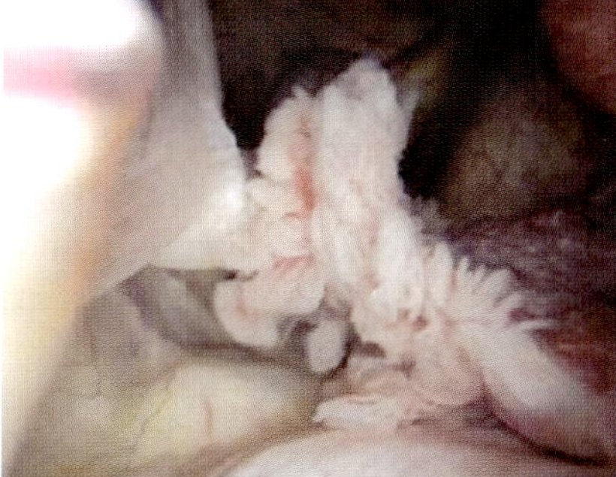

Figs 22.9 and 22.10: Healthy fimbriae

It is preferred to introduce the salpingoscope through the 5 mm midline secondary port, under vision from the primary telescope.

Fluid gently distends the ampullary portion of the tube and allows detailed assessment of the tubal endothelium.

There are usually 4-6 larger folds of endothelium which are described as major or primary folds.

In between two major folds, there are 3-4 smaller thin folds, which are minor or secondary folds.

Prof. Brosen has classified salpingoscopy into 5 grades depending upon the visual impression of the tubal endothelial folds which is modified slightly as follows.

Grade I (Fig. 22.11)

It is the normal, pink healthy looking major and minor mucosal folds. Major folds can be seen floating freely as the fluid passes through the tubal lumen.

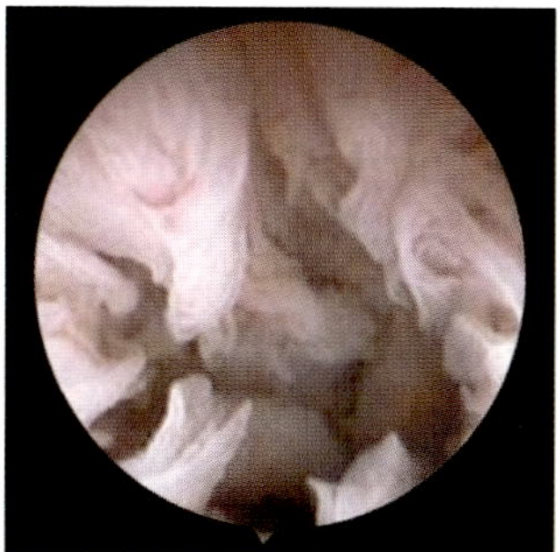

Fig. 22.11

Grade II (Figs 22.12 and 22.13)

Methylene blue is passed before salpingoscopy to confirm tubal patency.

Patchy staining of endothelial folds with methylene blue dye is seen and/or there is minimal flattening of major folds with separation of major and minor folds.

It indicates the inflammatory reaction within the endothelium.

This can be further divided in,

Grade II-A: Only staining of the endosalpinx (Fig. 22.12)

Grade II-B: Staining along with mild flattening of major folds with single band of adhesion (Fig. 22.13).

On contact micro-salpingoscopy with upto 150x magnification, inflammatory cells are seen as blue dots very clearly. They are nothing but the inflammatory cell nucleus which stains on methylene blue dye test (Fig. 22.14).

Rest of the mucosa appears healthy.

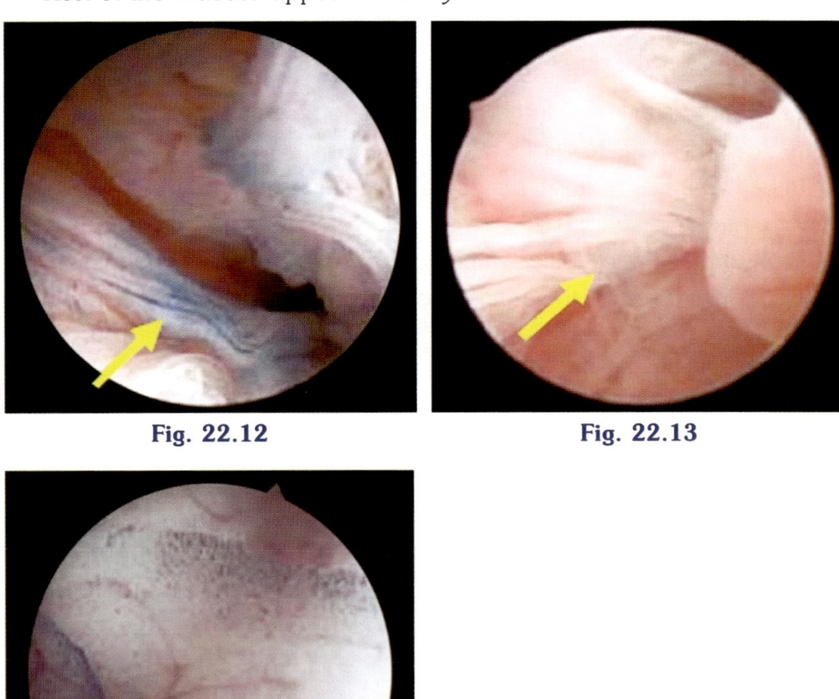

Fig. 22.12   Fig. 22.13

Fig. 22.14

Grade III (Fig. 22.15)

Variable degree of flattening of the endothelial folds with moderate adhesions between them. Flattening of endothelial folds give wide bore appearance of the lumen, and adhesions may cause restriction of free movements of major folds.

Grade IV (Fig. 22.16)

Severe degree of flattening with severe adhesions of the mucosa. Tube appears wide, rigid and bald from inside. It may be patent or even blocked.

Grade V (Fig. 22.17)

Lumen appears obliterated due to severe intraluminal cob-web type of adhesions. There is total destruction of endothelium leading to loss of the normal architecture and blockage of lumen at various sites.

These are totally dysfunctional fallopian tubes and they should be excised rather than conserved. Spontaneous intrauterine pregnancy is highly unlikely in these cases and if she conceives the risk of ectopic is significantly high.

Genital Tuberculosis (Fig. 22.18)

It often results in tubal damage. The external appearance of the tube may be normal. Often, tubes appear less supple, rigid and fibrotic. It may be patent or even blocked. It often shows the presence of small tubercles on the endothelium.

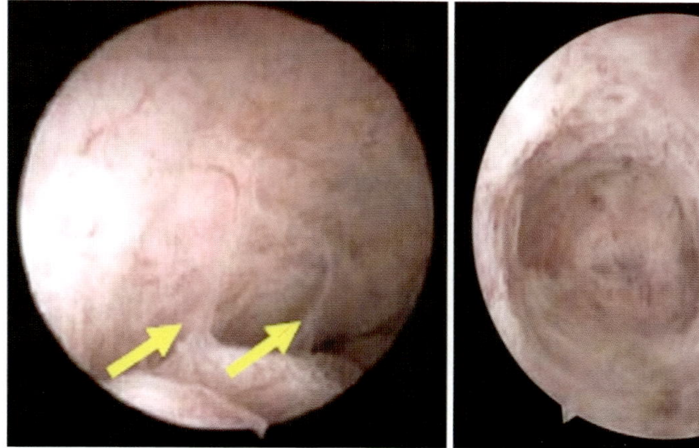

Fig. 22.15   Fig. 22.16

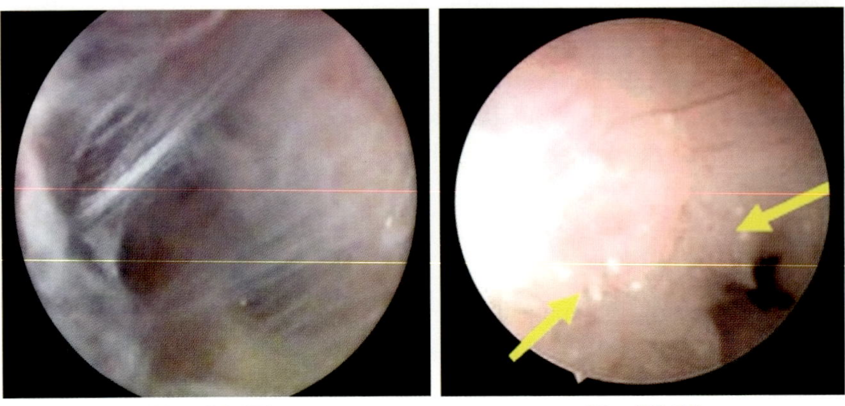

Fig. 22.17   Fig. 22.18

Endosalpingeal Polyp (Fig. 22.19)

Rarely small endosalpingeal polyps are seen, however, they don't seem to be of any significance.

Difficulties and Pit Falls

It is not always possible to perform salpingoscopy easily. The learning curve is steep and long. Fimbrial stenosis and accessory ostia can cause difficulty in performing the salpingoscopy.

Accessory Fimbrial Ostiae (Fig. 22.20)

Gentle fimbrial dilatation is recommended using Maryland grasper or retrograde dye pusher.

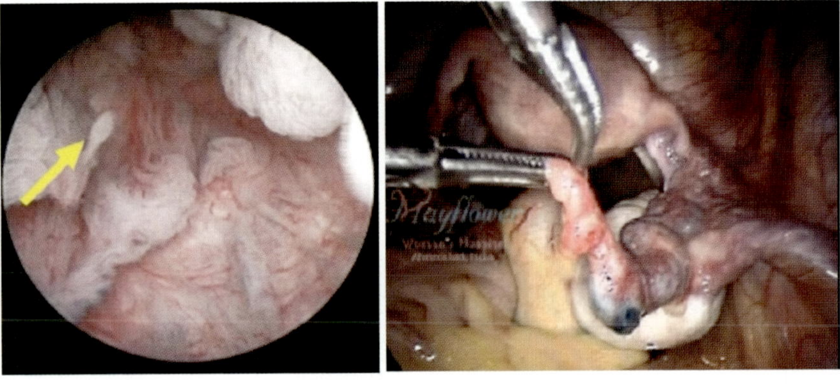

Fig. 22.19   Fig. 22.20

Occasionally a false passage (Fig. 22.21) may occur in the muscularis wall of the tube and it can appear like grade 5 salpingoscopy findings. However, it can be differentiated by identifying pulsatile vessels in between myofibrils.

It is recommended to use gravity-fall system to pass the fluid for distension. If it is allowed to flow under pressure, one can experience 2 problems.

1. It can result in tubal wall edema and
2. It causes temporary flattening of the folds, therefore giving false positive salpingoscopy findings.

Tubal Edema (Fig. 22.22)

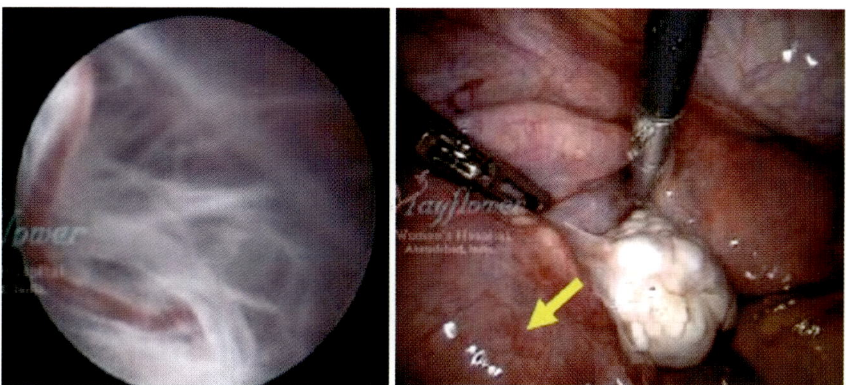

Fig. 22.21   Fig. 22.22

Generalised Endothelial Staining (Fig. 22.23)

However a pathological tube shows focal staining of endothelium.

Tubal Diverticulum (Fig. 22.24)

The fimbrial diverticulum is a normal anatomical variant and it may cause difficult introduction of the telescope.

If the telescope enters the diverticulum, it is a thin part of the tube and it may appear as severely flattened tube and may give false positive findings.

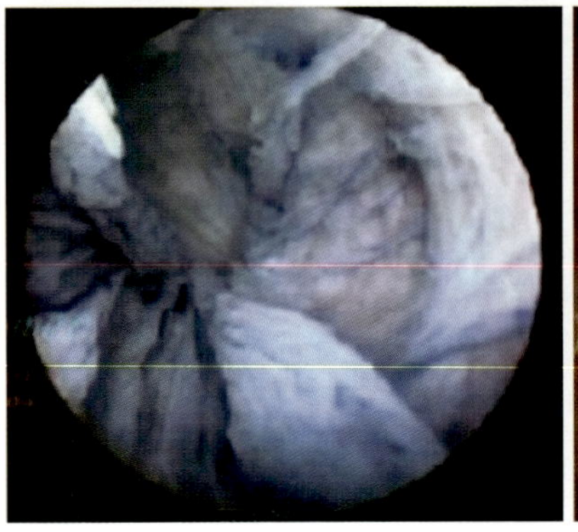

Fig. 22.23

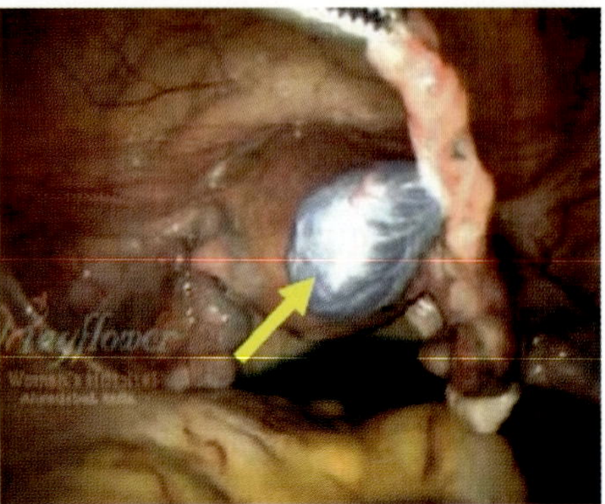

Fig. 22.24

TIPS

1. Dilute 3 drops of methylene blue dye into 100 ml of normal saline. If more concentrated methylene blue dye is used it may cause uniform staining of the endothelium giving false positive findings.
2. In cases with Grade III and more, IVF-ET is the preferable option rather than IUI. Spontaneous pregnancy or IUI would involve significantly higher ectopic pregnancy rate.

(Photographs Courtesy: Dr Sanjay Patel)

23 Laparoscopic Management of Adenomyoma

PREOPERATIVE EVALUATION

- History and clinical examination.
- Transvaginal sonography and Color Doppler. One needs an expert sonologist to differentiate it from myoma. Preoperative ultrasonic assessment for the location of the adenomyoma is the most important step in planning the surgery.
- Limited MRI of uterus is very useful.
- Rarely it may happen that adenomyoma gets diagnosed on table when patient is taken for myomectomy. Thus adenomyosis remains a difficult and challenging diagnosis and is often only established at hysterectomy specimen.

PREPARATION OF THE PATIENT

Usually no preparation. Bowel preparation may be advised in case of large adenomyoma to get better field of vision.

Instrumentation

1. Skilled laparoscopic surgeon; especially skilled in laparoscopic suturing and morcellation.
2. Anesthetist, skilled and trained assistant, nursing staff.
3. A complete set of Operative Laparoscopy instruments, 5/10 mm myoma screw, and electromechanical morcellator.
4. Both monopolar and bipolar cautery, Harmonic if available.
5. Proper suturing set with needle holders, knot pushers for extracorporeal knots and scissors.

Technique

- Placement of primary and secondary trocars depends upon the size and site of adenomyoma. As said earlier, preoperative ultrasonic assessment for the location of the adenomyoma is essential.
- Relation of adenomyoma with the uterus and fallopian tube should be carefully assessed after inserting primary trocar and then site of secondary trocars to be decided.
- It is possible to remove myomas without removing any normal uterine tissue during myomectomy. In contrast, adenomyoma is not a discrete tumor but rather a local swelling of the uterine wall as a result of the infiltration of endometrial tissue. Therefore it is not possible to remove tissue affected by adenomyosis without actually removing the involved myometrial tissues.
- Complete enucleation of adenomyoma is rarely possible and therefore wedge resection of the affected myometrium is done in elliptical strips manner using monopolar pure cutting current. One should aim at removing as much of adenomyotic tissue as possible.
- It is effective as the primary aim is to reduce the myometrial bulk, intra-myometrial tension and uterine vascularity. Adenomyotic tissue bleeds minimal on resection.
- The defect is sutured by intracorporeal slip knot technique.
- Thorough lavage is given at the end of surgery.
- Patient can be discharged on the same day.

TIPS

- Preoperative TVS/MRI diagnosis is a must.
- Suitable for patients with localized adenomyosis predominantly on one wall.
- Curved incision line may be more effective, as the Tension Per Linear Centimeter would be reduced.
- Expansible capacity of the uterus in pregnancy depends on increase in plasticity rather than elasticity. Plasticity depends on collagenous framework of connective tissue. Adenomyosis distorts this arrangement of microfibrils of collagen tissue. Hence, resection of adenomyoma helps in achieving higher pregnancy rates.
- One should always keep a close watch on uterine rupture in pregnant patients who have undergone adenomyoma excision.

LAPAROSCOPIC EXCISION OF ADENOMYOMA

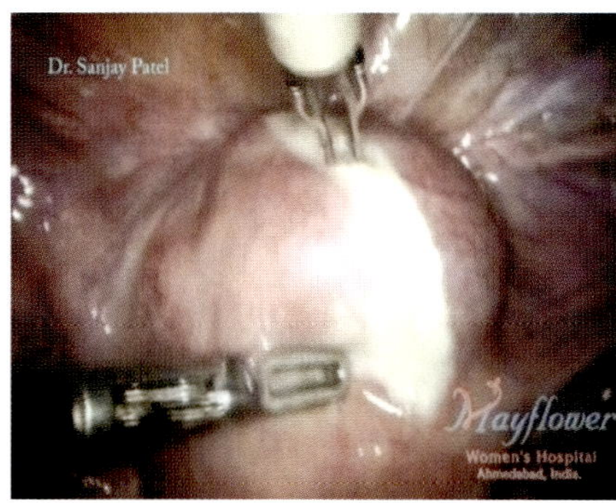
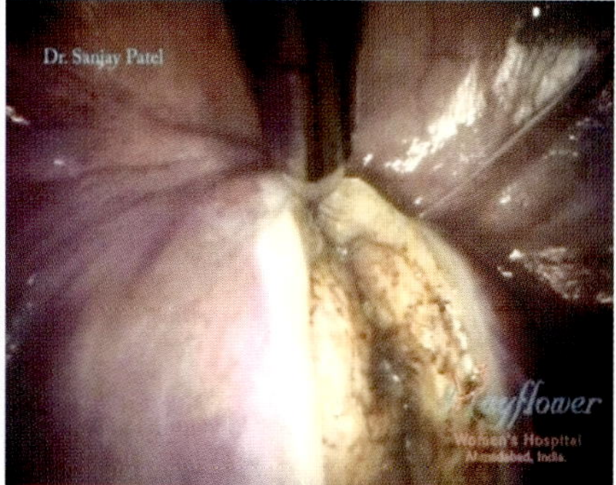

Anterior wall adenomyoma – incision with monopolar

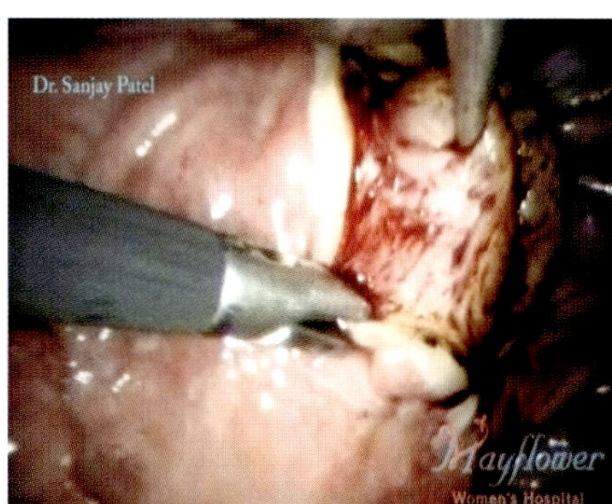
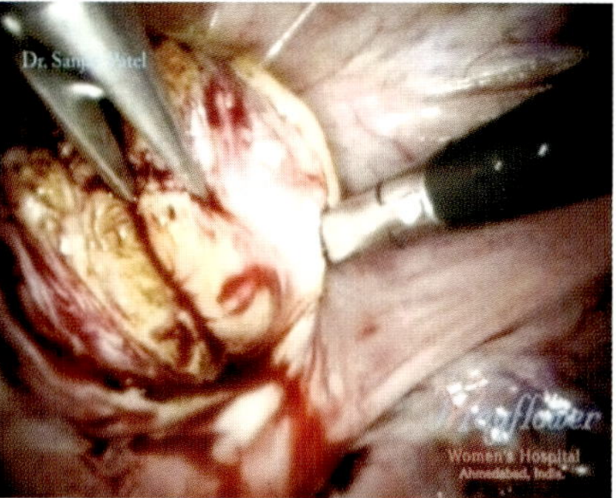

Adenomyomectomy with elliptical incisions in process

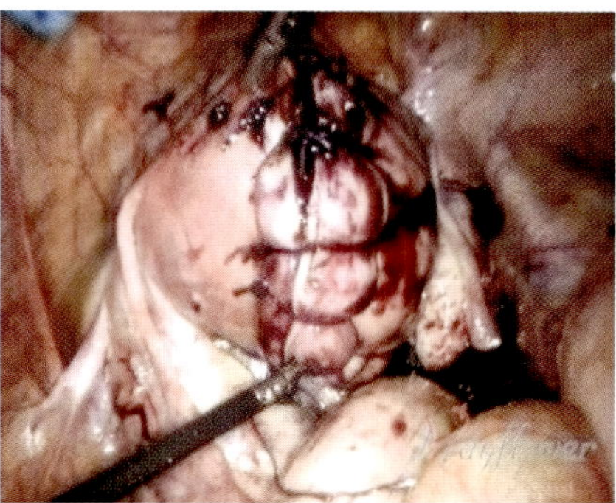

Defect sutured using vicryl

HYSTEROSCOPIC VIEW OF ADENOMYOMA

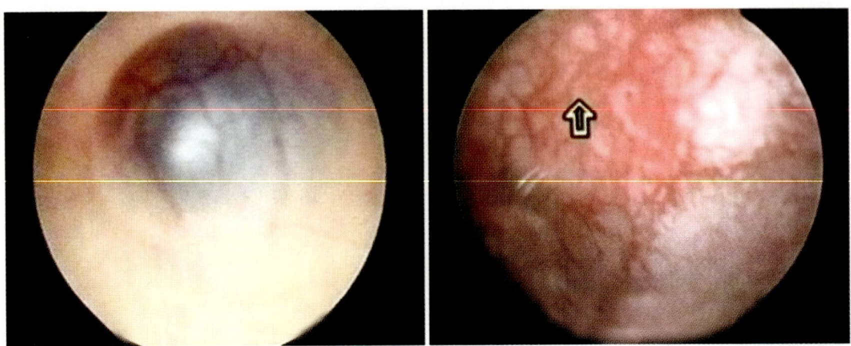

Adenoma on hysteroscopy | Hysteroscopy: increased vascularity

(Photograph Courtesy: Dr Sanjay Patel)

Section Four

Vaginal Surgery

24 Non-Descent Vaginal Hysterectomy

PREOPERATIVE EVALUATION

- Relevant indication
- Routine investigation
- TVS to know the exact size of uterus and the adnexal pathology
- To assess mobility of the uterus and vaginal laxity
- Decision to remove adenexa as per indication

PREOPERATIVE PREPARATION

- Vaginal disinfection
- Preoperative antibiotics
- Bowel cleansing

ANESTHESIA

- Spinal
- Epidural
- General

POSITION

- Lithotomy
- Modified lithotomy (refer to chapter laparoscopic hysterectomy)

TECHNIQUE

- Careful evaluation of descent of uterus and associated vaginal wall prolapse.
- Hold the cervix with two (preferably) long Allis' forceps.
- Saline adrenaline injection 50-150 ml as per the size of uterus and the comfort of the surgeon (Optional)

- Foley's catheterization.
- Transverse incision on the anterior lip.
- Pushing of bladder with wet gauze piece, perhaps in a single sweep upto bladder reflection.
- Posterior vaginal reflection over the cervix, identified and a bold transverse cut taken 1 cm below the reflection often opening the peritoneum in the same cut. Sim's speculum should compress the posterior vaginal wall so as to keep the bowel away from the incision line.
- Laterally, vaginal mucosa is not cut; in fact it is taken in the first clamp along with the uterosacrals.
- Uterosacral and Mackenrodts' are clamped, cut and transfixed and stumps kept long.
- Those trained in clampless surgery may directly ligate and cut.
- The bladder peritoneum if not opened, may be easily done at this step.
- Uterines are clamped, cut and ligated.
- Cornual clamps may be applied in case the adnexa are to be spared, after clamping, cutting and being held long.
- In case adnexa is to be removed, then begin with the routine round ligament, to reduce the bulk of tubo-ovarian pedicle and access the infundibulopelvic ligament.
- Seth's ovarian clamps are used to go beyond the ovaries. A poor cousin is usually the Kocher's at this stage.
- After a good review to rule out any bleeding from pedicles, vaginal closure is done.
- The vaginal angles are sutured, on both sides and one or two sutures are taken in between the two angles in the midline may be taken keeping opening for drainage.
- Vagina packed with betadine soaked roller gauze.

MODIFICATIONS

- In cases where there is fear of vault prolapse; simultaneous sacrospinous fixation may be done.
- Lateral vaginal mucosa should be taken with the uterosacrals.
- In case of long cervix, cut may be taken just below the bladder reflection.
- Cystocele may be repaired before mucosa closure.
- Excision of excessive posterior peritoneum during peritoneal closure cares for the enterocele.

- In cases of previous caesarean section. Adhesions are usually at the isthmus. So, sharp dissection should be done.

POSTOPERATIVE

- Ambulation out of bed after 12 hours.
- Pack removal after 12 hours.
- Fluids after 4-6 hours followed by a soft diet at night.
- Remove catheter after 24 hours.
- Antibiotics for 5-7 days.
- Discharge after 48-72 hours.

TIPS

- Careful evaluation of uterine size and mobility.
- Challenging to do size over 12 weeks and requires experience.
- Transverse breadth of uterus important while deciding the case.
- Associated adnexal pathology may decide in favor of LAVH or abdominal hysterectomy.
- Use of long narrow single bladed Sim's speculum for anterior retraction and broad long single bladed Sim's speculum for posterior retraction especially for removal of non-descent bulky uterus. Due to groove of Sim's speculum anteriorly the needle movement becomes very easy.
- No need to open the anterior pouch initially. Only confirm that the bladder is pushed up. After uterines, peritoneum will get opened up automatically.
- Closure of visceral peritoneum is usually not advocated.
- Continuous traction on cervix on contralateral side before applying clamp is very improtant.

Newer Concepts of Anterior and Posterior Vaginal Prolapse Repair

25

Kannan K, Fiadjoe P, Rane A

PELVIC ORGAN SUPPORTS

The pelvic organs are supported by pelvic floor muscles; such as levator ani and iliococcygeus, connective tissues such as cardinal (Mackenrodt's), uterosacral, pubourethral, pubocervical and puborectal ligaments, and a horizontal vaginal axis. These can all be disrupted by birth trauma. The vaginal axis is nearly horizontal when the woman is standing. Hence any intra-abdominal downward force will appose the vagina on the pelvic floor muscles preventing descent. This is aided by fascial and ligamentous support around the vagina (Fig. 25.1).

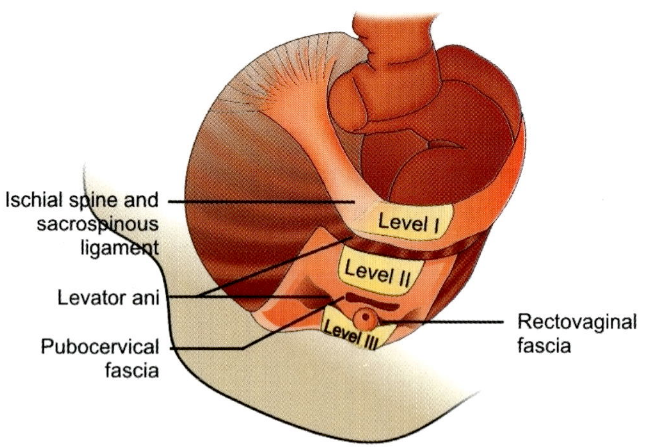

Fig. 25.1: Levels of fascial and ligamentous support (Reproduced from DeLancey JOL. 1992)

This support is divided into three levels:

Level 1: Includes uterosacral and cardinal ligaments supporting the upper vagina.

Level 2: Includes levator ani muscles via fascial attachments to the arcus tendineus ("white line") supporting the middle vagina.

Level 3: Includes the pubourethral and pubocervical ligaments supporting the lower vagina and posteriorly the perineal body.

Damage at different levels of vaginal support thus leads to different types of prolapse:

Level 1: Vault and uterovaginal prolapse,

Level 2: Cystocele and rectocele,

Level 3: Urethrocele and perineal body hypermobility. Therefore, treatment should aim to correct the specific anatomical defects in order to optimize outcome.

DIAGNOSIS

Prolapse is often asymptomatic and an incidental finding, and clinical examination may not necessarily correlate with symptoms. A comprehensive pelvic floor assessment should include a detailed history taking and POP physical examination that documents the maximum protrusion. There are validated pelvic organ prolapse questionnaires that may be used to assess patients' symptoms, bladder, bowel and sexual functions pre and postoperatively. There are specific questionnaires to address each of these functions separately.

In women with established POP, a standardized, validated system should be used. The traditional assessment tool is called Baden Walker Classification described in 1968. In this classification:

Level 1: Is described as prolapse extending half way to the hymen

Level 2: Extending to the hymen and

Level 3: Extending outside the hymen. This classification is simple and easy to follow but the drawback is that it is subjective. The POP-Q assessment was first described in 1996 (Fig. 25.2) and is more complex but objective, site specific, quantifiable and reproducible. This system is approved by International Continence Society and followed universally. There is still a 30 percent chance of under diagnosing prolapse in the clinic set up.

POP-Q SYSTEM

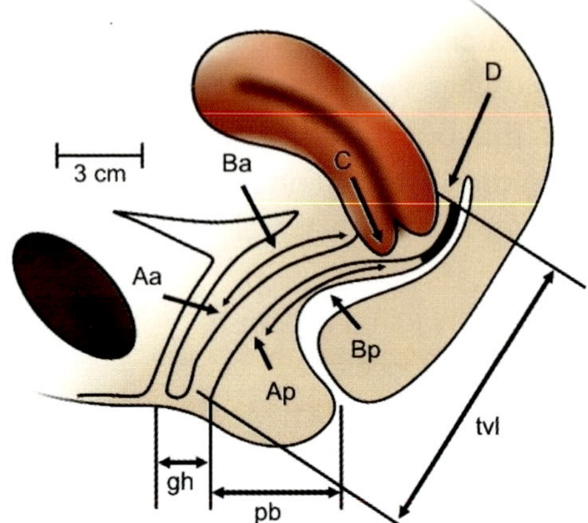

Fig. 25.2: POP-Q system

INVESTIGATIONS

Evaluation for research purposes is often different from evaluation of clinical care. While most of the clinical care worldwide is done by physical examination alone, additional tools are useful in complex patients and for research purposes. Some of these modalities are urodynamics and imaging.

URODYNAMICS

Urodynamic stress incontinence (USI) is diagnosed in 70-75 percent of these patients. Occult urodynamic stress incontinence (OUSI) is diagnosed in about 50 percent of the patients with genital prolapse not reporting stress incontinence before surgery. Performing urodynamic investigation in patients undergoing prolapse surgery may be valuable if diagnosing USI or OUSI results in the selection of the optimal treatment strategy. In women with severe prolapse ring pessary reduction of prolapse during urodynamics is useful to determine symptomatic and occult conditions.

IMAGING

Defecography or evacuation proctography is probably the most important imaging technique used in the assessment of POP. It is a study of voluntary bowel evacuation and therefore yields both anatomic and functional information. Traditionally defecography has mainly been used in the study of anorectal dysfunction as evacuation proctography. The equipment required includes a thick barium paste, a radiolucent toilet, and video equipment. Images are taken at rest, during straining effort, and during and after evacuation. Rectocoele is seen as an anterior rectal bulge and postevacuation barium trapping which may help to explain any evacuation dysfunction. It may suggest diagnosis of anismus as the main contributor to a patient's bowel dysfunction rather than rectocoele. The former is treated with biofeedback rather than surgery. An enterocoele is noted as a herniation of the small bowel into the cul-de-sac, into the vagina, rectovaginal space, or both.

ULTRASOUND

Over the recent years, there has been an interest in MRI and ultrasound of the pelvic floor using 3 D and quite a few papers have now been published. Using transperineal ultrasound, it is also possible to visualize the pelvic floor muscles in a dynamic fashion. CT scan also plays a role where there is any suspicion of associated pelvic pathology.

SURGICAL MANAGEMENT

There is no specific indication or standardization for treatment of POP. For the purpose of this chapter, we have restricted to mesh based pelvic reconstructive surgery. Since the introduction of the mesh over the last decade, there has been a steady increase in the types of mesh and different techniques associated with them. In this chapter, we discuss the transobturator mesh repair (Perigee) for anterior vaginal prolapse and transobturator sling (Monarc) and posterior defect specific repair.

TRANSOBTURATOR MESH (PERIGEE)

Instruments

- Perigee graft (large-pore polypropylene or a biologic porcine) has a tail that can be cut to fit the length of the patient's vagina and 4 arms that are attached to the pelvic sidewall.
- Needles used for anterior wall repair.

Procedure

- Patient is placed in modified lithotomy position.
- Local anesthetic can be injected into the anterior vaginal wall

- A midline skin incision is made and the bladder is dissected from the vaginal wall up to the bladder neck.
- The entry points for superior needles are marked at the lateral edge of the pubic ramus at the level of the clitoris just below the insertion of adductor longus tendon.
- The inferior needle entry points are also at the medial edge of the pubic ramus but at its inferior most point of the obturator foramen. The superior needles are identified by the pink color and the inferior needles are grey in color and sides are marked using arrows.
- The right superior needle is the first one to be inserted with the needle tip perpendicular to skin and handle positioned at 45°.
- The needle is advanced through the obturator muscle and membrane with gentle pressure and the needle tip should be palpated as it moves around the pubic ramus.
- The needle is then guided through the vaginal incision until the needle tip is through the incision.
- Before attaching the mesh, the mesh should be oriented so that the tail end is positioned down towards the table.
- The mesh is then attached to the needle tip and pulled through along with the sheath.
- The same is repeated on the other side.
- The right inferior needle is then passed with the needle perpendicular to the skin and the handle parallel to the vertical axis of the patient.
- The needle is then advanced through the obturator muscle and membrane.
- The needle handle is rotated upwards constantly palpating the tip of the needle until the handle is horizontal. The needle is then brought out in the vagina. Check should be made to detect fornicial puncture.
- The mesh is then attached to the needle tip and the mesh is pulled through.
- A Cystourethroscopy should be performed at this stage to ensure no mesh through the bladder or urethra.
- The mesh should be positioned to lie flat.
- Excess mesh should be trimmed.
- Skin closed with absorbable sutures.

Posterior Defect Specific Repair

- Patient positioning.
- Local anesthetic to skin.

- A midline incision on the posterior vaginal wall.
- Rectum dissected off the vaginal wall.
- The rectovaginal septum is identified at the lower end of the posterior vaginal wall.
- The septum is then attached to the iliococcygeus muscle on the lateral vaginal wall bilaterally using 2-0 PDS.
- A per rectal examination is performed to ensure no suture material is through the rectum.
- Skin is closed with absorbable sutures.

TRANSOBTURATOR SLING (MONARC)

- Patient positioned in open lithotomy position.
- Empty the bladder.
- Recommend local anesthetic injection into the anterior vaginal wall at the level of the midurethra.
- A 2 cm incision is made on the skin extending from about 1 cm from the external urethral meatus.
- Para urethral tunnels should be created.
- The Monarc needles are blue in color and sides can be identified by the direction of the arrow.
- The right needle is usually placed first with the handle at 45° and passed through gently around the pubic ramus.
- The tip of the needle should be felt through the vaginal incision and be guided through the incision.
- Ensure the fornices are clear and the sling is attached after orientation.
- The same is repeated on the other side too.
- Recommend check Cystourethroscopy for beginners.
- The sling should be placed relatively loose so as to avoid any voiding problems in postoperatively.
- Skin closed with absorbable sutures.

Postoperative Care

- Ensure adequate analgesia
- Postoperative antibiotics for 5 days
- Ensure spontaneous voiding with a trial of voiding prior to discharge
- Vaginal estrogen may be prescribed postoperatively.

Tips **in the Management of Pelvic Prolapse**

- *Anatomy*
  a. Surgeons should be familiar with the pelvic anatomy
  b. Bony landmarks: ischial spine, adductor longus tendon and ischial tuberosity
- *Patient positioning*
  a. Flexion of the hip by 45° decreases the incidence of perioperative neuropathy
  b. Avoid hyperflexion to prevent hip pain
- *To minimize mesh exposure*
  a. Preoperative (more than 2 fold decrease in mesh extrusion) and postoperative oestrogen cream
  b. Full thickness vaginal dissection
  c. Minimal vaginal skin excision
- *Minimize dyspareunia*
  a. Place the mesh tension free
  b. Ensure that mesh lies flat and not bunched up
  c. Release any bands of tissue under tension
- *Combined procedures*
  a. If performing Perigee and Monarc at the same time, leave the upper arms of the plastic sheaths of Perigee in situ and perform Monarc. Remove the sheaths of both Perigee and Monarc at the end
- *Mesh exposure management*
  a. Vaginal oestrogen
  b. Trimming in the clinic
  c. Excise only the exposed mesh
  d. Tension free suturing of the vaginal skin
- *Preventing complications*
  a. Preoperative evaluation
  b. Antibiotic prophylaxis
  c. Compression devices and/or clexane
  d. Patient positioning
- *Postoperative care*
  a. Early ambulation
  b. Pain control
  c. Trial of voiding
  d. Postoperative antibiotics/oestrogen
- *Avoid adductor* longus tendon to minimize groin pain
- If in doubt, take it out! (this applies to needles of monarc or perigee)
- Ensure objective and subjective follow up for up to three years.

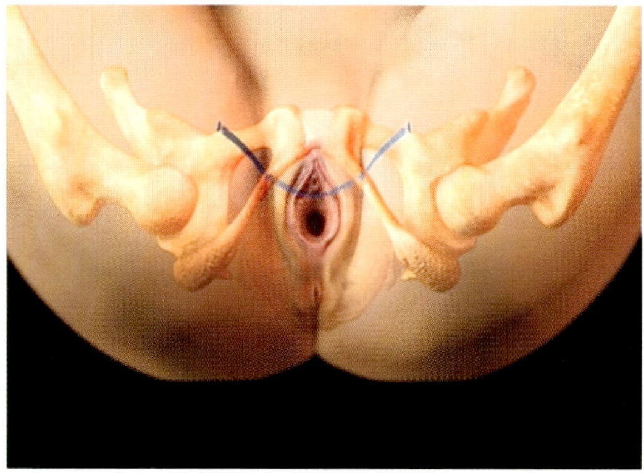

Fig. 25.3: Monarc

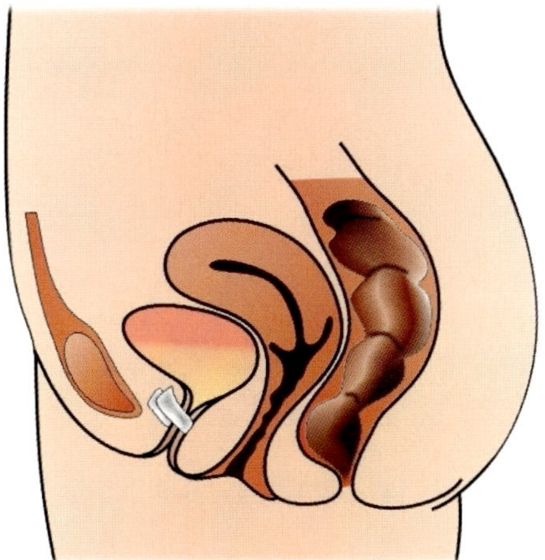

Fig. 25.4: Monarc

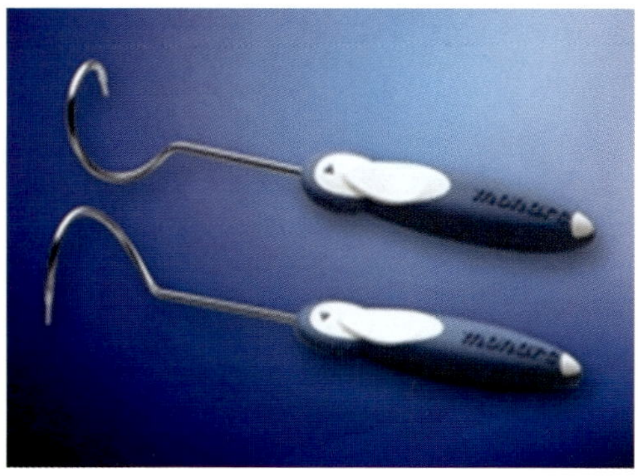

Fig. 25.5: Monarc

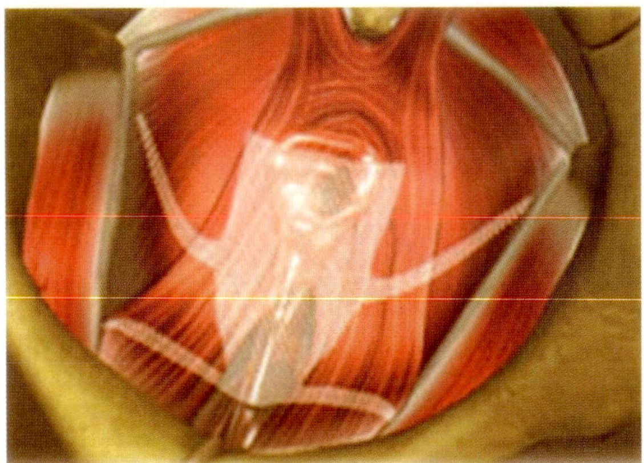

Fig. 25.6: Perigee

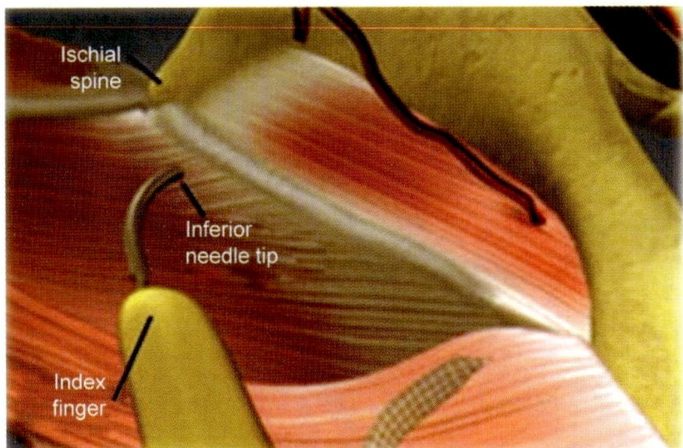

Fig. 25.7: Perigee

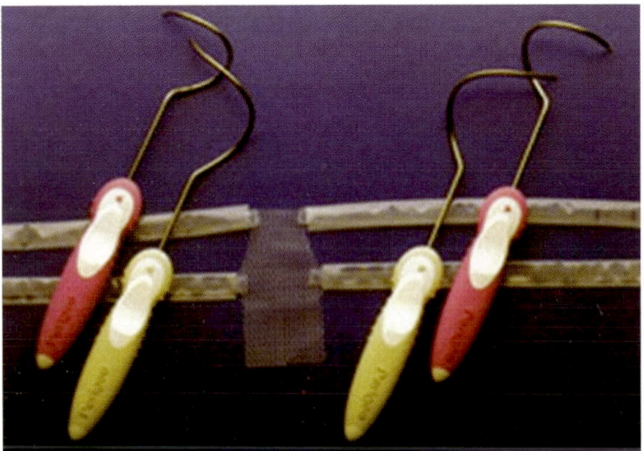

Fig. 25.8: Perigee

(Photographs courtesy: Prof Ajay Rane)

PREOPERATIVE EVALUATION

- Confirmation of diagnosis on table with full bladder. Bonney's and Marshall Marchetti test may help to give prognostic value of surgery.
- Urine routine, culture and sensitivity.
- Urodynamic studies.

PREOPERATIVE PREPARATION

- It is preferred to do the procedure in immediate post-menstrual period.
- Insert a urethral catheter with aseptic precautions to keep the bladder empty.
- Anesthesia - can be carried out under local/regional/general

IMPORTANT EQUIPMENTS

- TVT Obturator device
- TVT Helical Passers
- TVT Atraumatic Winged Guide
  (All come together in disposable packet)

PROCEDURE

- Position of the patient - dorsal lithotomy with hyperflexed hips over the abdomen and buttocks should be positioned flushed with the edge of the table. This position is very important as it gives better access to obturator membrane.
- Marking of the exit point - an imaginary horizontal line is drawn at the level of the urethral meatus and second line drawn parallel and 2 cm above the first line. Locate the exit point on the 2nd line 2 cm lateral to the folds of thighs. 5 mm incision may be made at each exit point at this stage or may be later.

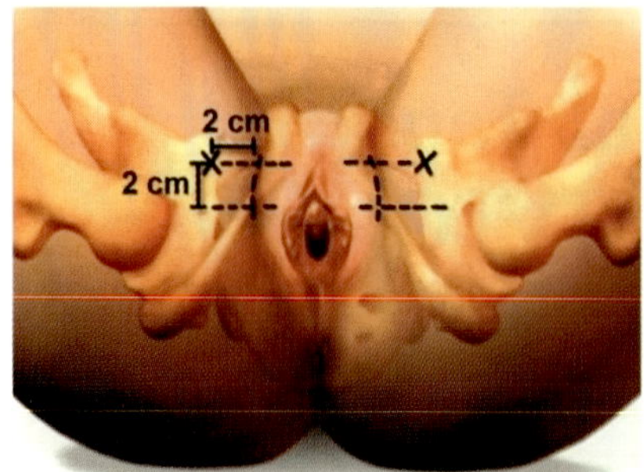

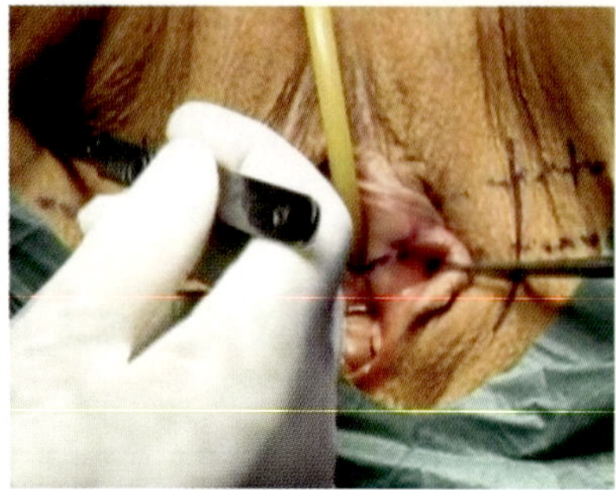

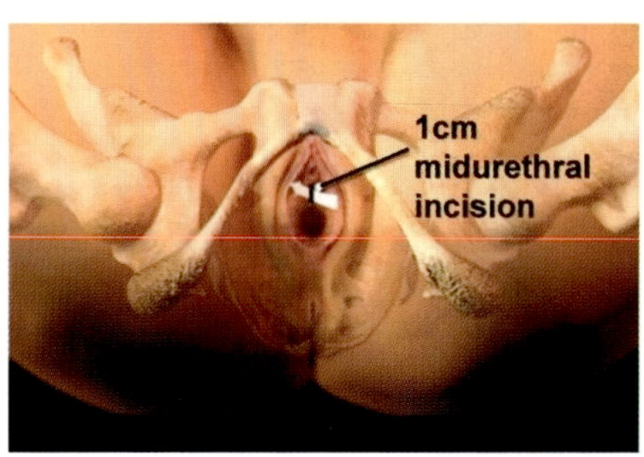

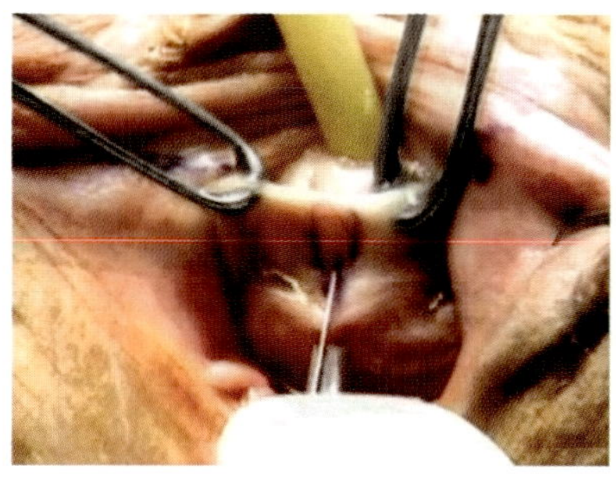

- Midline vaginal incision of 1 cm is made on the middle 1/3rd of the urethra (1 cm proximal to the external urethral meatus)
- With the help of pointed curved scissors, sharp dissection is done by using a 'push spread technique' through a path (should be approximately 5-7 mm in diameter and no deeper than 5 cm) which is as follows:

  1. First piercing the superior surface of perineal membrane and traveling underway from dorsal nerve of clitoris.

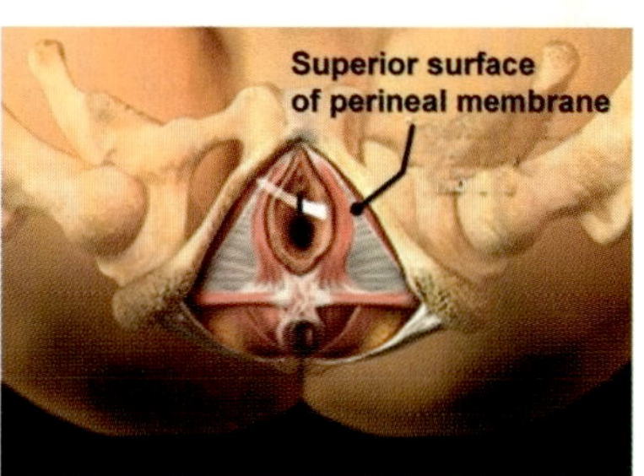

  2. Pathway continues through para-urethral connective tissue (path of lateral dissection should be oriented at a 45° angle towards the medial edge of the obturator foramen) towards inferior pubic ramus and origin of pubococcygeous and pubo-rectalis muscle.

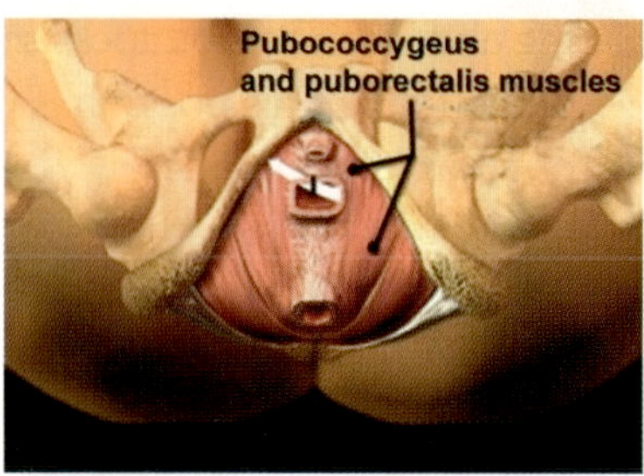

3. This continues below arcus tendinous, levator ani, obturator internus muscle through connective tissue and fat of the anterior recess of ischio-anal fossa, laterally along the inferior pubic ramus (Dissection beyond 5 cm may allow unintended entry into the retro pubic space).

4. When the junction between the body of pubic bone and inferior pubic ramus is reached, loss of resistance is felt when obturator membrane is perforated.

5. Path continues through obturator externus muscle, adductor magnus and brevis and the upper margin of gracilis muscle followed by fascia lata, subcutaneous tissue and skin at the exit point (which was marked previously).

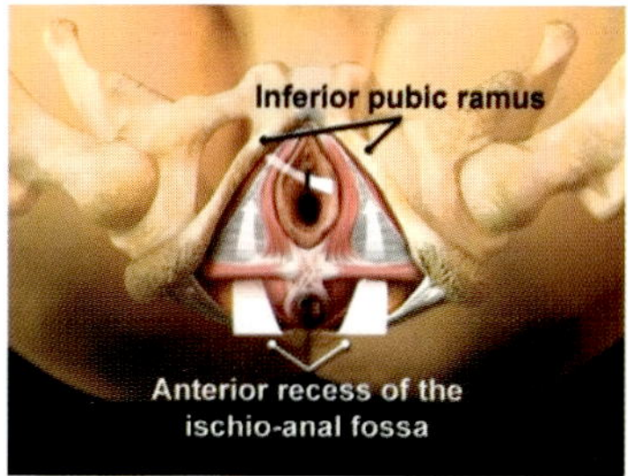

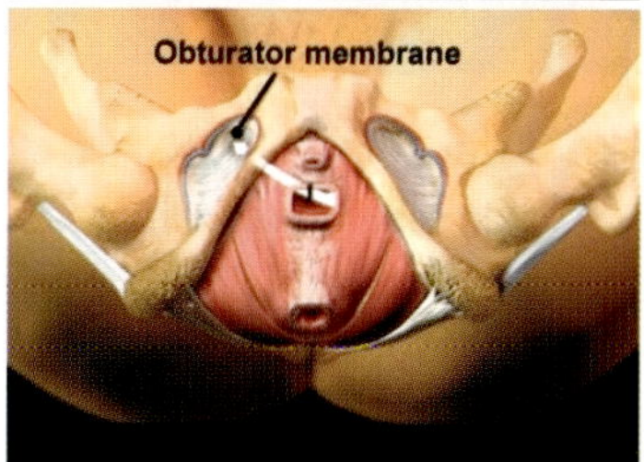

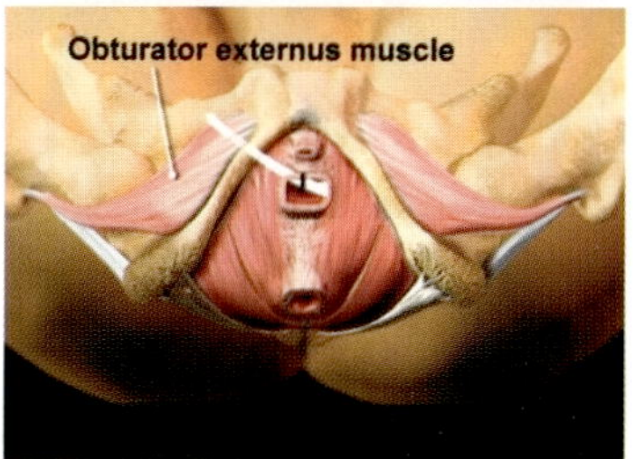

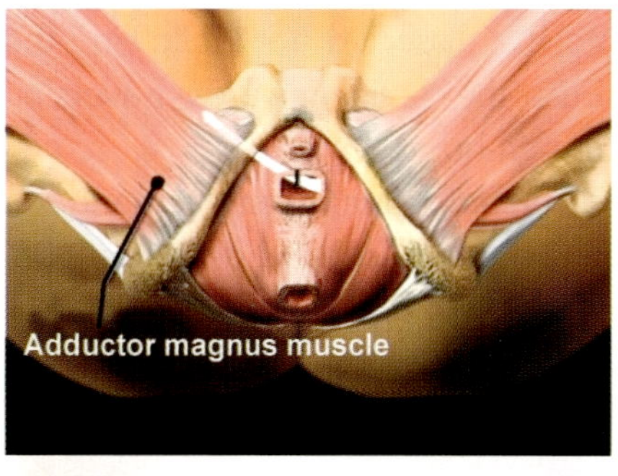

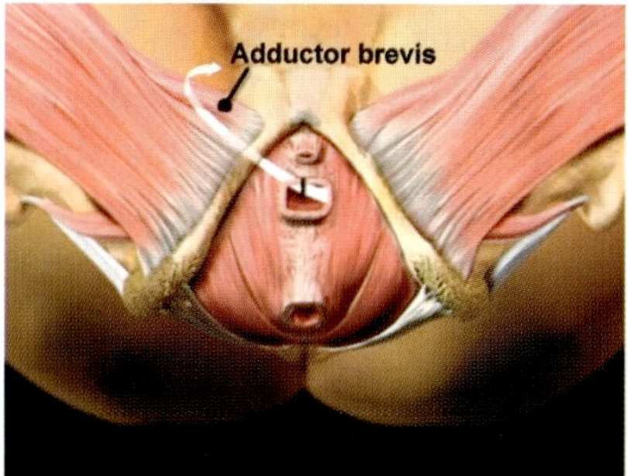

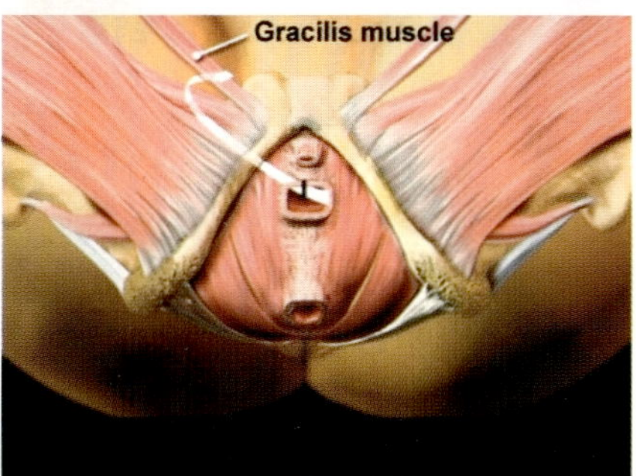

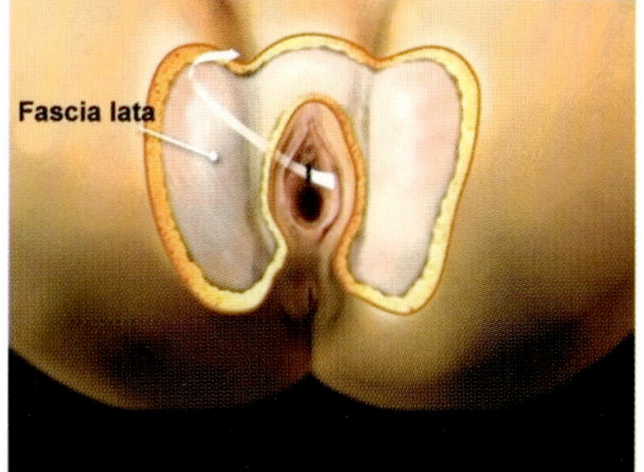

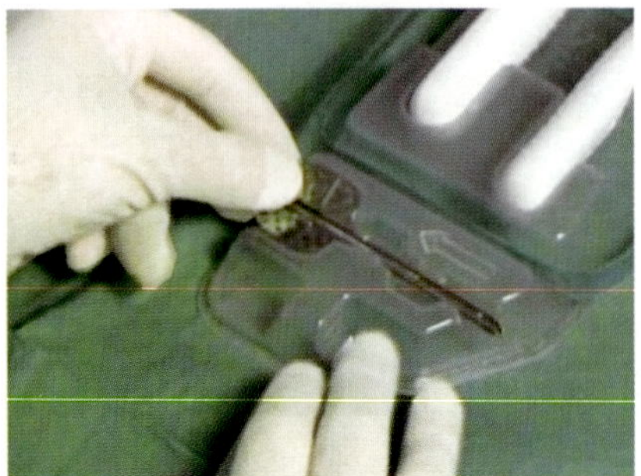
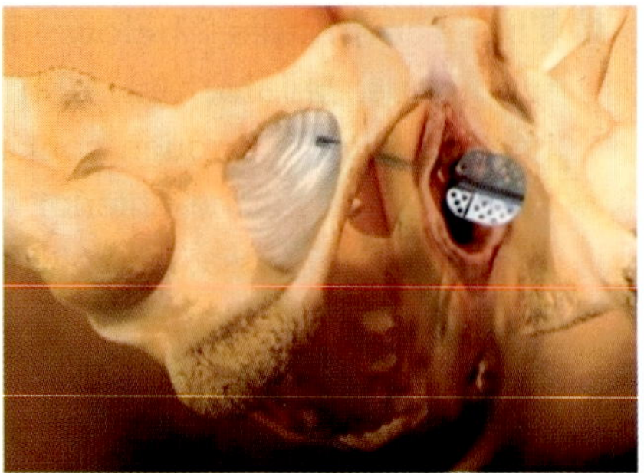

6. Insert the TVT winged guide into the dissected tract (after removing from the pack with aseptic precautions). If difficulty is encountered, reconfirm the direction of the tract with scissors.

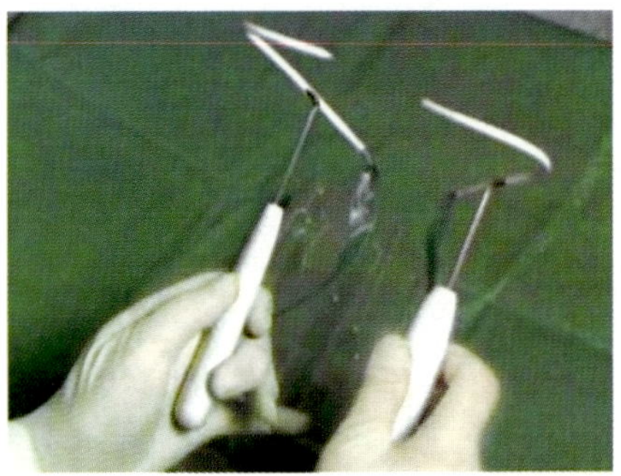
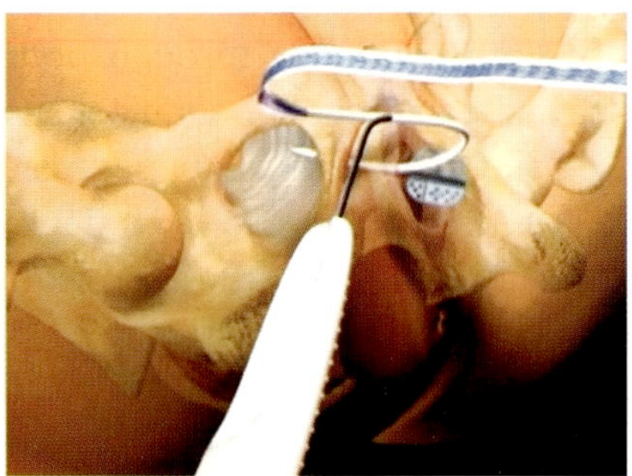

7. Insert the TVT helical passer into the dissected tract following the channel of TVT winged guide. Push the device inwards, traversing and slightly passing the obturator membrane.

8. Once in the above position, TVT winged guide is removed and the handle of the helical passer is moved towards the midline, until the handle is vertical to the floor.

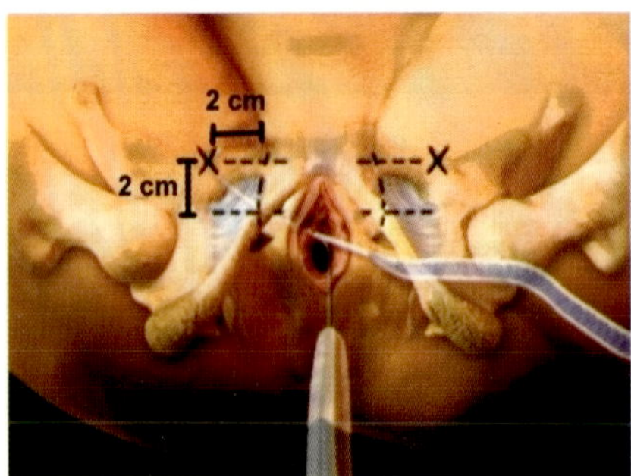

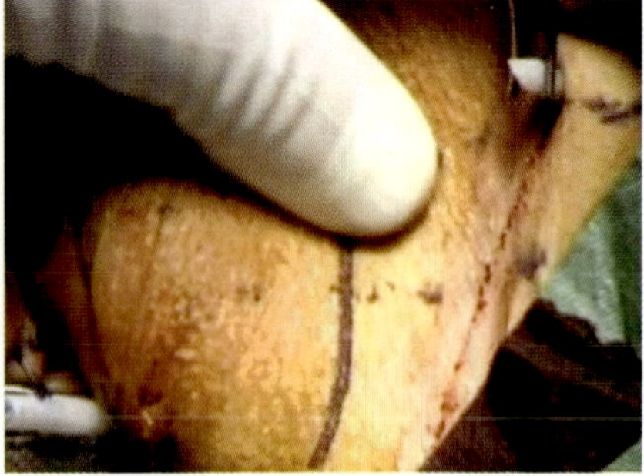

9. The point of the helical passer should exit near the previously determined exit points. When the tip of the plastic tube appears at the

skin opening, grasp the pointed tip of the plastic tube with a clamp while stabilizing the tube near urethra with thumb, remove the helical passer by a reverse rotation of the handle.

10. Pull the plastic tube completely through the skin until the tape appears.
11. Repeat the above technique on the other side, ensuring that the tape lies flat under the urethra.

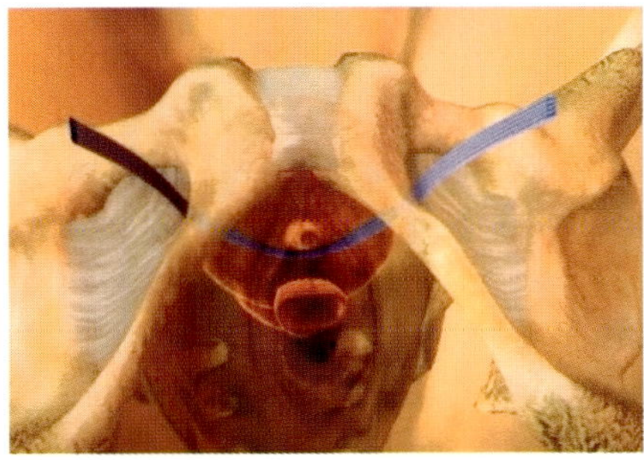
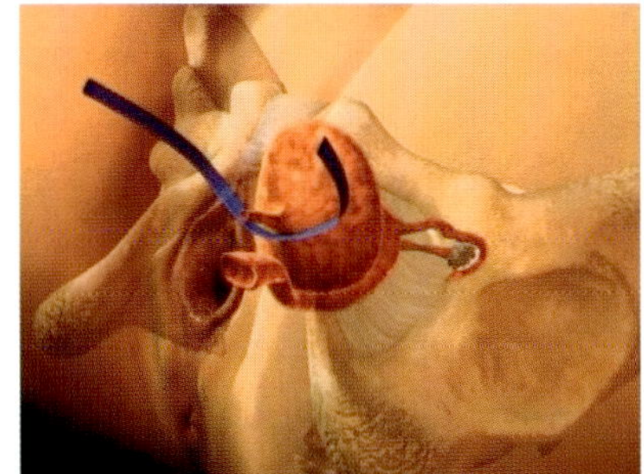

12. When both tubes have been extracted, through the skin incision, cut the plastic tubes from the tape and plastic sheath. Cough test can be performed at this stage which allows adjustment of the tape so that only a few drops of urine are lost during the cough.

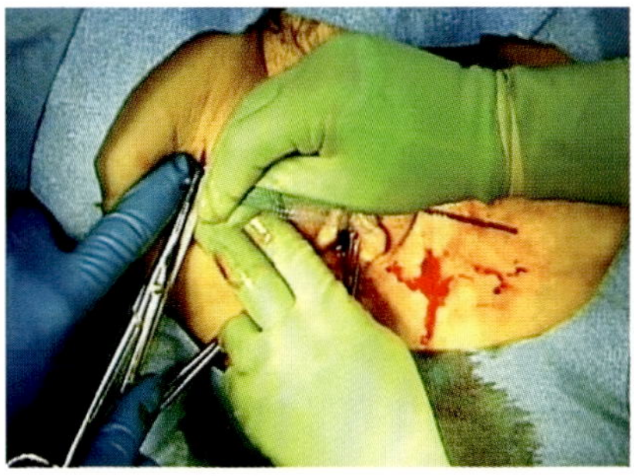

13. Remove the plastic sheath that covers the tapes.
14. Close the vaginal and skin incision.

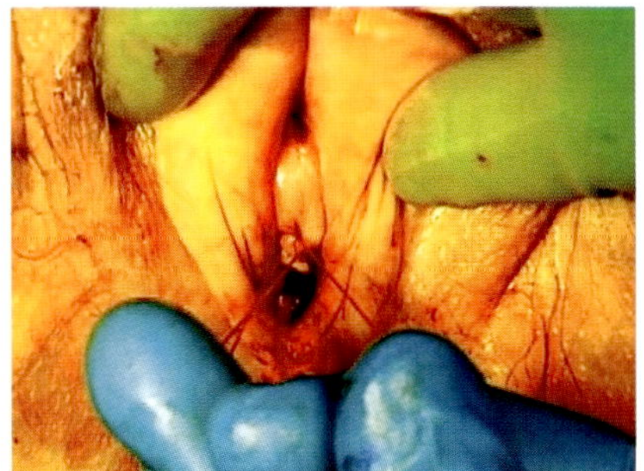

TIPS

- Dissection beyond 5 cm should be avoided as it will give unintended entry into space of Retzius.
- The open site of winged guide should always be facing the surgeon so that bendable tab can be bent to increase the length of the guide, (originally 6 cm) to 7 cm, if needed.
- Device insertion to be completed on one side before beginning the dissection on the other side.
- Ensure correct orientation of the helical passers and tape by identifying logo and thumb indent on the plastic handle, which should be facing surgeon. The helical passer in the surgeon's left handle must be used on the patient's right side.
- Never allow the handle of the helical passer to be oriented horizontal to the floor.
- Position of the tape should be loose without tension and flat under the mid-urethra.
- Blunt instrument like a scissor/forceps can be placed between the urethra and the tape during removal of plastic sheath to avoid tension over the sheath. Overcorrection (i.e. too much tension) may cause temporary or permanent lower urinary tract obstruction.
- Cystoscopy can be performed at the discretion of the surgeon.

(Photographs Courtesy: Gynecare, Johnson and Johnson)

TRANSOBTURATOR TAPE

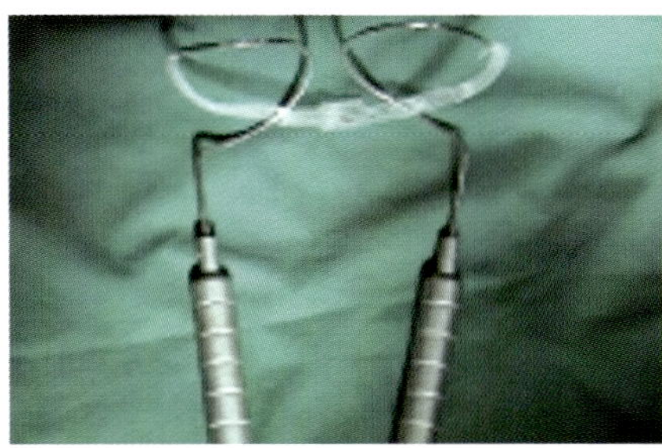

Tr-O tape and needle

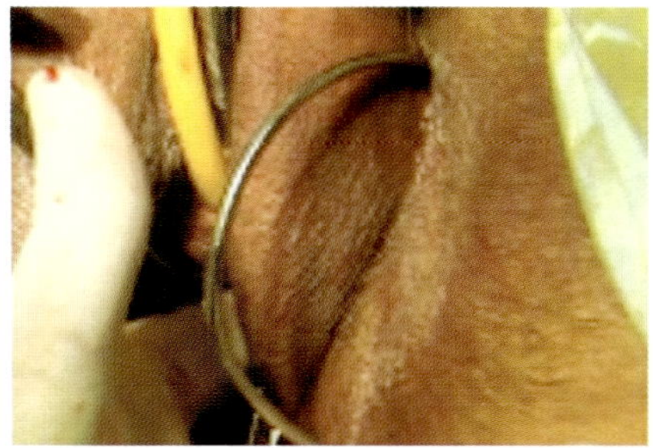

Left needle insertion at the upper and medial most area of obturation parameter

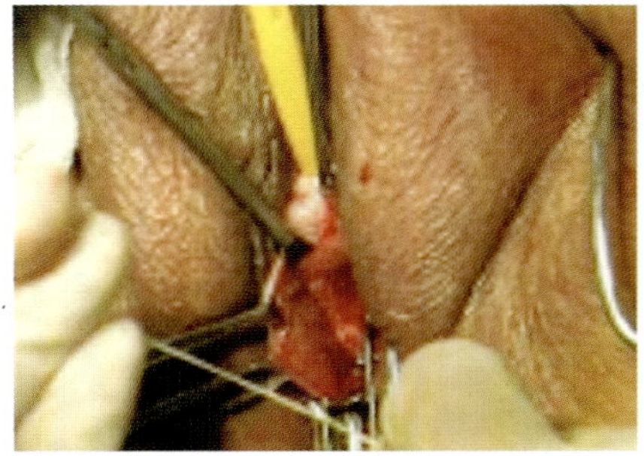

Needle seen coming out below the mid urethra

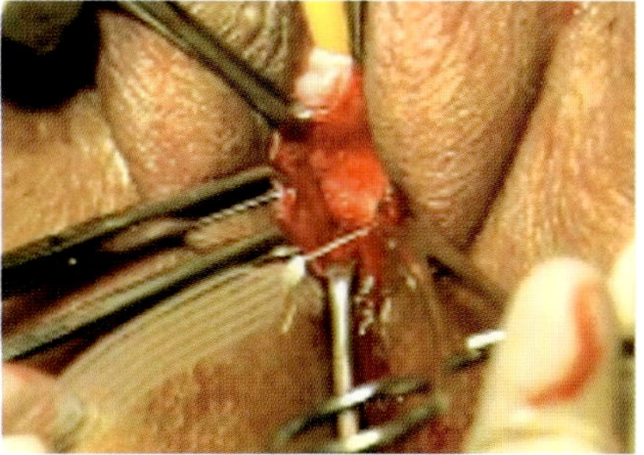

Loading of Tr-O tape on the TrOt needle's eye

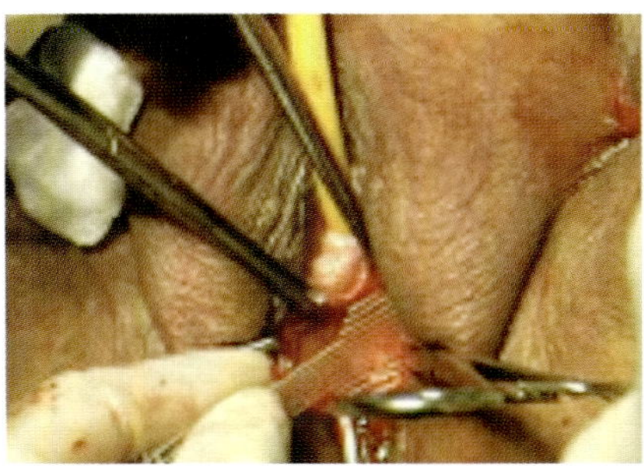

Withdrawing the TrOT needle pulling the TrOT sling

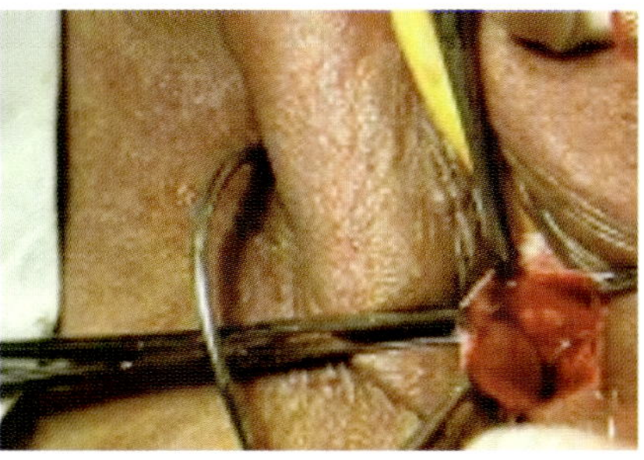

Right TrOT needle insertion

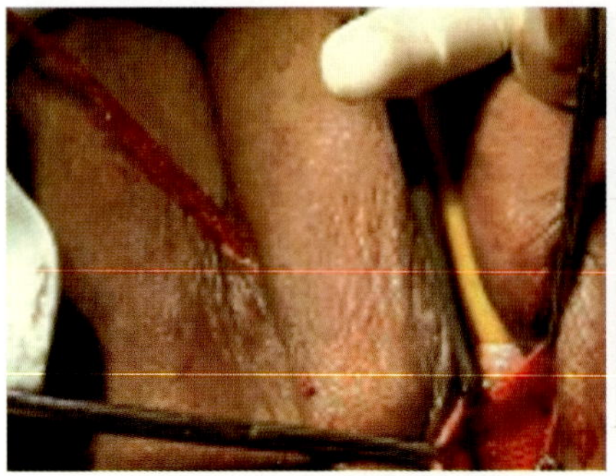

TrOT seen pulled out of the obturator foramen with tension free suburethral placement

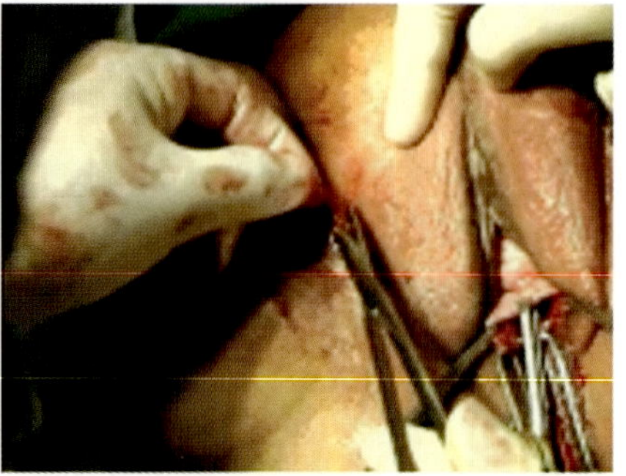

Cutting the extra tape at skin level

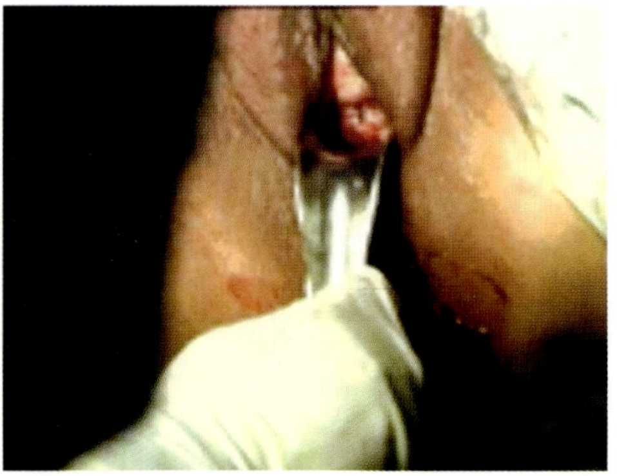

Final view after vaginal incision closure

(Photographs courtesy: Dr Prakash Trivedi)

T-SUIT

Dynamic Sling action of T-SUIT on muscle contraction

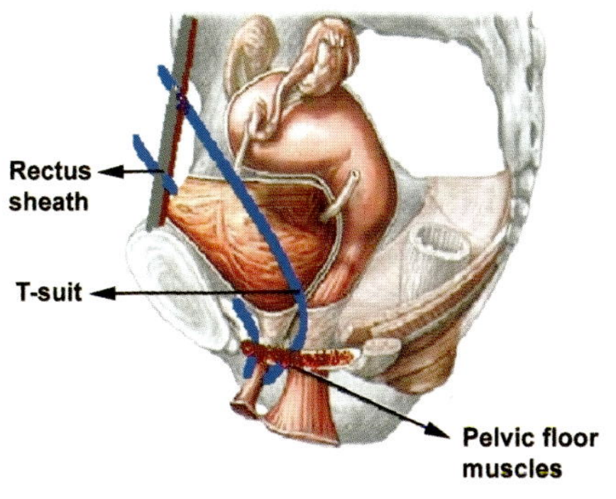

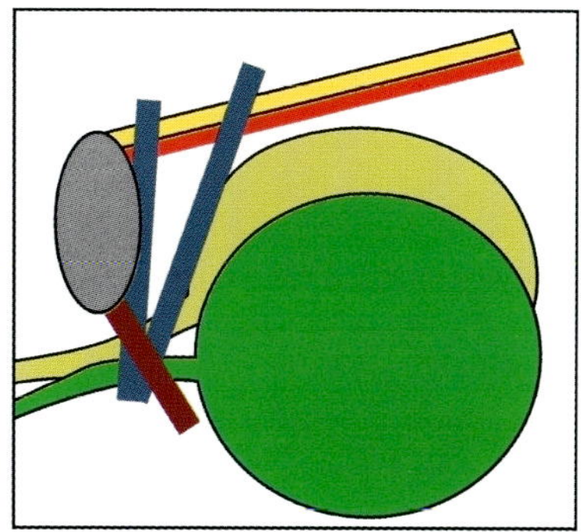

Narrowing of tape at pelvic floor and rectus

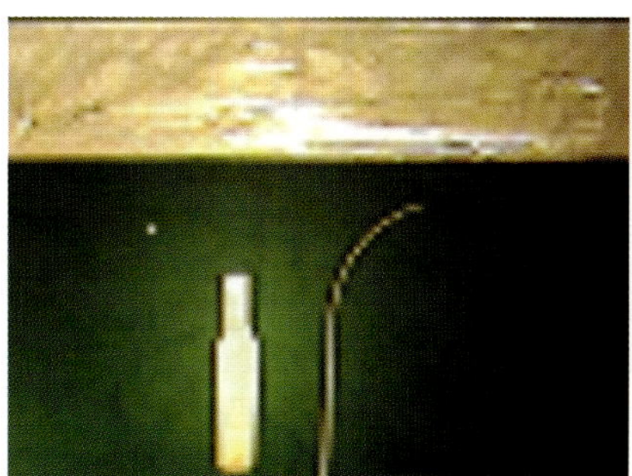

T-SUIT handle, needle and tape

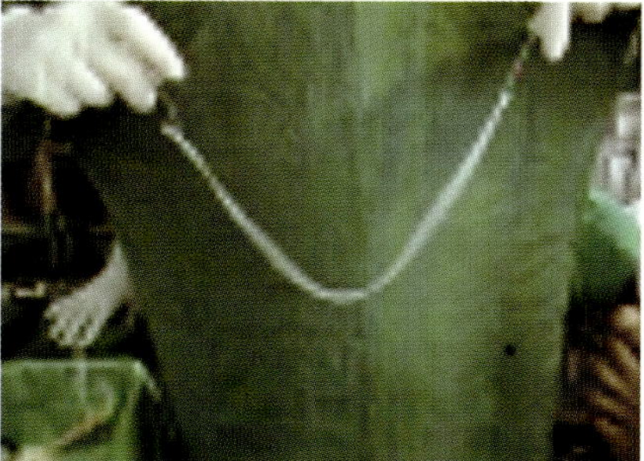

T-SUIT tape

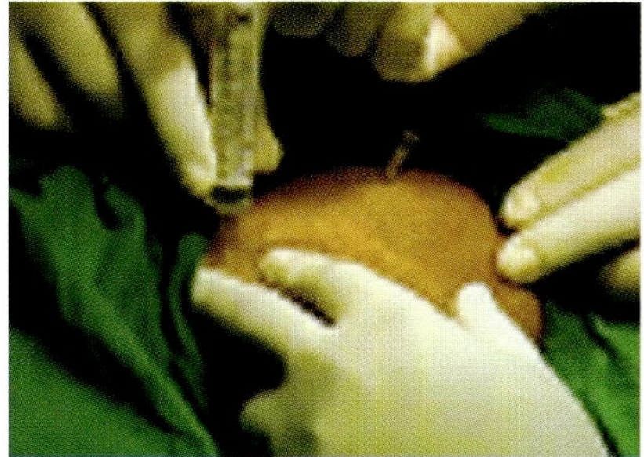

Suprapubic infiltration of 10-15 ml
2% lignocaine with adrenaline
3 cm lateral to the midline

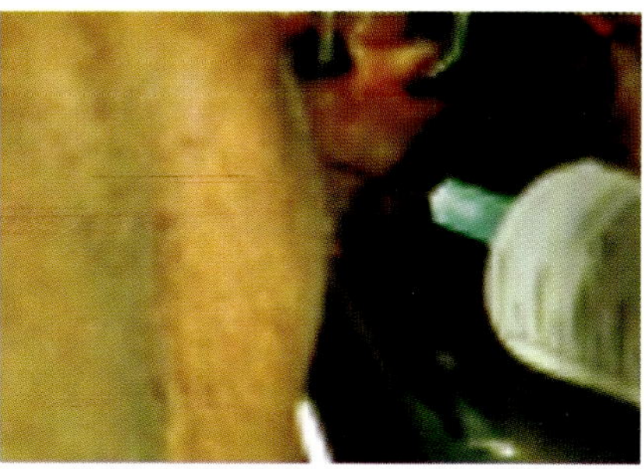

Anterior vaginal wall infiltration and
then 1.5 cm vertical vaginal incision
is made 1.5 cm from the
external urethral meatus

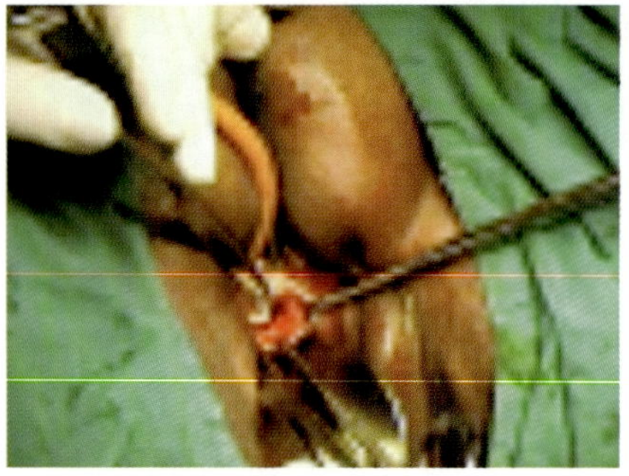

Para urethral dissection

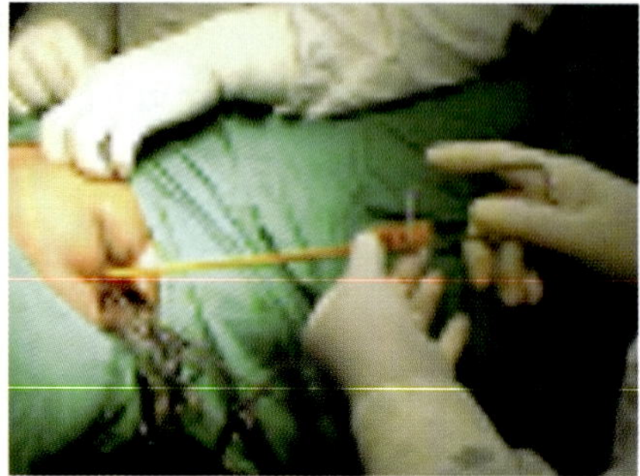

Insertion of metal guide
and pushing bladder neck

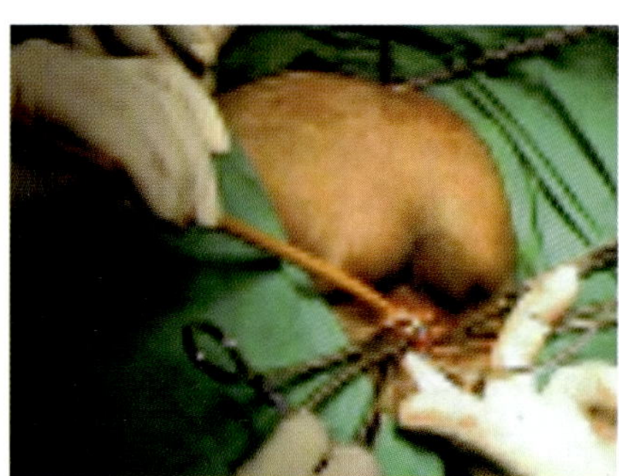

Insertion of left and right T-SUIT needles

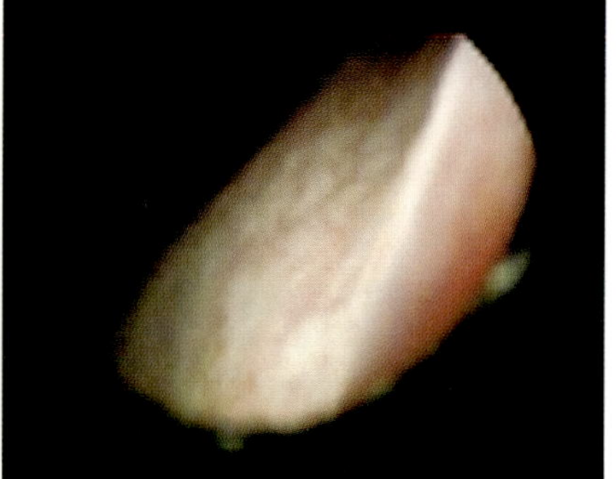

70° hysteroscopy/cystoscopy to
confirm correct placement of needles

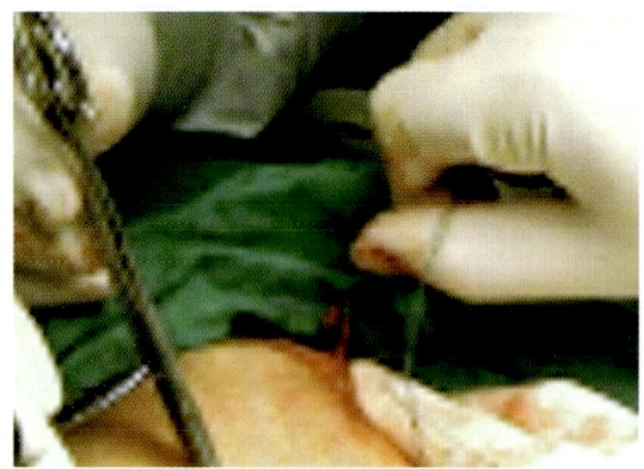

Pulling of left tape

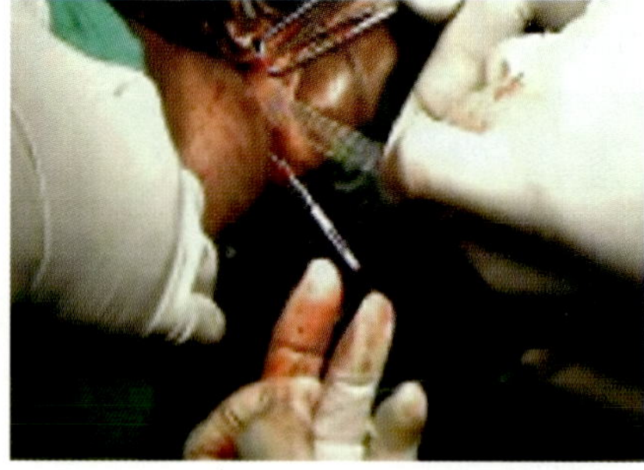

Loading of the sutures of T-SUIT

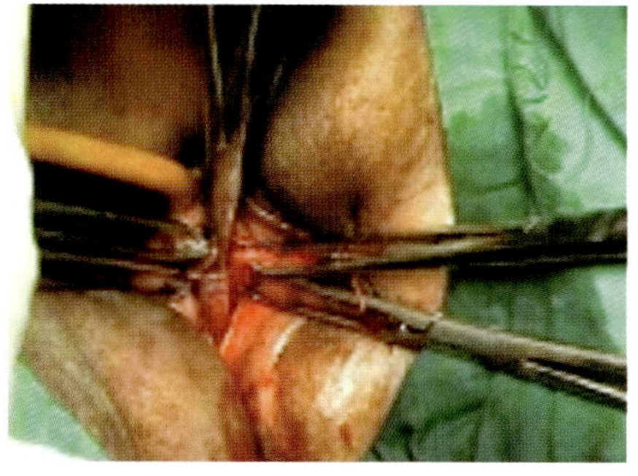

Tension free positioning of
T-SUIT with long artery forceps

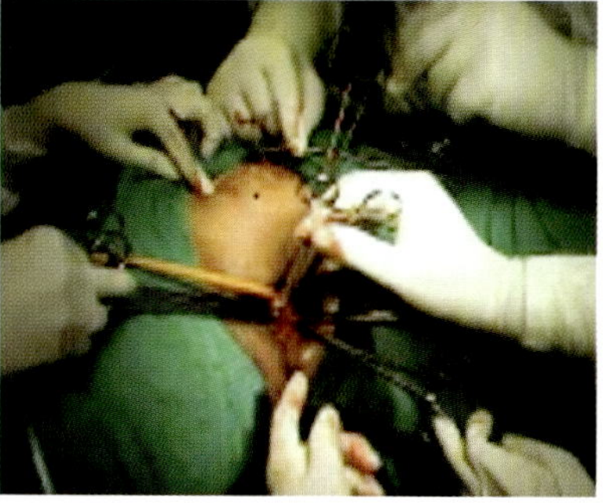

Both tapes pulled abdominally

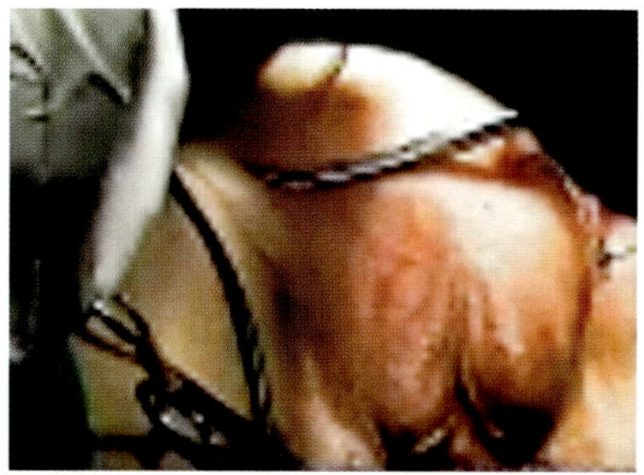

Cutting of the tape close to skin

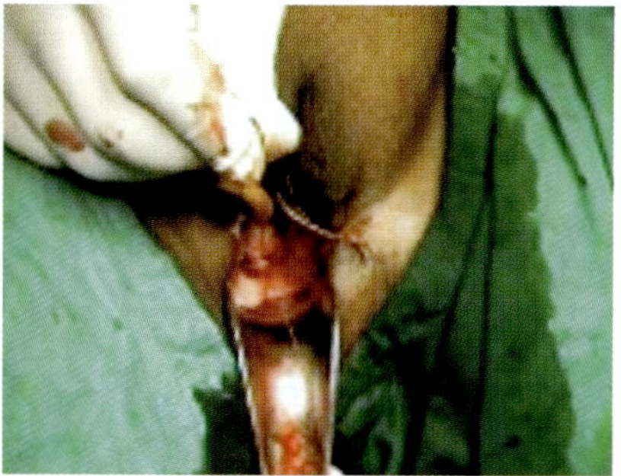

Closure of vagina

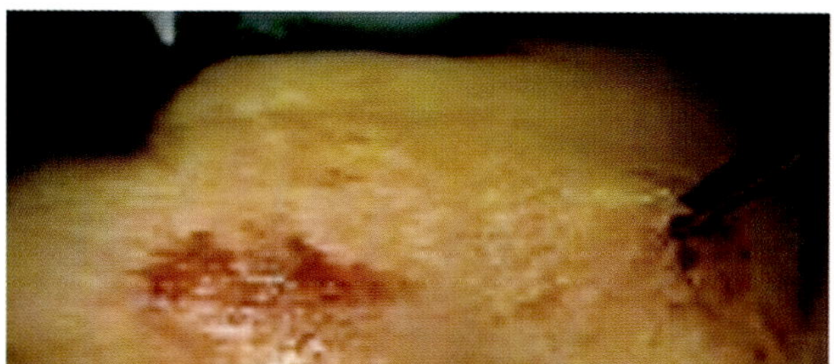

Sites of tapes after cutting

(Photographs courtesy: Dr Prakash Trivedi)

Section Five

Unusual Cases

Uterus Didelphys with Abnormally Placed Ovaries

30 years old female with primary infertility came to Ruby Hall IVF/ Endoscopy Center for evaluation.

TVS revealed uterus didelphys and inability to visualize the ovaries. Transabdominal USG revealed huge multicystic ovaries of approximately 10 × 15 cm each in lumbar region (as she had taken 3 cycles of clomiphene citrate outside). Findings were confirmed on MRI.

Patient was evaluated laparohysteroscopically- Uterus Didelphys confirmed. Both the ovaries were found in paracolic gutters and were multicystic (cysts ranging from 4-6 cm). Cysts were punctured. Ovaries could not be mobilized or transfixed in the pelvic region due to extremely short infundibulopelvic ligaments.

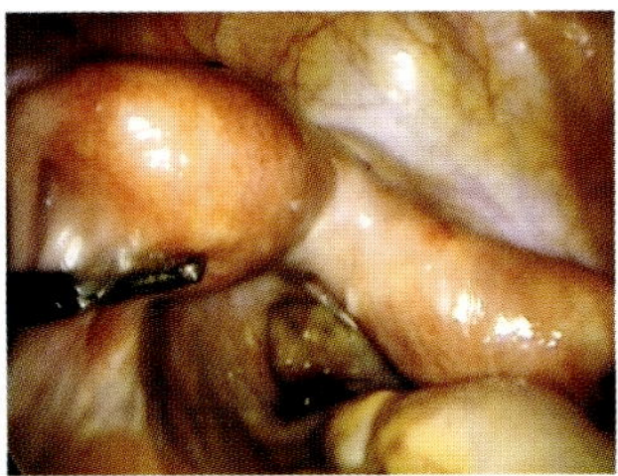

Didelphic uterus with absent ovaries in pelvis

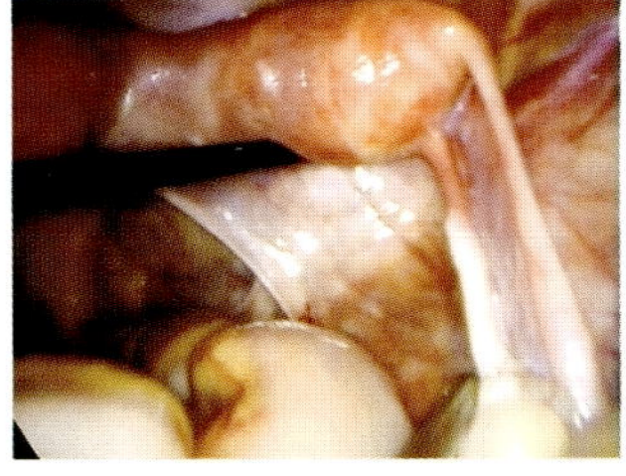

Lengthened right ovarian ligament

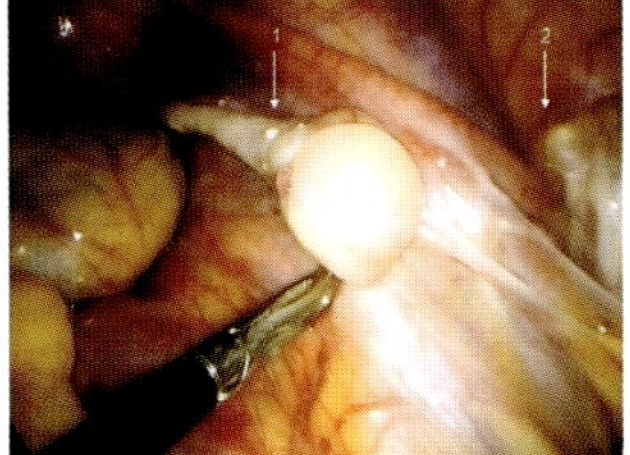

1 → small cyst at pelvic brim
2 → remaining right ovary in the lumbar region

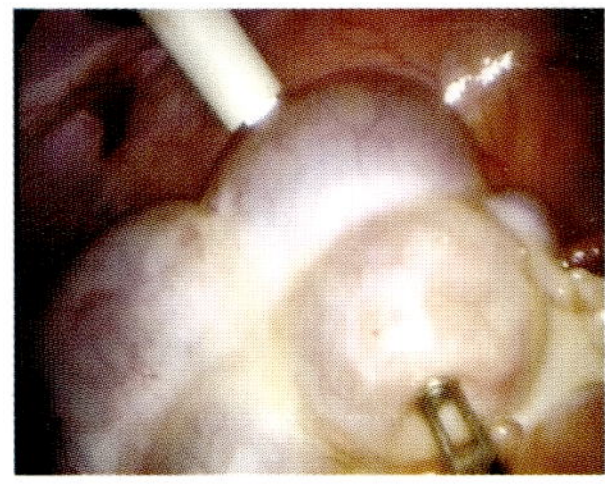

Panaromic view of left ovary

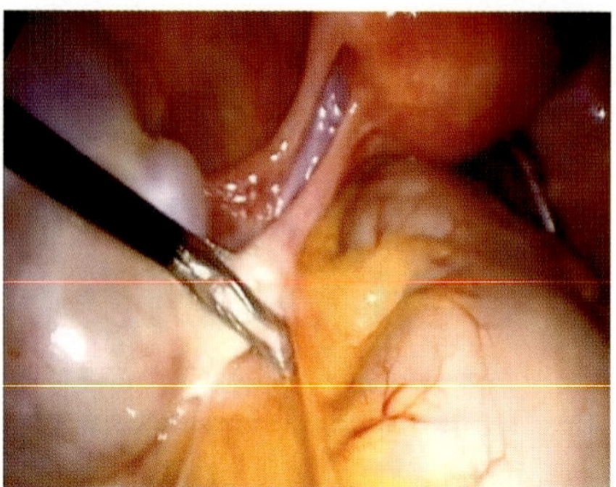

Left ovary in left paracolic gutter

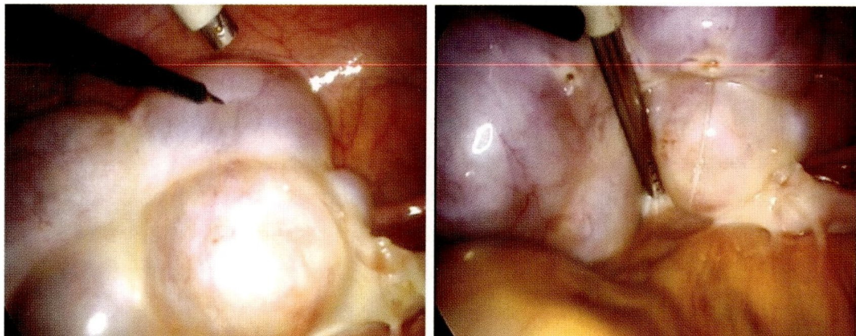

Drilling of cysts

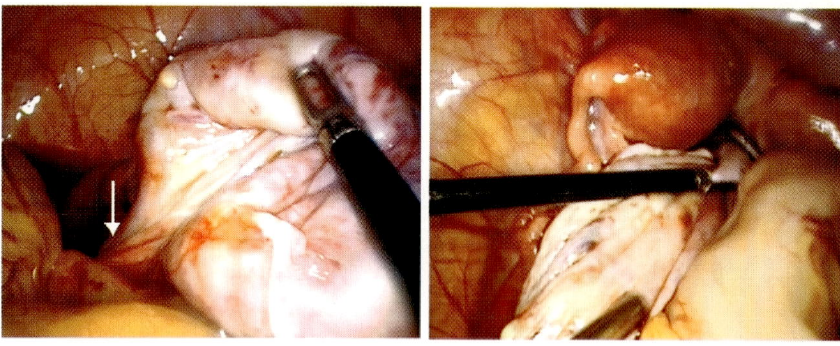

Short infundibulopelvic ligament   Collapsed left ovary

(Photographs courtsey: Ruby Hall IVF and Endoscopy Centre)

28   Case of Chronic Twisted Adnexa

A 30-year-old female had torsion of right adnexa. Patient refused surgical intervention and was managed with painkillers and serial USG and color Doppler studies. Over a period of time, the hydrosalpinx resolved and the ovary came back to normal size. But throughout, she had dragging pain in the lower abdomen. After 4 months, patient gave consent for laparoscopic evaluation.

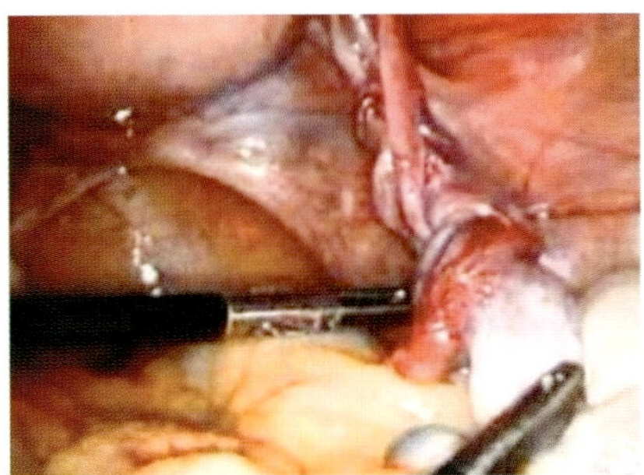

Twisted right adnexa

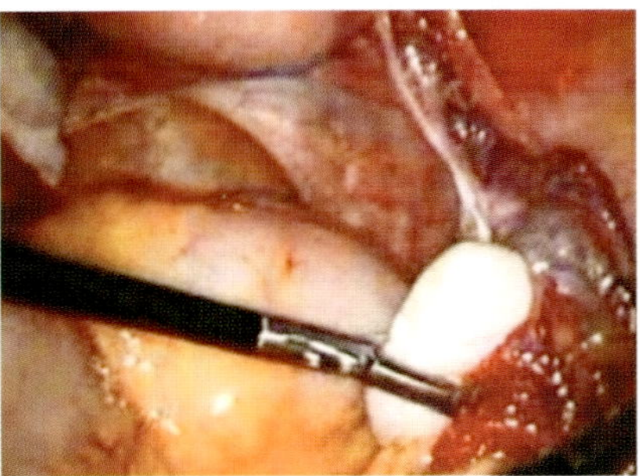

Detorsion done. Note the lengthening of the right ovarian ligament

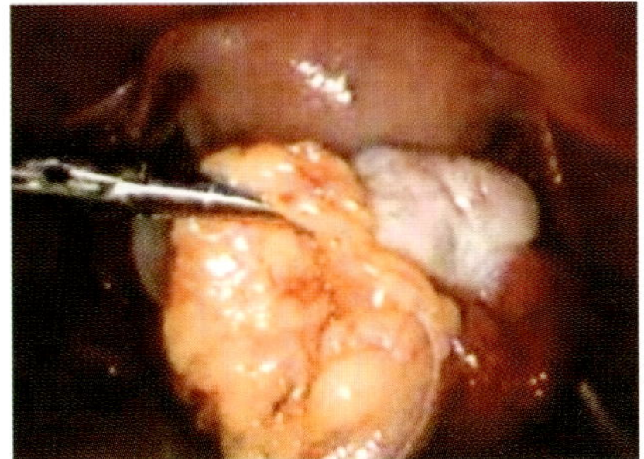

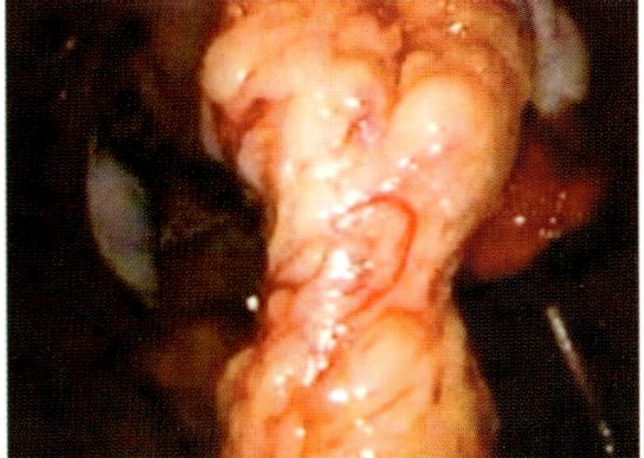

Omentum adherent to the lower pole of right ovary and twisted like a rope.

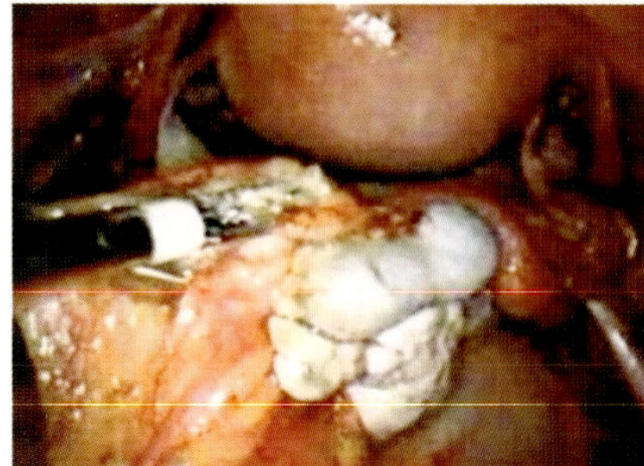 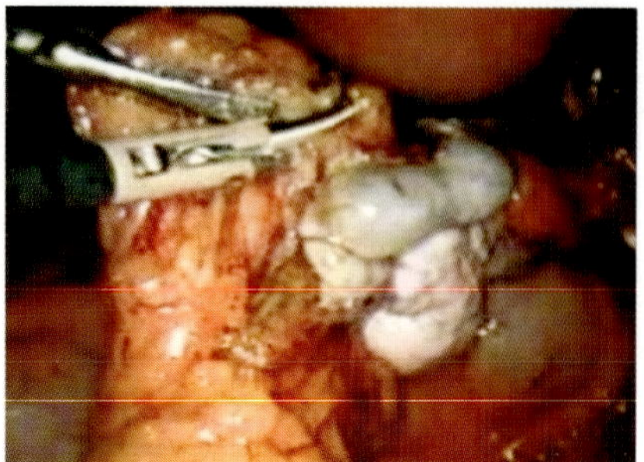

Omentum released from the lower pole of the ovary, keeping small portion
adherent to it, to be utilized later for anchoring it back to its ligament

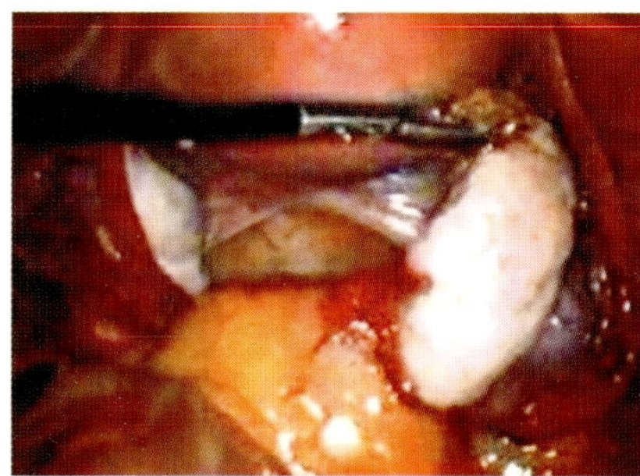 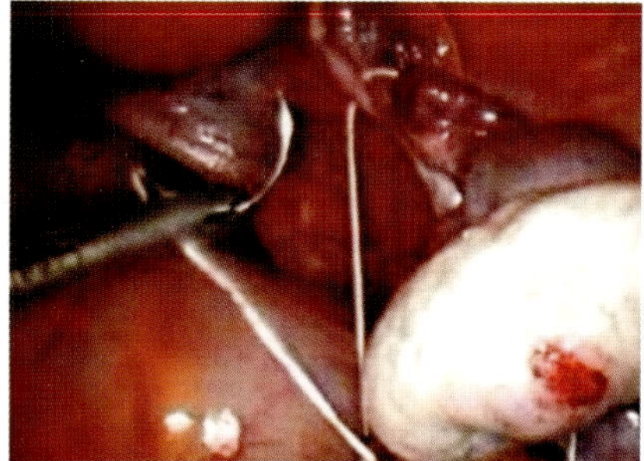

Ovary taken back in pelvis and sutured with nonabsorbable
suture material- Gortex

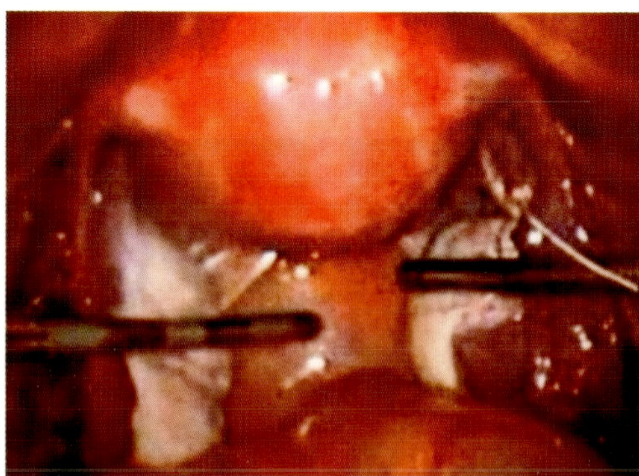

End result

(Photographs courtsey: Ruby Hall IVF and Endoscopy Centre)

29 27 Years Female with Bad Obstetric History with Unicornuate Uterus

27-year-old female has a bad obstetric history with recurrent abortions/ preterm deliveries between 12-24 weeks, last 2 abortions at 24 weeks inspite of cervical encirclage. She was diagnosed to have unicornuate uterus. The only alternative for her was to increase intrauterine capacity.

So we decided to perform metroplasty on her so as to convert tubular cavity into triangular one.

Patient was put on Tab Premarin 1.250 mg, 6 weeks + Duphastan 20 mg for latter 4 weeks.

Second look hysteroscopy was performed after 6 weeks to see the outcome of surgery.

It showed very good cavity with increased intrauterine capacity.

Patient conceived after 4 months and could continue pregnancy till 35 weeks.

We have performed 7 cases like this and quite satisfied with the results.

This surgery is not recommended for infertility.

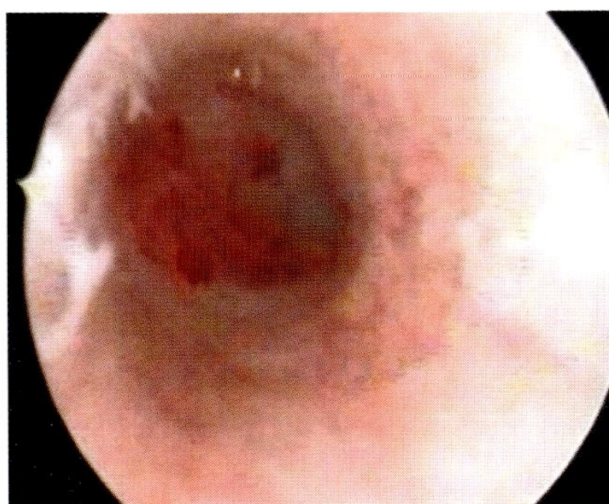

Unicornuate uterus

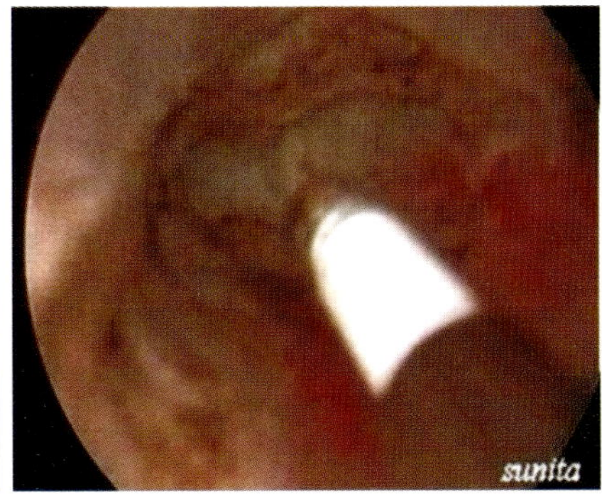

Metroplasty done with versa point so as to increase intrauterine capacity

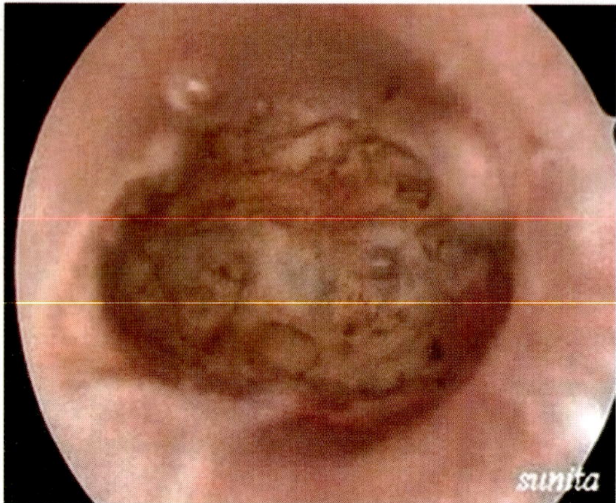

Good cavity formed as an end result

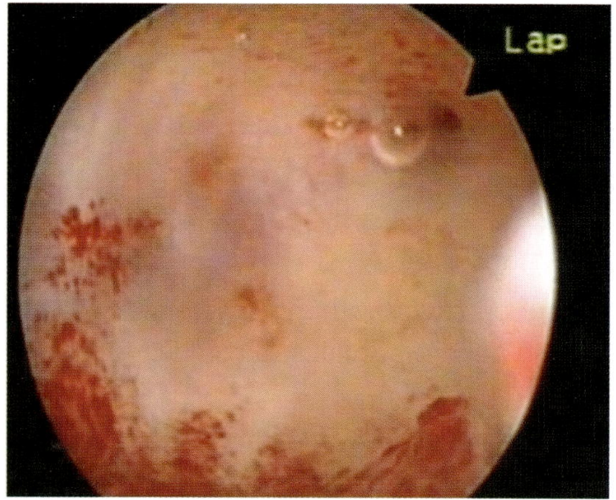

Second look hysteroscopy done after 6 weeks

(Photographs courtesy: Ruby Hall IVF and Endoscopy Centre)

Case of
Ovarian Fibroma

A patient schedule for Open Myomectomy and Laparoscopy done in view of age and future fertility. A large solid ovarian mass of 12.3 cm was identified the other ovary was normal. Oophorectomy done with 5 mm vessel sealing device. Specimen removed by electronic morcellator and histopath revealed ovarian fibroma. Postoperative period uneventful.

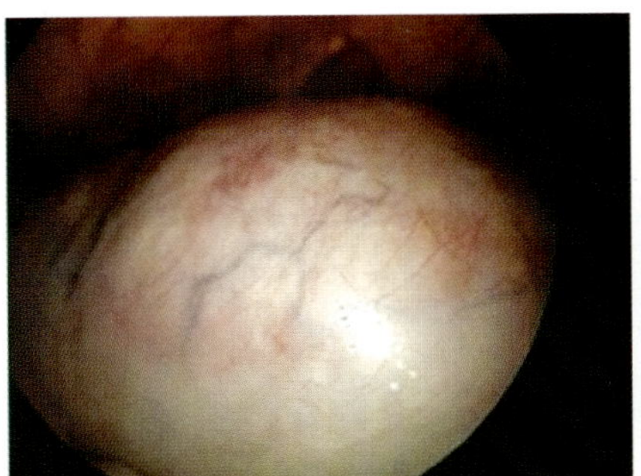

Large pelvic mass

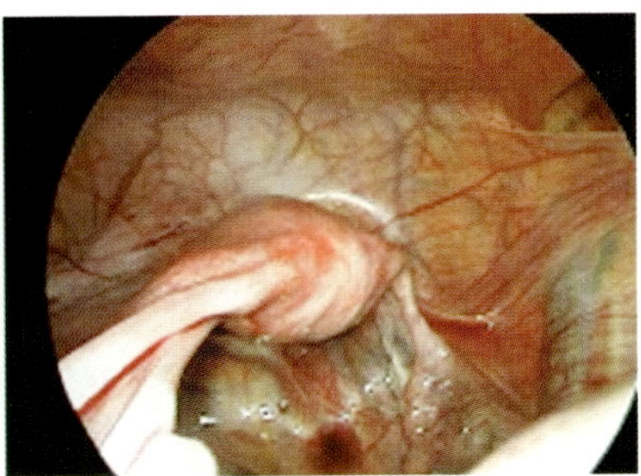

Small uterus seen

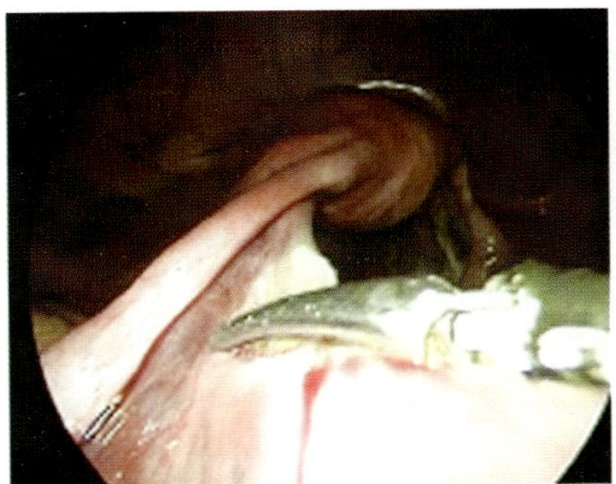

Base of left ovarian mass

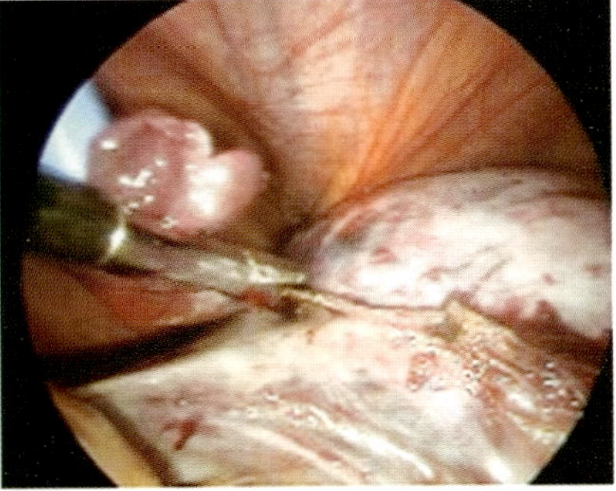

Mass separated by 5 mm
vessel sealing device

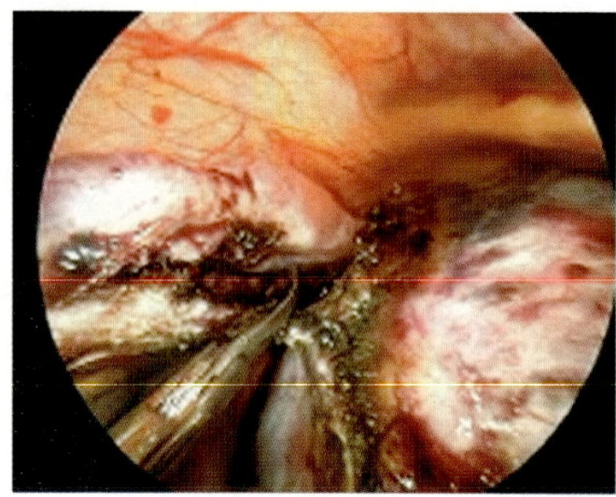

Mass separated by 5 mm
vessel sealing device

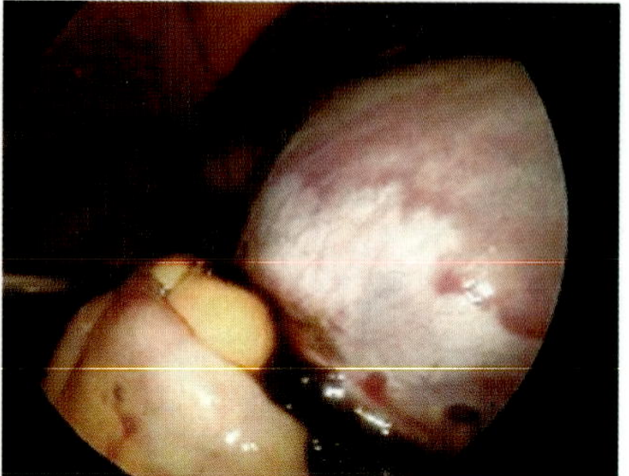

Ovarian mass detached

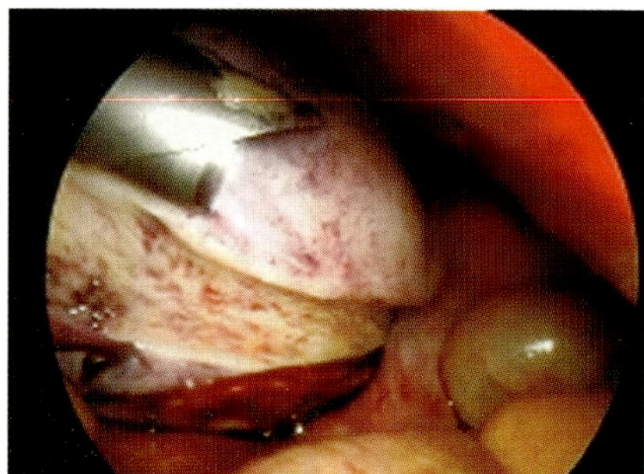

Morcellation of ovarian mass

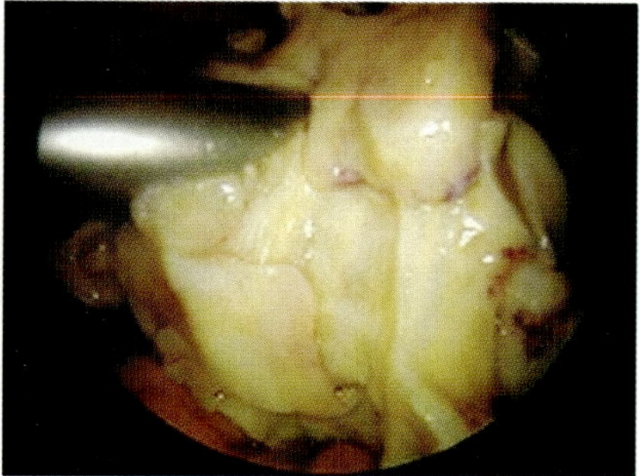

Last part of morcellation

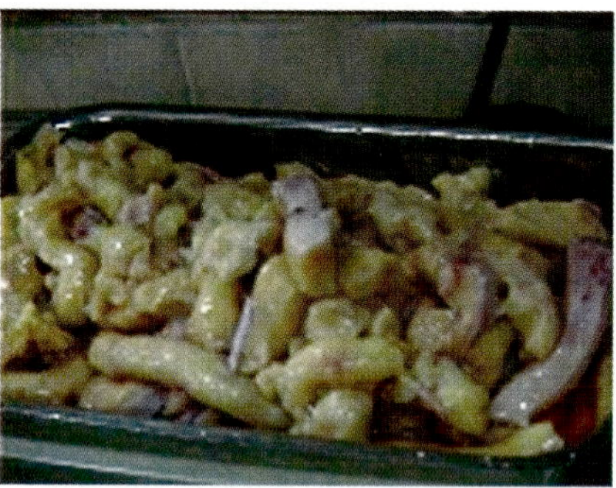

Morcellated pieces of ovarian mass

(Photographs courtsey: Dr Prakash Trivedi)

INDEX